Chemically Imbalanced

Chemically Imbalanced

The Making and Unmaking of the Serotonin Myth

Joanna Moncrieff

FOREWORD BY CHRIS VAN TULLEKEN

FLINT

This book contains advice and information relating to health care. It should be used to supplement rather than to replace the advice of your doctor or another trained health professional. If you feel that you are depressed or you are taking antidepressants, it is recommended that you seek your doctor's advice before embarking on or attempting to change any medical programme or treatment. All efforts have been made to assure the accuracy of the information contained in this book as of the date of publication. The publisher and author denies liability for any medical outcomes that may occur as a result of applying the methods suggested in this book.

First published 2025
This updated paperback edition first published 2026

FLINT is an imprint of The History Press
97 St George's Place, Cheltenham,
Gloucestershire, GL50 3QB
www.flintbooks.co.uk

British Library Cataloguing in Publication Data.
A catalogue record for this book is available from the British Library.

ISBN 978 1 83705 267 7

Typesetting and origination by The History Press
Printed and bound in Great Britain by TJ Books, Padstow, Cornwall

MIX
Paper | Supporting responsible forestry
FSC
www.fsc.org
FSC® C013056

The History Press proudly supports
Trees for Life
www.treesforlife.org.uk

EU Authorised Representative: Easy Access System Europe
Mustamäe tee 50, 10621 Tallinn, Estonia
gpsr.requests@easproject.com

Contents

Foreword by Chris van Tulleken

In 1998, in my second year at medical school, I attended a series of tutorials on depression. The pharmacology tutor began these by explaining that there was very little evidence that antidepressants improved the lives of most people who took them, and that we had little understanding of their effects on the brain and body. Refusing to believe this, I spent weeks looking through the literature for evidence to support the chemical imbalance theory of depression. I found instead inadequate trials, misinterpreted experiments, and huge gaps in logic. It was my first exposure to the gulf between what science shows and what happens in the clinic. But I was left confused. How had this theory, that depression is a chemical imbalance with a chemical solution, survived and spread to become one of the most pervasive cultural ideas of the last half century?

My confusion was finally resolved more than two decades later reading this book, which so elegantly describes the history of industry co-opting science and scientists against the interests of patients and public health to sell drugs that don't work, for conditions that we don't understand.

Yet, for me, reading this book wasn't just about finding the missing puzzle piece from my undergraduate essays; it has been a profound reimagining of my mind and brain.

In my fourth year of medical school, I had an episode of what everyone around me called depression. My pharmacology lectures meant that I was reluctant to use antidepressants so, instead, like some of the characters you'll meet in the pages that follow, I was forced to learn something about myself and my emotions, and I cobbled together a few crude strategies to cope with grief, loss and sadness. These have proved useful over the years, but I was left feeling vulnerable – as if I was, fundamentally, ill; someone with 'depression', a brain disease, that could, at any moment, come back unbidden. Despite all my reading, the chemical imbalance theory had somehow sunk in and coloured my idea of myself.

By the end of this book I had been gently released from this vulnerability. I finished reading and found it had been replaced with a much more nuanced understanding of myself and how I move through the world. It has left me empowered, with more and better tools to face the challenges that life throws at me.

Very few writers could pull this trick off, but Joanna writes with clarity, honesty and compassion drawn from years of work caring for people struggling with their emotions. This expertise shines through on every page so that at its heart this book is, for me, profoundly therapeutic. I hope you have the same experience

Preface

In the summer of 2022, I published a paper showing there is no convincing evidence that depression is caused by an abnormality of the brain chemical serotonin.[1] The paper consisted of a systemic review of the principal research in the relevant areas and I led the team that conducted the review. The theory that depression is caused by a deficiency of serotonin has been around for decades and most people believed it was proven. We showed it wasn't supported by scientific evidence after all.

This result had been suspected for years in the scientific community, but the public was shocked and shaken by the news. It turned everything people thought they knew about depression upside down. This brought home to me how the view of depression as a brain disorder has come to be accepted as the truth, with few being aware of its murky origins and shaky scientific foundations.

Doctors are good at making pronouncements as if they are 100 per cent certain, and these are amplified by the media. So, for decades, people have been told that depression is a biological condition and that antidepressants 'work' and 'save lives', as if these are indisputable facts. They are not. As I will show in this book, these beliefs are part of a myth – one that was constructed and is maintained to further various vested interests and bears little resemblance to the scientific reality.

The publication of our review ignited a process of questioning that started to unravel this myth. People wanted to know whether they had been given the wrong idea about depression. They asked why they should take antidepressants if there is so little evidence of a serotonin abnormality, and they were concerned about why they had been misled about this for so long. They wanted to know what antidepressants do exactly.

This book is an attempt to answer these questions, and to do so by presenting the relevant scientific evidence and philosophical concerns so that people can come to their own conclusions. It is an invitation to engage in an important debate that has a bearing, not just on how we understand and treat depression, but on how we think about ourselves and what it is to be human.

* * *

Antidepressants are some of the most used medicines in the world. They have been presented to the public as sophisticated and effective pharmaceutical weapons, but there is considerable research that questions this view, and there are legitimate scientific questions about their nature and effectiveness. Because most people are unaware of this, they are unable to make properly informed decisions about whether to take antidepressants or not – or if they are taking them already, whether to continue with them or not.

There is much in the following pages that is critical of antidepressants, because the evidence suggests they have little benefit and some concerning adverse effects that are only recently receiving the attention they deserve. However, it is not my intention to stop people taking antidepressants or starting them if they want to. My purpose is to ensure that people know exactly what they are doing and what risks they are running. If any readers are taking antidepressants and decide to stop them, it is important they do so slowly and carefully, preferably with the guidance of an informed doctor or prescriber, because severe withdrawal effects are one of the underappreciated hazards of using these drugs.

I trained as a medical doctor and then specialised in psychiatry. I have worked as a senior psychiatrist in the National Health Service (NHS) in England for over twenty years now, alongside my research and academic work, and I enjoy being a psychiatrist. I prescribe medication in some circumstances, and I know that most people who work in mental health services sincerely want to make patients' lives better.

There is no doubt that some people struggle with their mental health and need support and sometimes care. However, the idea that mental health problems are 'just like any other illness' has never been persuasive to me. Through my own experience (both personal and professional) and by reading critiques of psychiatry written by scientists, philosophers and psychiatrists, I came to the conclusion that there is a fundamental difference between what we sometimes refer to as 'mental disorders' and general medical conditions like arthritis or 'flu. When I was a young psychiatrist in training, this could be an uncomfortable view to hold, yet I knew I was not alone. In fact, there is a long tradition of critiquing psychiatry from within the profession and many psychiatrists, past and present, feel the same way. For this reason, I set up the Critical Psychiatry Network.

Members of this network, which now includes hundreds of psychiatrists from across the world, have a wide range of views. Most share a scepticism of claims that mental disorders like depression arise from simple biological causes that can be targeted by drugs or other biological interventions. That doesn't mean they disagree with the prescription of drugs in every situation. Many 'critical psychiatrists' adopt the 'drug-centred' approach that I have outlined in the scientific literature and set out in this book. This provides a new way of understanding what psychiatric drugs do that entails a more informed and cautious approach to using them.

In the wake of the publication of our paper, some mainstream psychiatrists weighed in to try to shut down the discussion and re-establish the status quo. Some members of the public were unsettled by the questions our paper raised too. When experts express contrasting points of view, it can be bewildering, especially if some of those are questioning a position that has been regarded as fact. That is why I have set out the evidence itself, in a digestible form, so that people can see the basis for my arguments and make up their own minds.

Many areas of science are not settled, and the story I am going to tell illustrates what can happen when people are misled into believing they are. Questioning and debate are key to making progress and avoiding mistakes in science and medicine, as in the rest of life. This book is intended to ensure these processes are not stifled and that everyone can take part.

Part 1

The Issues

1

How the Chemical Imbalance Theory Changed Our Lives

Mental health problems, as they are now referred to, are all around us. Whether it's depression, anxiety or attention deficit hyperactivity disorder (ADHD), you, or someone you know, probably has one. Generally, that means the person has been to see a doctor, the doctor has diagnosed them with one of these conditions and most likely recommended they take some medication. This reflects the fact that the predominant way of understanding these problems today is as medical conditions, and the predominant form of treatment is drugs. This medical view entails the idea that mental health problems arise from a malfunctioning of the body, particularly the brain, just like other medical diseases.

The nature of this malfunction has commonly been suggested to consist of a brain-chemical imbalance and drug treatment is proposed to correct the malfunction and restore the brain's normal chemical composition. In the case of depression in particular, it has been widely reported that an imbalance or deficiency of serotonin is the abnormality in question.

This message has been deeply absorbed into Western culture. The media and the internet are awash with news items, documentaries and articles about the importance of getting a medical diagnosis and treatment, and of how our brains are implicated in our problems.[1] People make songs, plays and works of art that express these ideas. In a song called 'Serotonin', a young Swedish singer tells listeners she doesn't have enough serotonin, that this chemical imbalance is messing her up and she needs medicine to fix it.[2] You can also buy a variety of antidepressant-themed paraphernalia, which joke about the normality of antidepressant use. Vendors on Redbubble do a range of Prozac cushions, for example, and some on Etsy sell T-shirts, keyrings, fridge magnets and bags carrying slogans such as 'if you're happy and you know it, thank your meds' and 'today's good mood is sponsored by antidepressants'. For all the tongue-in-cheek humour, such items display the depths to which the idea that we are chemically imbalanced and need to be corrected with medication has become part of our psyche.

What is happening here? Have we always been this ill and just not known about it before, or has some mysterious disease come out of nowhere? Or might there be another way of understanding these problems and, with it, another way of helping and supporting people?

This book will reveal that the idea of a chemical imbalance is a myth. The strongest candidate for this idea – the theory that depression is caused by low serotonin – is not supported by consistent or reliable evidence. The emperor has no clothes, and this matters, because our widespread use of antidepressants and other drugs for mental health problems is grounded in this idea.

I will focus mainly on depression, since depression is where the idea of the chemical imbalance has played out most clearly. Depression is strongly linked with anxiety, however; therefore, so much of what I have to say will also apply to anxiety, as we understand it now. It is recognised that there is considerable overlap between anxiety and depression. Most people with depression have some symptoms of anxiety and vice versa.[3] It has also been suggested (based on the history we will delve into later) that most people in distress have elements of both, and whether they are deemed to have anxiety or depression is determined more by what set of drugs are being marketed than what people actually experience.[4]

Our understanding of anxiety piggy-backs on the conventional view of depression. Like depression, it is now most commonly treated with antidepressants, and these are implicitly presented as working in the same way as in depression – that is, by correcting an underlying brain abnormality, although the nature of that abnormality is not often specified in the case of anxiety.

Being depressed in the 1980s

When I was a precocious 14-year-old, I had a period of what might have been called depression. I don't want to claim this was a really serious situation, but I had several of the classic symptoms: difficulty sleeping, loss of pleasure, waking up with a sinking feeling every morning when I realised I had to face another day, and doubts about whether I really wanted to carry on living. I had some idea of what was making me feel that way, but I didn't know what I could do about it, and I worried that I was naturally susceptible to depression. I felt I was odd and different. I found it difficult to find people who shared my passions for philosophy and punk music, especially in my slightly stuffy girls' school, although admittedly I had cultivated interests my classmates didn't share. Looking back, I was a pretty stereotypical teenager: full of burning questions about the meaning of life that I felt no one else cared about, but still desperate for friends and companionship like everybody else.

I never saw a doctor about it, and no one suggested that I should. Maybe my parents knew what sort of reaction they would get; I was terrified of being told to take a drug that would cloud my mind. Despite the fact I was unhappy being me, I didn't want to take anything that would stop me reading my philosophy books and, more importantly, prevent me from working out what I could do about my situation. I expect my resistance was coloured by my parents' general stoicism.

In the end, I changed schools, found some more like-minded friends and a lovely boyfriend, and I was happy again. For years afterwards I felt vulnerable, though. I was concerned that I would slip back into a depressed state – that my recovery was precarious. I can't remember at what point I stopped worrying about it, but at some point I did.

I wrestled with writing this autobiographical sketch because I know I will be criticised for trying to generalise from my situation. And I agree that none of us can speak for anyone else about the nature of our feelings. But I wanted to make some important points. One of them is that depression is a near-universal experience. We have this idea that there is ordinary low mood or sadness, and then there is this different thing called 'clinical depression' or 'major depression'. We have been told there is a difference between these two situations, but, in fact, there is no dividing line. There is no test that can tell us who has the 'ordinary' version and who has the 'real' medical condition. Researchers in New Zealand, for example, followed people from birth until middle age and found that 86 per cent of people fulfilled official diagnostic criteria for some form of mental disorder before they reached the age of 45, and 70 per cent for anxiety or depression.[5] Not having emotional problems is the exception not the rule in life.

Back in the 1980s, my reaction to my difficulties was common. Research conducted in 1991 showed that people were reluctant to consult their doctor about emotional problems and the majority thought depression was primarily caused by adverse life events such as unemployment or divorce. They also shared my worries about taking antidepressants. They didn't think depression should be treated with drugs and they worried that antidepressants were 'addictive' and 'dulled the symptoms rather than solving the problem'.[6]

Changes were afoot, however. In the 1990s, an onslaught of advertising campaigns that accompanied the introduction of the Selective Serotonin Reuptake Inhibitor (SSRI) antidepressants started to change people's previous understanding of depression. This, in fact, was exactly what the campaigns were designed to do. But where did these drugs come from and what evidence suggested they were effective and useful? Why was so much invested in promoting them, and why was the chemical imbalance theory so critical to that effort?

Being depressed in the twenty-first century

In the 1990s, a slightly geeky boy with a talent for maths was being bullied at school. It was an all-boys' school and he happened to be the youngest and shortest boy in his year. Despite the sharp wit he developed to deflect the bullies, the experience sapped his confidence and left him feeling pessimistic and despondent, which continued when he left school and went to university to study medicine. His penchant for existential philosophy filled him with further doubts about the direction of his life and the course he had chosen, and by 2002, having been posted to a remote town away from family and friends, he started to spiral downwards. Too ashamed to talk to anyone about the state he was in, he sneaked books about cognitive behaviour therapy (CBT) out of the hospital library in a furtive attempt at do-it-yourself therapy. When this didn't work, he decided to see a doctor.

Like me, he came from a medical family: his father was a doctor and his mother a pharmacist. Medications were as plentiful in the family home as books, he told me, so seeking medical attention seemed like a natural thing to do. By the time he saw his general practitioner (GP), he was so desperate for relief he was excited to try the sample pack of antidepressants he was offered.

This was the start of a nineteen-year career of taking psychiatric medication, over the course of which he took five different antidepressants. When he subsequently developed problems with fatigue, concentration and memory, most likely as a consequence of the antidepressants, he was prescribed further drugs, including a stimulant to keep him awake and a tranquilliser to send him to sleep. Overall, at one time or another, he was prescribed twenty different medications, and at the height of his treatment he was on five drugs at the same time. Despite these difficulties, he graduated from medical school, became a doctor and subsequently managed to complete a PhD; but he was so debilitated by fatigue and concentration problems, he could only work part time for much of his career.

This doctor is my colleague, Mark Horowitz, who was one of the co-authors of the paper on the serotonin theory of depression. As a medical student, he had absorbed and accepted the message that there was something wrong with his brain that was making him depressed. He remembers being impressed by lectures about how antidepressants compensated for various brain chemicals, including serotonin, that were said to be deficient or awry in people with different sorts of depression. While he was conducting research for his PhD, he delivered lectures in which he told students that serotonin is involved in causing depression.

It was when he experienced severe withdrawal symptoms while trying to discontinue his antidepressants that Mark started to re-evaluate the drugs he had been taking for so many years, and the messages he had absorbed along with them. He had been told that antidepressants were safe and easy to stop, but he quickly found out this was not the case, at least not for him. This led him to wonder what else he had been led to believe that wasn't true.

He also remembered how he had been asked by a psychiatrist in the past, 'When did all this begin?' For the first time, he realised the question had a clear answer: when he was being bullied at school. Slowly, the story he had been telling himself – that he was someone with a broken brain – unravelled. In its place, he began to think of himself instead as someone who had responded, perhaps quite normally, to a difficult period in his life.

By this time, however, Mark had been on medication for so long that withdrawing from it had become an excruciatingly difficult process. He had to make tiny reductions in his dose to prevent uncomfortable and disabling withdrawal symptoms, and it was clear that stopping his medication would take years.

Back in the 1980s, I managed to get through my troubles, work out what I needed to change and move on with my life. Mark, on the other hand, entered a spiral of pharmaceutical interventions, which left him in a worse state than he had started in. He went from having existential problems, which only slightly dented his ability to function, to having significant physical symptoms, which prevented him from working full time, destroyed his hopes of a conventional medical career and prevented him from enjoying many of the usual life experiences of a young adult. 'Fifteen years of my life have been damaged because of unnecessary and unhelpful medical treatment for a problem that was never medical to begin with and could have been solved – as it was over time – by better relationships and making sense of who I was,' he told me. 'And,' he added, 'I have had five more years disrupted by trying to come off that treatment.'

* * *

Not everyone's experience of antidepressant treatment works out as badly as Mark's, of course. Many people feel they have been helped by antidepressants; although whether antidepressants are actually effective and useful is, it turns out, uncertain. Not everyone experiences major difficulties with withdrawal, either; but many do, along with other complications, including significant sexual dysfunction, which is sometimes enduring.

Yet, the point of this book is not to tell you how bad antidepressants can be. It is not a catalogue of side-effects or a reproach for how the mass use of antidepressants has abolished sadness, as previous critiques have been.[7] The effects of antidepressants are not as simple as this idea implies in any case. My aim is to reveal that people have been profoundly misled about the nature of antidepressants. In fact, there has been a systematic programme to mislead the public about the nature of depression and the action of antidepressants. Not only have antidepressants never been shown to rectify a chemical imbalance or any other underlying brain abnormality, but there is another, more intuitive and scientifically supported way of understanding what antidepressants do. This alternative view of them highlights how they interfere with the normal state of the brain, just like alcohol and other mind-altering drugs. This explains how they can produce the uncommon but potentially devastating side-effects that are beginning to emerge.

I have no problem if people choose to take antidepressants, and I know that among people who read this book, there will be many who do. But I do want people to be properly informed about what they take. This book will show that trusting doctors or purported scientific experts is not enough – people need to inform themselves.

Over the last twenty years, I have also been on a journey to appreciate the full nature of drugs like antidepressants, and particularly to understand their potential to cause lasting damage and consequent suffering in some people. The best evidence on this has come from people like Mark, who use or have used antidepressants themselves. I am deeply indebted to all those who have bravely shared their experiences of drug-induced harm, and if this book achieves anything, I hope that it will reduce the number of future victims.

The story I am going to tell has echoes of the way the pharmaceutical industry deceived people about the non-addictive nature of OxyContin to create a mass market for a highly addictive drug, igniting the United States' twenty-first-century opioid crisis.[8] In the case of antidepressants, the myth that they normalise an underlying brain dysfunction has facilitated the successful promotion of a range of highly profitable drugs, whose full range of harmful effects was never properly investigated. This book tells the story of how the quest for money and professional status, the hubris of the scientific community and the quiet desperation of so many people combined to create one of the most widespread and harmful delusions of recent times: the idea that emotional problems can be resolved with a pill.

2

Justifying Antidepressants: The Purpose of the Chemical Imbalance Theory

The first part of the twenty-first century has witnessed a rising epidemic in the use of antidepressants and other drugs prescribed for psychological problems, including depression and anxiety. Data from England show the number of prescriptions issued for antidepressants has been rising year on year for over three decades now. The number almost doubled between 2011 and 2022 and has increased more than eight times since 1990.[1]

In 2022, 8.6 million people in England were taking an antidepressant: almost 19 per cent of the total adult population and 23 per cent of adult women.[2] In the USA in the same year, 23 per cent of the population had taken a drug for some kind of mental health problem.[3]

The number of people who have taken antidepressants at some point in their lives is likely to be higher still. We also know that increasing numbers of people are using antidepressants on a long-term basis, often for years on end.[4] Eighteen per cent of people who start an antidepressant in England end up taking it for more than a year, and at any one time, two-thirds of those who are taking antidepressants have been taking them for over a year.[5] The use of other drugs prescribed for psychological problems has also been rising.[6]

The official view is that these drugs are treating a variety of previously unrecognised diseases that afflict a substantial proportion of the population. Public information emanating from pharmaceutical companies and medical organisations has informed people that depression is, or is likely to be, caused by an abnormality of brain chemistry – that it is due to a chemical imbalance. This message has encouraged people to take antidepressants and other prescription drugs intended to modify their moods and emotions, something they might otherwise have been reluctant to do.

My team and I started working on the serotonin review in 2019, and the paper was published in July 2022 in the academic journal *Molecular Psychiatry*.[7] We showed that, despite heavily funded research taking place over several decades, there is no convincing evidence that serotonin is linked with depression. Specifically, there is no evidence for the hypothesis that depression is caused by low serotonin. The paper has become one of the most widely read and influential papers of modern times (it is ranked in the top 5 per cent of all scientific papers ever written by Altmetric, an online influence tracker, and in the top 1 per cent of papers the same age).[8] The interest the paper inspired around the world demonstrates how deeply convinced people were that the link between depression and serotonin had been scientifically demonstrated. Some were literally stunned to find out this was not true: it 'blows your mind,' said a presenter on ITV's *This Morning*.[9]

The serotonin paper was news because the idea that depression is caused by a deficiency of serotonin, or some other sort of chemical imbalance, has been intimately entwined with the justification for using antidepressants. Millions of people have been told by their doctors they have a chemical imbalance in their brain and they require an antidepressant to fix it.

In the hullaballoo that followed the publication of the paper, it became clear to me that there are facts about antidepressants that the psychiatric establishment and sections of the media do not want people to know. From the beginning, high-profile psychiatrists lined up to tell the public we had no right to raise questions about antidepressants. Antidepressants work, they said, and it doesn't matter how. They played down the significance of the paper, and when that didn't work, they tried to discredit it. Some insisted no one believes the serotonin theory of depression in any case, while others claimed serotonin *does* play a role in depression but couldn't specify what that might be.[10] They accused us of irresponsibly discouraging people from seeking treatment, of putting people at risk of relapse and of causing people to attempt suicide.[11] Sections of the media aligned with this position suggested we were putting 'millions in danger' and tried to paint us as right-wing extremists and conspiracy theorists.[12]

Leaders of the psychiatric profession were on the defensive. No one actually contradicted our conclusions, but they didn't like them. The strategy was to stifle the message and impugn the messenger.

These attempts to manipulate the information that reaches the public are the tip of an iceberg. A tangled web of misconceptions has been disseminated over many years, starting with the over-optimistic view that we understand the links between brain chemicals and emotions, and including the unwarranted presumption that drugs like antidepressants target the underlying biological basis of depression and other unwanted mental states. Exposing that the chemical imbalance theory of depression is not supported started to unravel this edifice. It challenges the view of depression as a brain disorder and calls into question our use of antidepressants. It also raises the issue of what antidepressants are doing to us exactly, if they are not correcting a chemical imbalance.

Before I go on, I want to stress that I am not against the use of drugs for psychological problems in any circumstances. I believe some psychiatric drugs (drugs prescribed for psychiatric or psychological disorders) can be useful in some situations. However, the way these drugs are currently presented as working is fundamentally incorrect. And because of this, they have not been properly researched and we therefore do not understand the full consequences of taking them.

The downsides of antidepressants

It goes without saying that we need to be cautious about using chemicals that modify the normal state of the brain, which is what antidepressants do. At the very least, we need good-quality information about all the consequences of taking a particular drug over the sort of period that people commonly use it for – that is months and years in the case of antidepressants. Yet, no such research was conducted before modern antidepressants were released into the world, soon becoming some of the most widely prescribed medicines of their generation. What took place were short-term trials typically lasting eight weeks. There has been little interest in establishing the adverse effects of these drugs past ensuring they don't immediately kill or maim people.

Modern antidepressants are safer than older generations of these drugs, in the sense that it is more difficult to die if you overdose on them. However, they do have harmful effects on the body. SSRIs are known to prolong bleeding time and have been linked to an increase in haemorrhages, birth complications and strokes (which may be caused by bleeding).[13] Evidence also suggests they reduce bone mineral density, causing osteoporosis and fractures.[14] In younger people, antidepressants can cause a state of agitation and impulsivity that has been linked to suicidal behaviour and aggression.[15]

Over recent years, further disturbing complications have been coming to light. Severe and prolonged withdrawal reactions are one of these. Although we have known about antidepressant withdrawal for decades now, it was thought to be mild and short-lived. We used to think the brain quickly returns to normal after people stop using whatever substance they are using, but it is becoming clear this is not always true. Antidepressants, and benzodiazepines in particular, produce withdrawal symptoms that can last for months and sometimes years after they are stopped, causing considerable suffering and impairment. There are now huge online communities of people, who, like Mark, are struggling to get off these drugs, many of whom have lost jobs and careers, suffered relationship breakdowns and become suicidal as a consequence of severe and protracted withdrawal reactions.[16] Yet, despite this, persistent withdrawal has not been widely acknowledged by the medical community.

The gravity of this problem was brought home to me when Ed White, an IT executive and researcher with whom I was collaborating, sadly and shockingly took his own life in 2021 at the age of 57. He had suffered severe and incapacitating withdrawal symptoms since stopping his antidepressants some years earlier. Despite this, he had dedicated much of his time to helping others in the same boat, as well as contributing to research intended to improve our understanding of protracted withdrawal.[17]

Another potentially devastating complication that is emerging is persistent sexual dysfunction. It has long been known that antidepressants, particularly SSRIs, cause sexual dysfunction while people are taking them, but it was assumed the problems resolved when people stopped them.[18] However, accumulating evidence suggests the sexual side-effects persist in some people. Internet-based support groups have campaigned to raise awareness of this problem, with men and women describing their experiences on social media. A typically sad post from a young man reads, 'No more love, no more sex, no more feelings'.[19]

No one currently knows exactly how common it is for people to experience severe and protracted withdrawal or persistent sexual dysfunction. However, millions of people now take antidepressants, so even if these conditions only affect a small minority of users, they still amount to a colossal public health problem and many individual tragedies. No one should be prescribed antidepressants any more without being warned about these effects in the strongest possible terms, yet the medical community has not been quick to publicise them.

Fudging the issues

For more than three decades now, people have been misled about the origins of depression and what antidepressants do. Judging by reactions to our paper, some psychiatrists and sections of the media want this situation to continue. They want to replace the idea that depression is caused by low serotonin with vague suggestions that depression is caused by a complex interaction of many brain chemicals and systems, including, but not limited to, serotonin; or they want to persuade people that depression is something to do with abnormalities in the generation of new nerve cells and nerve cell connections; or that it is connected with the disruption of other brain chemicals. Yet none of these theories, nor others like them, are supported by robust evidence either.

Essentially, all these theories are ways of persuading people to take prescription drugs. A new array of substances derived from or related to recreational drugs is currently being developed and promoted for the treatment of depression and anxiety disorders. These include ketamine, and its close relation esketamine, psychedelics, benzodiazepine-like drugs and even opioids.[20] These are all claimed to counteract an underlying biological abnormality or deficiency, often by people with links to companies that are marketing them.

Whatever the details, the message is the same: depression is in the brain and can be targeted by drugs. The pharmaceutical industry and its allies need business to go on as usual. People must be convinced there is something wrong with their brains and that antidepressants and other drugs prescribed for common mental health problems rectify the biological nature of the problem in some way. Then the market will be sustained, and people won't pause to think that they are taking foreign chemicals into their bodies – chemicals we understand little about and which are unlikely to be harmless, especially if taken, day in, day out, for years at a time.

I will come back to these subjects, but the point is we have been far too blasé about the use of antidepressants. We have not appreciated the full implications of taking drugs that change the normal state of the brain, partly because we have not acknowledged that this is what drugs like antidepressants do. I don't want to alarm people, but it is essential that everyone understands exactly what they are doing when they take an antidepressant, or any other drug prescribed for a mental health problem. To put it bluntly, they are tinkering with their brain in ways we do not fully understand – and we mess with the brain at our peril.

Chemical imbalance messaging

I set out to do the serotonin review because I was aware that most of the public had come to believe causal links between serotonin and depression were an established scientific fact. This came home to me when I gave a presentation in 2014 at a seminar organised by members of the University College London Centre for German Studies. The audience of professors, lecturers and

PhD students were shocked when I suggested that the biological basis of depression had not been established. They believed the science was settled, and that biochemical abnormalities, including those involving serotonin, had been clearly demonstrated to play a causal role in depression. Yet, I knew that people who were familiar with the research recognised this was not true.

Surveys conducted in the USA around 2006 and Australia in 2011 showed that almost 90 per cent of the public believed depression is caused by a chemical imbalance.[21] The idea is frequently referred to as a fact in the press and on the internet. In 2014, a British radio presenter said depression was when 'all the goodness is flushed out of the brain [and you have to] top it up now and again; that's why you need medicine'.[22] An internet blogger put it like this: 'Literally, we depressed people don't have the "happy" chemicals that the rest of the world operates with.'[23]

It is not surprising people think this. The pharmaceutical industry has been bombarding the Western public with the idea that depression is the result of a chemical imbalance for decades. In the USA, where pharmaceutical companies can advertise directly to the public (unlike most of the rest of the world), television advertisements beamed this message into people's living rooms, illustrating their claims using scientific-looking pictures of nerve cells and serotonin molecules. A now infamous television advertisement for the antidepressant Zoloft (sertraline) featured a sad, blob-like creature who takes Zoloft and then miraculously cheers up. A voiceover told people, 'Depression may be related to an imbalance of natural chemicals between nerve cells in the brain' and 'prescription Zoloft works to correct this imbalance'.[24]

Websites set up by drug companies conveyed the same message worldwide, as illustrated by the examples provided in Appendix 1. Time and again, the public were told that people with depression had a brain-chemical imbalance, involving serotonin and sometimes other chemicals (depending on the drug being advertised), and that they needed to take an antidepressant to 'restore the brain's chemical balance'.[25]

Medical institutions have been busily disseminating the idea too. In 2024, eighteen months after our paper was published, the American Psychiatric Association was still telling people that 'differences in certain chemicals in the brain may contribute to symptoms of depression'.[26] In April 2023, the then president of the association, psychiatrist Rebecca Brendel, told a podcaster, 'We know that serotonin has been strongly associated with depression' and antidepressants 'work on neurotransmitters, the chemicals in our brain, to rebalance the relative levels'.[27]

Up until 2022, the Royal Australian and New Zealand College of Psychiatrists informed people that medications 'work by rebalancing the chemicals in the brain. Different types of medication act on different chemical pathways.' The page was subsequently taken down for 'review'. The UK Royal College of Psychiatrists' public information on antidepressants has become more circumspect in recent years, due to pressure to moderate its claims from academics and people who had experienced the harmful effects of antidepressants.[28] It has made similar claims in the past, however, and in its information on antidepressants, it continues to imply that they rectify a chemical imbalance without stating this explicitly. 'We don't know for certain,' it reads, 'but antidepressants do affect the activity of certain chemicals in our brains called neurotransmitters ... The neurotransmitters most affected by antidepressants are serotonin and noradrenaline.'[29] A further selection of the many institutions that have promoted the chemical imbalance theory of depression is provided in Appendix 1.

Professional positions

When challenged, leading psychiatrists have long admitted there is no good evidence to support the theory that depression is caused by low serotonin or any other chemical abnormality. They don't tell the public this, however; at the same time, they are unable to give up on the theory altogether and instead reassert that it is true, or likely to be true, or that something similar is the case.

In 2005, two American academics published a paper called 'Serotonin and depression: a disconnect between advertisements and the scientific literature'.[30] It pointed out that messages in pharmaceutical advertisements and promotional websites were out of step with the views of leading scientists, who admitted there was a lack of evidence for a chemical imbalance in depression.

The article received attention because it was the first time the media had got wind of the possibility that the serotonin theory might not be supported by evidence. Like our paper, it provoked a defensive reaction from the psychiatric profession, who insisted at one and the same time that no one believed the serotonin theory anyway, yet it was still true in some form. Even if it was not true, they said, it was useful.

Academic psychiatrist and then Chair of the USA's Food and Drug Administration's (FDA) Psychopharmacological Committee, Wayne Goodman, for example, conceded to a reporter that evidence of a chemical deficiency in people with depression was 'elusive'. However, he described the chemical imbalance idea as a 'useful metaphor' that represented a 'reasonable short-hand' to describe how depression 'is a chemically or brain-based problem and that the medications are normalizing function'.[31] He failed to mention that the basis for these suppositions was the very evidence for a chemical imbalance that was in question.

In 2011, another leading US psychiatrist, Ronald Pies, wrote an article in the widely read professional magazine *Psychiatric Times* (of which he had been the chief editor until 2010), in which he dubbed the chemical imbalance theory of depression an 'urban legend'. Pies claimed that no well-informed psychiatrist believed the theory was true.[32] A few months later, when readers wrote in to tell him they had, in fact, been told by their doctors they had a chemical imbalance, he had to row back on his words. In a follow-up article, he admitted that psychiatrists might tell this to their patients, but they don't really believe it. They only say it to make patients feel better or to save time. He spent the rest of the article reassuring readers that there are lots of 'sophisticated, modern theories' about the biology of depression, including the idea that 'certain psychiatric illnesses probably involve abnormalities in specific brain chemicals'. He even presented the 'biogenic amine hypothesis' of depression (more commonly referred to as the monoamine hypothesis)[33] as a credible hypothesis, even though, as we will see, this *is* the chemical imbalance theory that he was trying to disown.[34]

Therefore, at the same time as Goodman and Pies acknowledged the chemical imbalance theory was unproven, they were quick to provide the public with reassuring messages that this didn't change the narrative about the biological origins of depression. It seems that some in the profession want people to go on believing that depression is a brain disorder, and don't want people to ask questions about the scientific justification for the use of antidepressants.

A different story

Consequently, as well as looking at the science itself, this book is also about exposing the institutions and vested interests that distort medical science and co-opt the media, so that the public receives a select and one-sided story about research on the biology of mental health. Most people know about the influence of the pharmaceutical industry by now, but the interests of the medical establishment and how these are exerted are less well documented. My account will raise questions about whether we can really trust our doctors and other medical authorities to know and recommend what is best for us. For, although I don't doubt they have patients' best interests at heart, the information they have access to is already partial and distorted and, like all of us, they operate with unconscious biases that incline them to take a rose-tinted view of the things they have to offer.

Many doctors and members of the public now assume that depression is a biological disorder, but there are other ways to think about it. I will suggest that emotions and moods are better characterised not as brain events, but as the distinctive reactions of intelligent creatures to their circumstances – a view that is aligned with our intuitive understanding of the nature of human feelings. There are more obvious ways of understanding what drugs like antidepressants do to our feelings, too. We naturally understand that using drugs to drown our sorrows or obliterate our worries is at best a temporary distraction and, at worst, an act of self-harm.

The pharmaceutical industry had to actively suppress these understandings when it started promoting its new range of antidepressants back in the 1990s. Preceding this, the scandal of the mass prescribing of benzodiazepines (drugs like Valium) and the revelation of their addictive properties had brought the use of drugs to numb and suppress emotions into disrepute.

A new narrative was needed if drugs were to continue to be marketed for psychological problems. The chemical imbalance was that narrative. It enabled the SSRIs and the antidepressants that followed them to be presented in a way that suited the new times. These were not emotional anaesthetics, the marketing went, and they would not get you addicted. They were sophisticated medical agents that targeted an underlying 'disease' – the disease of depression. This disease was common and caused by an imbalance in brain chemicals and this could, by happy coincidence, be reversed by the new drugs. How could people resist this sort of message, especially when it was delivered not just by drug companies, but by national medical institutions and by their own doctors?

Yet, this narrative is a myth – one that was woven to support a particular view of human emotions; a view that just happened to coincide with the interests of the multibillion-dollar pharmaceutical industry and some in the medical profession.

3

So, What is Depression?

When I was interviewed about the serotonin paper I was frequently asked, 'If not serotonin, then what?' When I tried to explain that we don't have to think of depression as something caused by a particular biological mechanism, several of my interviewers were perplexed.

This is not surprising. The idea that depression is a biological condition has been presented for decades as if it is an established fact, with few of its promoters acknowledging that it is not a universal or necessary way of thinking about depression. In 2008, the prominent psychiatrist and researcher David Nutt, who is currently championing psychedelics, declared that the 'origins' of depression and related psychiatric disorders 'are clearly explained by altered brain functions'.[1] In 2023, another senior psychiatrist told the BBC's *Naked Scientist* programme, 'Different underlying abnormalities in the brain' can lead to the symptoms of depression, although we don't know exactly how.[2]

There are two versions of this idea. The first is that everything can be explained by biology. Human beings can be understood as complex machines and, ultimately, everything we do, say or feel is determined by a particular biological process (even if it may be triggered by something else).

The second version is that depression is different from normal feelings. It is the result of the brain malfunctioning in some way. This is the argument that depression is a disease, just like other medical conditions. 'Depression is a real illness, with real physical causes' was how one psychiatrist summed it up.[3]

The simplest response to both these positions is that there is no good evidence from neuroscience or medicine to support either of them. Indeed, the point of this book is to reveal the lack of scientific evidence that depression is related to any specific brain process or abnormality. But first, I want to suggest that both positions fundamentally fail to grasp the nature of human feelings and behaviour and, specifically, that they fail to explain depression.

An alternative approach to understanding mental characteristics, including emotions like depression, acknowledges that humans are biological organisms and that our biological make-up determines the extent and limits of our physical and mental capacities. Yet, it is a mistake to think of feelings such as happiness, sadness, pride, disappointment, fear, guilt, jealousy *and* depression, even serious depression, as states of the brain or of the body. They are attributes of human beings and that means of *whole* human beings, with their individual histories, personalities, desires and values. It is not my brain that feels happy because it's a sunny day or dejected because it is raining, it is *me*.

A painting, such as the *Mona Lisa*, provides a useful analogy. The painting would not exist without the materials used to create it, but we cannot understand the picture by examining the nature of the paint or the type of canvas used. We recognise and understand the image because of what it means to us as human beings, living our lives in the world we share with other human beings.

In the last few years, I have had the pleasure of getting to know Dr Cathy Wield, who works in accident and emergency medicine and whose story illustrates some of the points I am going to make in this chapter.[4] When Cathy was a junior doctor in the 1990s, she became profoundly depressed and suicidal and she was hospitalised for long periods on a number of occasions over the course of seven years. She was given every medical treatment in the armoury, including multiple different antidepressants, other sorts of drugs, electroconvulsive therapy (ECT) and ultimately brain surgery (she had a procedure that, like the once-dreaded lobotomy, aims to destroy small parts of the brain). None of these had a lasting effect.

Initially Cathy had thought her problems were caused by a confluence of stressful circumstances – she was working long hours, had four children at home and her daughter being admitted to the Royal Ballet School had brought back memories of her own 'horrendous' experiences at boarding school. But the doctors kept telling her she had a serious medical illness that required physical treatments to correct her malfunctioning brain. Cathy and her family accepted what they were told – why wouldn't they? She followed her doctors' advice, she took the antidepressants and, despite some misgivings, she became convinced that her 'depression was caused by a physical phenomenon such as a chemical imbalance, which science had not yet fully elucidated'.[5] It was difficult to resist this point of view, she told me in an email, because the 'biological illness model was reinforced throughout'. 'It's almost as if I became conditioned into believing the opinion of the day,' she continued. 'I was in awe of these experts who kept on telling me how I had a uniquely severe endogenous [biological] depression.'

During a period of remission, Cathy took a job as a junior doctor in a psychiatric ward. Previously, her doctors had told her she was unusually 'resistant' to treatment, so she was surprised to find she was far from alone. 'Few if any of the patients on my ward got better,' she recalled. This was the beginning of a process of questioning the narrative she had been fed and of revisiting her past in order to, as she put it, 'relearn how to see myself as a good person who had a right to feel the way I felt'.[6]

In the end, Cathy would come to see her depression as she had at the beginning: an understandable, if extreme, reaction to events in her life. To comprehend depression is to know how individual people react when faced with the challenges life can throw up. Cathy's story, like Mark's and mine, is the story of a life, not a brain process and not a diagnosis.

Humans are not just complex machines

A common modern point of view is that we can understand human beings as if they are sophisticated machines and each one of our thoughts, feelings and actions can be traced back to a particular configuration of our brain chemistry or activity. This idea has been encouraged by neuroscientists and the media, who frequently claim that one emotion or another has been linked with a particular brain chemical.[7] It has also become deeply embedded in our culture. Referring to serotonin and dopamine when talking about our feelings or habits is now commonplace. On social media, people post pictures of their 'serotonin moments', a phrase that has become synonymous with happiness or serenity (though the derivation of the word serotonin has nothing to do with serenity).[8]

Although many people feel uneasy about the 'reductionism' of this perspective, few have had the courage to challenge it. One of those who has is the contemporary philosopher Peter Hacker, who teamed up with distinguished neuroscientist Max Bennett to mount a 'withering attack' on the conceptual basis of modern 'cognitive neuroscience' (the neuroscience of thinking).[9] I have been lucky enough to get to know Peter Hacker recently and the following account is deeply indebted to him.[10]

Like other animals, human beings operate on biological principles. However, we are distinguished among animals for having particularly complex nervous systems, including our large brains that enable us to perceive and react to the world around us. Importantly, we have the capacity for rational thought and sophisticated emotions, and for language on which these are based.

The feelings we call emotions and moods are a reflection of our ability to evaluate the world and they entail that we care about things. Emotions and moods manifest our reactions to events or circumstances from the past, the present or the future. This is integral to the way we understand the concepts of emotions and moods, and it is evident from the way we use the related vocabulary: I am sad that my dog ran away; I am happy to see my friends; I am disappointed I failed my exams.

Hacker describes moods, specifically, as 'frames of mind' that infuse everything we think and do and that last for a significant period of time. Like other types of emotion, moods are not neutral and they are, by and large, a response to the world around us.[11] Negatively inflected moods and emotions, such as sadness, disappointment, anger, fear, worry, despair and depression, are reactions to circumstances that threaten our welfare, comfort, future hopes and peace of mind. They also relate to our previous experiences, which colour the way present-day circumstances affect us.

Emotions and moods are not the same as freely willed thoughts and actions. We do not choose to feel happy or sad or depressed like we choose to go for a walk. Although we have some degree of control over them, we cannot simply will them into being or will them away. Nevertheless, emotions are not the same as physical sensations, such as pain, or biological 'appetites', like hunger, thirst and sexual desire. They are not biological reflexes. They are the reactions of an individual with a particular history and character. For this reason, emotions need to be explained in terms of reasons rather than mechanical causes, such as brain events.

The reasons for our emotions can be complex, however. They relate to our current needs and desires, but also to the predispositions we have developed over the course of our lives; and, therefore, they relate indirectly to everything that has ever happened to us and, in turn, to the history of our society and culture. Partly because they are so complex, we are not always aware of the reasons why we feel something or we might be mistaken about them. Sometimes, we only become aware of the most likely reasons for our feelings later in the day, when we have a different perspective on our previous situation. Unlike Cathy, who at least had an inclination about the source of her troubles, some people cannot figure out why they are depressed, especially when they are in the depths of despair. Yet, that doesn't necessarily mean there is no reason.

Going back to our analogy with the *Mona Lisa*, we understand the picture, not through our knowledge of the chemical composition of the paint, but because we recognise the image as a whole, with reference to our prior experience of what women look like, what a smile looks like and, crucially, what it means. We understand the picture because we recognise our fellow creatures and we have learned that their expressions manifest their feelings about the world around them. Looking in the brain to understand depression is like dissecting the canvas rather than seeing the picture.

I am not denying that activity is taking place in our brains when we have feelings, what I am arguing is that what is happening in the brain does not *explain* those feelings. In fact, we know that quite different emotions can be accompanied by the same biological changes. Fear, anger, excitement and surprise, for example, are all associated with the physiological state of arousal we call the 'fight or flight' response, which is characterised by the release of adrenaline, among other things. Yet they are different sorts of feelings, and their nature can only be described with reference to the context that provoked them.

To argue that depression is not rightly thought of as a brain process, therefore, is not to say that human experiences and actions are disconnected from the body, the brain and the material world. It is to suggest that depression, along with other emotions and moods, has to be understood at the level of the person as a whole, not the brain. Our emotions and moods are a characteristic feature of the way that intelligent beings with large brains, like us, respond to the world. They are reactive and understandable, and they reflect the individual desires and concerns of each one of us. They are an integral part of who we are, and they have meaning.

This view of depression is how people have understood it for most of human history. It is a reflection of our intuitive understanding of moods and emotions as expressed in the way we use the language that describes them.

Physical influences on emotions

Saying that emotions are meaningful reactions to our circumstances doesn't mean our physical make-up has no influence on them at all: there is a biological component to our personality. It is our individual biology, determined by our genes interacting with the circumstances we grow up in and the choices we make, that forms the person we become. And some people, through a combination of their biological inheritance and their life experiences, will be more susceptible to depression, anxiety and other mental health problems than others.

As well as this, there are times when things that happen in our bodies or brains determine our emotions and moods. We might feel sad or irritable because we are tired, for example, and we often feel better after exercise. Drugs like interferon (used in multiple sclerosis and liver disease) can make people depressed, and the withdrawal or 'come-down' from other drugs (notoriously stimulants, like cocaine) can do the same.

Some medical diseases also impact our emotions. Brain diseases like dementia and Parkinson's disease can make people depressed, although people usually become more apathetic than sad. Thyroid disease can also make people sluggish and depressed. These situations are exceptions to the general nature of moods and emotions, however. They are equivalent to there being a mark on the painting that modifies the image.

An influential report called *The Power Threat Meaning Framework*, written by prominent psychologists from the UK, argued that 'there are important differences between forms of distress and troubling behaviour that are *enabled and influenced* by our biology – as all human experience is' and states in which 'there is evidence for a *primary causal role* for biological disease processes'.[12]

This is a key distinction. Depression is 'enabled and influenced by our biology' but not caused by it in the way that the symptoms of Parkinson's disease are caused by progressive degeneration of parts of the brain. A meaningful emotional reaction is different from feelings or behaviour that are generated by a disease mechanism or by another specific biological process (such as in drug-induced states).

Is depression a medical condition?

In contrast, the second biological position I outlined at the beginning of this chapter attempts to identify depression as a disease or a disease-like condition. Although people who make this argument might accept the account of 'ordinary' emotions I have just presented, they suggest there is something distinctive about depression and that we can distinguish a medical form of 'clinical depression' from normal depression or sadness. This is just not true.

When a doctor makes a diagnosis of depression, it is a fundamentally different process from when they diagnose a physical condition, such as rheumatoid arthritis. In rheumatoid arthritis, people have swollen and painful joints that indicate something is wrong with a particular part of the body. In this situation, examining the mechanics of the body, like the pigments in the painting, makes sense. The combination of the symptoms (the painful joints) with certain abnormalities in laboratory tests enable doctors to identify the underlying biological process, which distinguishes rheumatoid arthritis from other conditions that produce joint symptoms. This is what the term 'diagnosis' usually means. It means you have identified the source of the problem.[13]

Nothing like this happens when a doctor diagnoses depression, or any other mental health problem for that matter. A diagnosis of depression is made on the basis of what people say about how they feel and how they are doing. Although psychiatrists have tried to make the process *look* scientific by drawing up criteria that specify the number and duration of symptoms required to qualify for a diagnosis, in reality, diagnosis in psychiatry is simply the act of applying a label to what the person reports they are experiencing. The criteria set out in diagnostic manuals, such as the American Psychiatric Association's *Diagnostic and Statistical Manual of Mental Disorders*, the *DSM*,[14] for example, specify that a low mood that lasts for more than two weeks is 'clinical depression', but there is no scientific basis for this. There is no evidence that depression that lasts longer than two weeks is different from depression that lasts for a shorter time – that it has any special characteristics or that it has a physical basis. Two weeks is just the arbitrary cut-off, after which psychiatrists have agreed it is no longer reasonable or normal to feel unhappy.

Many people do not realise it but diagnostic terms, such as 'depressive episode', 'major depression', 'clinical depression' or 'anxiety disorder', do not *explain* anything in the way that medical diagnoses generally do. They are not the cause of someone's symptoms. A psychiatric diagnosis is like diagnosing someone as having a headache. The term 'headache' doesn't tell you anything about the underlying problem, it just names the symptom the person has described. In the same way, when the doctor tells you that you have a diagnosis of depression (or anxiety, or any other mental disorder for that matter), the doctor is effectively saying, 'You have told me your problems, now let's call them this'. The diagnosis does not identify the origin or cause of the symptoms, it is simply a label for them.

Unlike in medicine, where there are usually physical signs, such as swollen joints and laboratory tests to go on, whether to apply a diagnostic label to emotional or psychological problems is a highly subjective decision that depends on how the individual conveys their problems, as well as how the person making the diagnosis interprets them. Someone who displays their emotions conspicuously may appear to be more depressed than someone who is more inhibited or stoical, for example; but who is to say they really are? We cannot measure our emotions or moods with a ruler or a pair of scales and draw a neat line between what is normal and what is a medical problem. The person who is given a diagnosis of depression has just come across as more distressed than their particular doctor thinks is usual on that particular day.

Understanding depression as an emotional reaction or 'frame of mind' makes it clear that it is a different sort of process from the identification of a physical condition, like rheumatoid arthritis. The first is equivalent to recognising the image of the *Mona Lisa*, the second is analogous to detecting a blemish in the picture that has been produced by a defect in the paint or the canvas.

Biological research on depression

The importance of the serotonin story and other biological interpretations of depression is that they enable depression to be portrayed as a physical condition or disease. They give the impression that we have identified an underlying physical process, which gives rise to depression in the same way that we have identified the biological mechanisms that produce the symptoms of rheumatoid arthritis, Parkinson's or thyroid disease. They have persuaded people to discard their natural inclination to see depression as a meaningful, emotional response to life and embrace the medical concept instead.

This is why it is so important to clarify that we have not established any underlying biological dysfunction in depression – not in the serotonin system nor in any other system or process. We will look at evidence for the serotonin theory and some of the other leading theories later; but, before that, let me tell you about a large review published in 2019 of evidence on the proposed biological mechanisms of depression. The authors of the review looked for studies that specifically explored whether certain proposed biological abnormalities ('biomarkers') *preceded* the onset of depression – that is, whether they could genuinely be a cause of depression, rather than just a correlation. They didn't look at serotonin research because none of it has examined whether changes in the serotonin system occur prior to someone becoming depressed. They identified seventy-five studies that had assessed the volume and thickness of different parts of the brain; brain 'connectivity' (meaning the correlation of activity in different brain regions); chemicals involved in inflammation; aspects of gut activity; various hormones, including stress hormones; and other chemicals. They found no evidence that abnormalities in any of these areas or systems might be causing depression and concluded, 'There is a lack of evidence for leading biological theories for onset and maintenance of depression'.[15]

Social influences on depression

In contrast to the weakness of biological research, there is abundant evidence that depression is associated with traumatic or upsetting events and unfavourable social and economic conditions – just as we would expect if depression is a meaningful response that relates to an individual's experiences and character.

British social scientist George Brown was one of the first people to conduct research on the relationship between depression and social conditions. In the 1970s and 1980s, Brown surveyed working-class women in London and showed how depression was strongly related to the occurrence of stressful life events, such as marriage breakdown or the loss of a job. In one of his surveys, 91 per cent of the women who became depressed during the course of a year had experienced a stressful life event, compared to only 23 per cent of those who did not become depressed.[16] Another study showed that having lost a parent early in life, not having close friends and having young children at home made women more vulnerable to depression when faced with a stressful event.[17]

Brown's findings that depression is a response to negative life events, and that past events and current circumstances influence people's vulnerability to depression, have been replicated many times. Studies have demonstrated that low income, financial strain, unemployment, lack of social support, living alone, poor working conditions, poor housing and exposure to crime or discrimination all increase people's chances of becoming depressed.[18] Being the victim of child abuse or neglect, witnessing family conflict or violence and being bullied make people more vulnerable to depression later in life and the effect is cumulative.[19] The more adverse childhood experiences you have, the greater your subsequent likelihood of suffering depression.[20]

It is not controversial to say that mental health is strongly influenced by people's social conditions. A joint report by the United Nations (UN) and World Health Organization (WHO) published in 2023 made the point that 'Mental health and well-being are strongly associated with social, economic, and physical environments, as well as poverty, violence, and discrimination'.[21] What is more contentious, however, is to point out that if depression is a meaningful reaction to events and circumstances (like other moods and emotions), it cannot simultaneously be a brain condition, in the sense of being something such as Parkinson's disease, which is caused by a particular brain process.

Why depression can't be both biological and social or psychological

Many people acknowledge the role of social adversity but believe there is still a biological component to the causation of depression and other common mental health problems. This hybrid view – that the causes are a bit biological, like a brain disease, but also a bit psychological and a bit social – is sometimes referred to as the 'biopsychosocial model'.

The trouble with this position – appealing as it sounds – is that, where a biological process is genuinely responsible for producing symptoms of depression, such as when depression is caused by thyroid disease or Parkinson's disease, it trumps other causes. This is because, as I wrote in a paper about the general nature of mental disorder published in 2020, 'bodily processes are biologically programmed in ways over which human beings have limited control'.[22]

What happens in our bodies and brains follows the laws of biological science, not the interests or values of human beings. A heart attack is the predictable outcome of the occlusion of the blood vessels supplying the heart. When the vessels get blocked to a certain extent, a heart attack occurs, however the individual feels about the situation. We can modify our bodies to a degree through our behaviour, for better or worse, but we cannot escape the inexorable logic of biology, which inevitably involves ageing, disease and death. We cannot cure ourselves of cancer through positive thinking, unfortunately.

On the rare occasions when a physical disease or process *is* found to be the cause of depression or another mental condition, we do not need other explanations. If someone with depression is found to have an underactive thyroid gland, then they will be treated with supplementary thyroid hormone and that would be that. We wouldn't also wonder about the state of their marriage or whether they were unhappy at work, as we would if we thought this was a typical case of depression. It would be as if we discovered the *Mona Lisa*'s ambiguous smile was the result of a crack in the painting. If this were the case, we wouldn't ponder, as we do, on the artist's intentions and the model's state of mind.

Because biological events are determined primarily by the laws of biology, not by human concerns and interests, something that arises as the direct result of a biological process cannot be 'psychological', in the sense of being the expression of one's character. It also cannot be social, in the sense of being an understandable response to one's social circumstances. It sounds nice to have a halfway house, where personal and biological factors mingle equally, but when biological processes are genuinely causal, they override human inclinations.

Since we have no grounds to believe that depression and related states are the result of a specific biological abnormality or variation, it follows that they must be meaningful emotional reactions – that is, part of the range of ways that human beings make sense of their world.

Support for the alternative view of depression

The view I have put forward here is not new. There is a long tradition of critiquing the 'medical' model of mental health problems[23] and, recently, leading UK psychologists have put forward similar views to those I have out outlined here in several influential reports, including the *Power Threat Meaning Framework* and a 2019 report by the British Psychological Society entitled *Understanding Depression*. In the latter, depression is described as 'an experience, or set of experiences, rather than as a disease' and one that 'like other emotions, is often an understandable human response to the world around us that involves complex evaluations of events'.[24] The UN special rapporteur on mental health, Dainius Puras, has also expressed concern that there is too much emphasis on the 'biomedical model' of mental disorders, which 'has led [...] to the medicalisation of normal reactions to life's many pressures'.[25]

Popular writers, such as Johann Hari, have suggested that depression should be understood as a 'signal' that something is wrong in life and the conditions that produce this signal in the modern world consist of a lack of social connection, meaningful work, shared values, security and experiences of trauma or abuse.[26]

An important theme of these critiques is how the medicalisation of mental health problems, such as depression, diverts attention from the social, economic and environmental issues that make people distressed and unhappy in the first place. The joint WHO–UN report, for example, observed that the current 'focus on diagnosis, medication and symptom reduction' neglects 'the social determinants that affect people's mental health'.[27]

Severe depression

Sometimes, people who are depressed end up in an extreme state of inactivity, withdrawal and negativity. They might not be able to get out of bed, sometimes they stop eating and drinking, and some develop morbid delusions, such as thinking parts of their body are missing or not working, or that they are guilty of terrible things they haven't done. This pattern usually occurs in the elderly, and up until the mid-twentieth century it was called 'involutional melancholia' (melancholia of old age). Some psychiatrists agree that the majority of people currently being treated for depression do not have a brain abnormality, but argue that the small number of people with this more severe condition do. It has been suggested that we rename this situation 'melancholia' to distinguish it from more usual forms of depression.[28]

Severe depression like this does sometimes turn out to be the prelude to a neurological disease such as dementia; but for the majority of people, severe depression, as with milder cases, is a reaction to depressing events, such as loss and loneliness. In older people, it is frequently precipitated by bereavement or retirement, and it is associated with having suffered stressful life events in the recent past and adversity or abuse in childhood.[29] In other words, although the manifestations are extreme, severe depression is also, usually, a meaningful response to one's life course and circumstances. And as we will see later, the evidence shows that antidepressants are no more successful in severe depression than they are in any other type of depression.

Why it matters

How we think about depression is not just an academic or philosophical exercise. It profoundly affects how we understand and cope with our own emotions, and how we respond to other people's emotions. These, in turn, affect the whole trajectory of our lives.

Cathy, whom we met earlier, was conditioned into thinking she had a problem with her brain. Her belief that her difficulties were an understandable reaction to her previous experiences was overridden by constant authoritative assertions that she had a biological condition, reinforced by the daily act of taking pills.

She was expressly told that if she discontinued her medication she would relapse, so she dared not stop. 'Fear secured my compliance,' she said.[30] How could she develop confidence and resilience in the face of such messages?

An experiment conducted by academic psychologists from the University of Wyoming demonstrates the powerful influence that ideas about the biological or chemical origins of depression exercise over people. They recruited students who had had an episode of depression and gave them a fake test for serotonin levels. After having the test, half the students were told they had a serotonin deficiency and were presented with a made-up graph showing a low level of serotonin compared to other brain chemicals. The other half were told all their brain chemicals were normal. The people who were randomised to the news they had a serotonin imbalance were more pessimistic about their chances of recovery and less likely to believe they could do anything to improve their mood themselves.[31]

Another group of researchers from McLean Hospital, Boston, found similar results in people enrolled in a therapeutic programme for the treatment of depression. Patients who believed that depression was due to a chemical imbalance had lower expectations of recovery and were less likely to improve.[32]

Negative expectations and outcomes are not inevitable: many people who believe they have a chemical imbalance recover and do well. In Cathy's case, however, the idea that her problems were located in her brain may have contributed to making her depression more prolonged and severe than it might otherwise have been.

One of the attractions of the idea that depression is caused by a brain process, whether that is thought of as a disease or as a variant of normal brain functioning, is that it relieves us from responsibility for our feelings and actions. This alleviates the guilt we might feel for not being able to fulfil our usual obligations – for letting other people down or for making them or ourselves unhappy. But although telling people that depression is a biological state may seem like a kind thing to do, Cathy's experience and the Wyoming research suggest it isn't. It may ease feelings of guilt and shame for a brief time, but in the long run, it traps people in a sense of impotence; it saps people's confidence and weakens their autonomy; it gives people unrealistic expectations about the power of medicines; and it undermines people's own efforts to change their lives. Cathy eventually concluded she had been 'absolutely and utterly misled in the worst possible way'.[33]

Saying that depression is linked with character is not to blame people for how they feel, it is to empower them to realise that feelings have meaning. They are a barometer of our lives; they tell us that something needs changing. People who promote the biological or disease model offer a false binary choice between blaming the person with depression and blaming the brain. But no one needs to blame anyone: we are all human; we all struggle; we all need help from time to time. For a myriad of reasons that we can all sympathise with, some people struggle more than others.

This chapter has been a diversion to try to persuade you that we do not need to think of depression as being the consequence of a particular brain-chemical reaction or pathological process. I have argued that it is more appropriate and useful to think of it as a meaningful emotional response – a view that is more intuitive and enduring. Unfortunately, however, this view has been suppressed by the increasingly dominant biological model of depression, which empties depression of its significance and its power to help us to change. In the rest of the book, I will explain how this situation came about and what its consequences have been.

4

What are Antidepressants?

Before we proceed with the story, some further clarification is required, this time about antidepressants. Just as we have developed an inadequate and misleading picture of depression, we are fundamentally confused about the nature of antidepressants.

Let me illustrate the different ways of explaining what antidepressants do. On the one hand, there is the view espoused by Dr Rebecca Brendel of the American Psychiatric Association that antidepressants 'rebalance' particular chemicals that are awry in people with depression, or that they correct some other underlying brain abnormality.

On the other hand, Annie Corcoran, who described her experiences in *The Independent* in 2018, was struck by the way that taking antidepressants caused mental and physical changes to her normal self. Although initially she had been happy to take the tablets, it was only after stopping them that she became fully aware of how they had affected her. She came to the conclusion that the changes they produced were not, in fact, helpful: 'What I didn't realise was that rather than lifting my mood, my antidepressants just made me feel numb. In all honesty, I felt a bit like a zombie, just going through the motions.' She stopped her antidepressants, lost the weight she had gained while taking them and 'started to feel again'. The experience worried her, though. It made her realise the drugs were affecting her body and brain in ways that should not be 'taken lightly'.[1] Although not everyone finds the experience of taking antidepressants as unpleasant as Annie, the point is they made her feel different from usual.

Dr Brendel articulates the widely accepted view that antidepressants are drugs that reverse or ameliorate an underlying brain disorder – a view that makes them sound welcome and necessary. I have been challenging this position for almost twenty years now and explaining that there is an alternative understanding of the action of drugs like antidepressants; one that is reflected in Annie's experience and that doesn't make them sound so benign. I am going to summarise my work on this subject because it is critical to understanding the nature of antidepressants and why their use has become so hotly contested.[2]

The disease-centred model of drug action

Since the 1960s, the conventional notion is that antidepressants and other drugs prescribed for psychological or psychiatric problems work by targeting the biological mechanisms that produce the disorder or symptoms they are intended to treat. Hence, 'antidepressants' are thought to counteract the mechanisms proposed to underpin depression or the symptoms of depression; 'anxiolytic' drugs are thought to modify the biological basis of anxiety; 'antipsychotics' are thought to reverse the biological origins of psychosis or schizophrenia;[3] and drugs for ADHD are thought to correct the suggested mechanisms of ADHD.

In my previous work I have called the idea that drugs work by targeting an abnormal brain process that is presumed to produce the symptoms of a disorder or disease the 'disease-centred model' of drug action. The disease-centred model is based on the way that drugs work in the rest of medicine, in most instances. Some medical drugs work by attacking the ultimate source of the disease, such as antibiotics. Many are what we might call 'symptomatic' treatments, but these also work in a disease-centred manner by targeting the biological mechanisms that produce symptoms. The common asthma drug salbutamol (likely the one in your inhaler, if you have asthma), for example, doesn't affect the fundamental causes of asthma, but it works by relaxing the constricted airways in the lung and thereby counteracts the mechanism that produces the main symptom of asthma: wheezing. Painkillers, like paracetamol and aspirin, also work by modifying biological processes that give rise to pain, although they don't usually target the ultimate cause of the pain.

It is no accident that medical drugs act in a disease-centred way: they are developed to target identified disease processes. Even if we do not fully understand their mechanisms of action, as is the case with paracetamol, for example, we can reasonably assume they act in this way because in most cases there is no other plausible way they could be having their effects. But this is not the case with psychiatric drugs, where there *is* an alternative.

This disease-centred view of how drugs work underpins the way psychiatric drugs are presented in the medical literature, marketing and the media, and is used to justify the use of these drugs in most situations in which they are used. Sometimes, the message is explicit, as when antidepressants are said to rectify an underlying chemical imbalance, but sometimes it is left implicit.

We will look at the evidence for this view of antidepressant action in detail in the rest of this book, but in my previous work,

I have documented that *no* psychiatric drug has been demonstrated to work in this way. Moreover, there is an alternative way to understand what antidepressants and similar drugs are doing, which is both plausible and scientifically corroborated.

The drug-centred model of drug action

The other way of explaining the effects of psychiatric drugs is what I have called the 'drug-centred model'. The drug-centred model suggests that psychiatric drugs, like antidepressants, affect our feelings and behaviour in the same sort of way that alcohol and recreational drugs affect them. It emphasises the obvious fact that psychiatric drugs are drugs and that drugs are chemicals that change our biology. Drugs that enter the brain, such as psychiatric drugs and recreational drugs, change the normal state of the brain. Far from correcting an underlying chemical imbalance or abnormality, psychiatric drugs change our normal brain chemistry, and this influences the way the nerves in the brain communicate and can modify the very structure and organisation of the brain itself.

These changes lead to alterations in our mental activity: they change our sensations (the way we perceive things), and the way we feel, think and behave. These effects occur in everyone who takes the drugs, and although there is always a degree of variation between individuals, they are not restricted to people who have a particular disorder or diagnosis. The effects can also be observed in animals. The idea that is sometimes proposed that antidepressants only affect people who have depression is incorrect.

We sometimes refer to drugs that change our normal mental states as *psychoactive* drugs or, more colloquially, as 'mind-altering' drugs. Although we commonly apply this term to recreational drugs, psychiatric drugs can also be thought of as having psychoactive properties, meaning they produce characteristic mental alterations that are different from our usual state of mind – that is, when we are not under the influence of a drug. Each drug that enters the brain, whether it is a recreational substance or a prescribed medicine, produces its own distinctive effects depending on how its particular chemical make-up impacts on the brain and the body.

Certain psychoactive drugs cause more profound changes than others. The effects of caffeine are relatively mild, for example, whereas alcohol and heroin have more obvious effects (although dose also plays a part). Like recreational drugs, some psychiatric drugs produce alterations that are subtle, whereas some produce more noticeable changes. Bearing in mind that people have different tastes and preferences, by definition, recreational drugs have effects that some people enjoy, at least in the short term. Several drugs prescribed for mental health problems do, too, such as benzodiazepines and amphetamine; therefore, they are also used for recreational purposes. On the other hand, some psychiatric drugs, including most antidepressants and antipsychotics, produce states that vary from mildly unpleasant to very unpleasant for most people.[4]

Whereas the disease-centred model assumes that psychiatric drugs alleviate psychological problems by restoring normal brain functioning, the drug-centred model suggests the alterations produced by drugs are superimposed onto the individual's state of depression, anxiety or other troubling or unwanted feelings and thoughts. Taking the drug substitutes a drug-induced state for the original emotional state. If the underlying distress and disturbance is severe, being in the drug-induced state may be regarded as preferable by the sufferer, or by people who are trying to help them.

We can understand this if we think about the familiar effects of alcohol. Alcohol changes our usual mental state and behaviour, and it produces broadly the same characteristic changes in everyone – and in animals. By and large, alcohol makes us calm and relaxed, and it has the effect of loosening our inhibitions. These effects can bring relief to someone who is acutely anxious and help those who are extremely shy – people who might be diagnosed with 'social anxiety disorder'. Alcohol doesn't do this by rectifying an underlying chemical imbalance, it does it by superimposing its calming effects onto the individual's anxiety, and these calming effects are a consequence of the way that alcohol interferes with normal brain functions. We also recognise how the intoxicating effects of alcohol can temporarily replace underlying feelings of sadness or despondency. We have a phrase for this situation in English: 'drowning our sorrows'.

Changes produced by psychiatric drugs

With the drug-centred model, therefore, what we want to know about a particular drug is how it changes our biology and how those changes impact our thoughts and feelings. Only when we understand what these changes consist of can we evaluate how the drug might impact on someone in distress and whether it is likely to be useful or not. A difficulty we immediately encounter, however, is that there is little relevant research. We lack good-quality animal studies and studies with volunteers who do not have mental health problems that could establish in detail how they influence ordinary mental activity and behaviour. This should surprise and concern us. It means millions of people are taking substances that affect the brain without us understanding how their biological effects impact on our mental functions.

The alterations produced by some drugs, such as benzodiazepines, are well known because they are immediate and obvious. This makes it relatively easy to understand their effects from a drug-centred perspective. Benzodiazepines are fundamentally sedative drugs. In a similar way to alcohol, they reduce arousal levels and inhibit nervous-system activity, inducing drowsiness and sleep and slowing down reaction times. They act as a muscle relaxant and they produce feelings of calmness and relaxation. People who are feeling intensely anxious or agitated often welcome their effects.

We know that benzodiazepines work by enhancing the activity of a brain chemical called gamma-aminobutyric acid (GABA). GABA acts as a general inhibitor of activity in the brain and nervous system. However, the body soon adapts to counteract their effects, and therefore become weaker. These adaptations are also what lead to the well-recognised withdrawal effects associated with benzodiazepines.

The immediate effects of benzodiazepines and some of their withdrawal effects are predictable from their effects on GABA, but they have other unexplained effects after long-term use, such as cognitive impairment and persistent neurological and emotional effects following withdrawal.[5] These illustrate how even drugs whose actions are relatively well understood can have unpredictable and surprising effects, and not in a good way.

Changes produced by antidepressants

We know considerably less about the mental and behavioural changes produced by antidepressants and the mechanisms behind those changes. First, I should explain that antidepressants come from a variety of different chemical classes; so, unlike benzodiazepines, which all have the same basic action, it is impossible to describe the overall alterations produced by antidepressants.

Like benzodiazepines and other drugs that affect the brain, antidepressants modify the action of a class of brain chemicals known as neurotransmitters. Neurotransmitters, which include serotonin, GABA and other chemicals, such as noradrenaline, dopamine and glutamate, help to transmit the electrical impulses that travel through the brain from one nerve cell to another. When the impulse arrives at the terminal of a nerve, the nerve releases the neurotransmitter chemical into the gap, known as the synapse, between that nerve cell and the next one. The chemical travels across the synapse and activates a receptor on the adjacent nerve. The activation of this receptor then propagates the electrical impulse along the second nerve cell or, as is mostly the case with GABA, this process inhibits the transmission of the impulse.

After the neurotransmitter chemical has enabled or inhibited the transmission of the nerve impulse, it is taken back out of the synapse (where it is active), into the nerve cell (where it is not) and it is stored in the nerve cell until it is released into the synapse again. This process is referred to as reuptake and it is facilitated by proteins called transporter proteins, which literally transport the neurotransmitter out of the synapse. Serotonin, for example, is reabsorbed back into the nerve cell by a protein called the serotonin transporter (shortened to SERT). Figure 1 illustrates this process in relation to serotonin.

SSRI antidepressants inhibit the action of the serotonin transporter, and this is the mechanism by which they are thought to increase the amount of serotonin available in the synapse and increase serotonin-related transmission of nerve impulses. Exactly what their final effects on serotonin activity are remain uncertain, as we will see later. Moreover, although they are

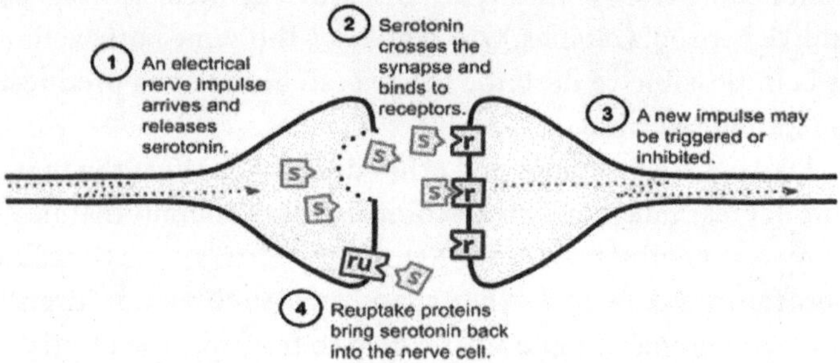

Figure 1

intended to target serotonin specifically, SSRIs, like other types of antidepressant, also affect a range of other brain chemicals, including noradrenaline, GABA, glutamate and the body's natural opioids (the endorphins).[6]

The disease-centred model of the action of SSRIs suggests they correct an underlying deficiency of serotonin in the synapse. The drug-centred perspective, in contrast, suggests that what we need to know is how the neurochemical changes wrought by SSRIs and other types of antidepressants change our level of arousal, sensations, thoughts, feelings and behaviour in general – not how they adjust a hypothetical, but unproven brain-chemical abnormality (or other biological dysfunction) and not just how they affect low mood or anxiety or some other condition.

Common alterations produced by antidepressants

ANTIDEPRESSANT	ALTERATIONS
SSRIs	Drowsiness, fatigue and lethargy of varying degrees (depending on the individual agent and dose); emotional numbing; sexual dysfunction; agitation, especially in younger people; nausea; dizziness; weight gain; insomnia.
SNRIs	Drowsiness, fatigue and lethargy; emotional numbing; sexual dysfunction; agitation, especially in younger people; nausea; dizziness; weight gain; insomnia.
Mirtazapine	Drowsiness, fatigue and lethargy; emotional numbing;[7] significant weight gain; increased sleep.

Bupropion	Mildly stimulant, can cause agitation across age groups; weight loss or no effect on weight; insomnia; anxiety; seizures (at high doses).[8]
Vortioxetine	Not clear – drowsiness, emotional numbing, irritability and agitation reported;[9] sexual dysfunction; nausea; diarrhoea, vomiting, constipation; itching; dizziness; insomnia.[10]
Tricyclic antidepressants (e.g., imipramine and amitriptyline)	Significant drowsiness, reduced reaction times and cognitive test performance; emotional numbing not well studied; sexual dysfunction (depending on the individual agent); weight gain; increased sleep.
Agomelatine	Less significant mental alterations than other antidepressants. Can cause drowsiness and fatigue. Less emotional numbing than with some other antidepressants.[11] No or minimal effect on sexual function. Nausea, dizziness, minimal weight gain.
Reboxetine	Mildly stimulant, can cause agitation; dizziness; nausea; decreased appetite (no weight gain); insomnia.

I have summarised the changes induced by different classes of antidepressants in the table. There is variation within the classes of antidepressants as well as between them, however, especially the SSRIs. Some SSRIs, such as fluoxetine (Prozac) and citalopram, have relatively mild effects and people taking them may not feel particularly different from usual, whereas others, such as sertraline, have more obvious effects.

Many antidepressants make people feel tired and lethargic. People taking them describe 'feeling groggy' or 'sleepy all the time' and as experiencing 'constant fatigue' and 'listlessness'. Linked to these effects, people have problems with concentration and mental acuity and describe feelings of 'fogginess', 'slowness, 'lack of clarity and 'fuzzy thinking'.[12] The Mayo Clinic warns people that 'Fatigue and drowsiness are common, especially during early weeks of treatment with an antidepressant'.[13] Despite this, SSRIs and SNRIs are not typical sedatives and are more likely to cause insomnia than to increase sleep.[14] The older tricyclic antidepressants and the newer agent, mirtazapine, have more usual sedative effects, and all these antidepressants have a tendency to make people put on weight (some more than others).[15] In contrast, two antidepressants, bupropion and reboxetine, have some stimulant properties.

Mark's experience of the initial effects of antidepressant effects is fairly typical. He told me that when he started them:

> The drugs made me feel woozy and a bit out of it and I returned to my doctor twice to try a different one because the effects were unpleasant. On the third one I also felt woozy and funny but I just gave up trying to find one that had fewer side effects and thought this is as good as it gets.

We know that SSRIs and many other antidepressants commonly have an adverse effect on sexual function and desire. It is also apparent that they can reduce the intensity of emotions in general. People describe how they feel less sad and less anxious, but also that they no longer feel pleasure, happiness, joy or excitement. A former user of antidepressants described the experience this way, 'It "blunts" me – no extreme laughter or tears. [...] I don't feel fully myself.' Another said, 'The drugs make me totally disconnected from everything and lifeless.'[16]

The withdrawal symptoms that can occur when people stop taking antidepressants, and the persistent sexual dysfunction that has recently been identified, reflect the fact that these drugs modify many biological systems and that these modifications may take a long time to normalise again when the drugs are stopped. It is only when we appreciate all the ways in which a drug changes our mental activity, emotions and bodily functions, both in the short term and over longer durations, that we can evaluate whether taking it might conceivably be worthwhile. We will come back to this question when we have looked at evidence from clinical trials of antidepressants and the nature of the emotional changes they produce in more detail. But for now, it is important to understand the principle that this is what antidepressants do.

The drug-centred model *has* to be our default way of understanding what psychiatric drugs do because it is undeniably the case that they change the normal state of the brain. As a consequence, they influence the feelings and behaviour of everyone who takes them, just as they are temporarily altered by the use of alcohol and other recreational drugs. Most doctors don't talk about antidepressants in this way, however. Although antidepressant-induced alterations are recognised, they are designated as 'side-effects', which makes them seem incidental and unimportant.

So, if you are prescribed an antidepressant, you may be told (depending on the type of antidepressant you are given) that it can make you tired, that it can cause sexual dysfunction and possibly even that it can dampen emotions. Yet, because the disease-centred model still predominates, these effects would most likely be presented as irrelevant to the drug's intended impact on your mood and mental symptoms – as something you just have to put up with while you wait for the real action of the drug to kick in.

The drug-centred model is the most plausible way of accounting for the effects of antidepressants and other psychiatric drugs.

The idea they work in a disease-centred way, by targeting an underlying mechanism is merely an assumption, and one that ignores the reality that these are drugs which have brain- and mind-altering effects that influence people's underlying emotional state in one way or another.

Reactions

I am not the first person to express these ideas about what psychiatric drugs really do. US psychiatrist Peter Breggin has been highlighting the way that psychiatric drugs change normal brain functioning and mental activity since the 1980s. In his book, *Toxic Psychiatry*, published in 1991, he suggested that all psychiatric drugs work by producing 'brain dysfunction'.[17] Mild degrees of brain dysfunction impair the most sophisticated mental capacities, such as emotions, sensitivity, initiative and creativity. Commenting on antidepressants, he suggested that far from correcting serotonin deficiency, they cause 'extreme imbalances in the [serotonin] system' and he warned that 'we are in no position to safely tamper with the extraordinarily complex activities of the brain' – prophetic words in the light of the enduring complications of antidepressant treatment that are coming to light.

An increasing number of practising psychiatrists embrace the drug-centred explanation of what psychiatric drugs do. They use it as the basis for conversations about the sort of mental and physical alterations patients might expect with any given drug, the positive and negative consequences of such alterations, the physical risks associated with taking a brain- and mind-altering substance and then how these considerations play out in the patient's individual situation.

On the other hand, academic psychiatrists and leaders of the profession have studiously ignored the drug-centred approach. Even when they suggest that psychiatric drugs might not be as useful as claimed, they fail to question the presumption that these drugs work by targeting biological mechanisms.[18] In contrast, other professions have embraced the drug-centred model. It is covered in numerous psychology textbooks, reports and university courses, for example.[19]

In a rare example of engagement with the debate about drug action, two British psychiatrists have attempted to offer an alternative to the disease- and drug-centred models. They called this the 'outcome' or 'pragmatic' model of drug action and explained it as pertaining when 'research has shown medications to be effective for certain clinical indications but how this effect is achieved is uncertain'. In a survey of their colleagues, they found the majority subscribed to the 'outcome-centred' model in preference to the disease- or drug-centred models.[20] This view is also implied by the many responses to our serotonin paper that suggested it doesn't matter what antidepressants do exactly, only that they have been shown to work.

But the outcome model is not a model of drug action at all. It has nothing to say about how drugs might modify unwanted feelings, thoughts and behaviour. It just means doctors can go on behaving as if the disease-centred model were true, while knowing it can't actually be substantiated. Yet, the matter of how psychiatric drugs work cannot be brushed aside in this way because the different possibilities – the disease- and the drug-centred models – have starkly different implications.

People who are recommended to take a prescription drug within the disease-centred framework, whether this is made explicit or kept implicit, are essentially being told they have an abnormality in their brain and the drug will help put it right. In this situation, other things being equal, it makes sense to take it. Who could reasonably refuse the opportunity to correct their brain deficiency if the tool to achieve it is on offer?

The drug-centred model, on the other hand, highlights how drugs are chemical substances that, far from returning anything to normal, induce an artificial physical and mental state by interfering with the normal functioning of the body and brain. Sometimes, this will be preferable to the distress someone is going through, and sometimes, the benefits will outweigh the inevitable negative consequences. But often, taking a drug in this situation will do more harm than good, especially if it is taken, day in, day out, for years on end.

Taking a drug that affects the brain is an inherently risky process, as Peter Breggin pointed out. When you put a foreign chemical into a highly complex and finely balanced chemical and electrical system, it disrupts it. This results in immediate alterations to people's mental capacities and experience, and it has downstream effects that may take weeks or months to develop and may only be revealed when the drug is withdrawn.

The drug-centred model provides a scientific and common-sense explanation for what psychiatric drugs do. There is no need to presume they work in a disease-centred manner, and there is no evidence that they do so either.

Part 2

The History

5

The Origins of the Chemical Imbalance Theory and the Early History of Antidepressants

The idea that psychiatric drugs change our normal feelings and behaviour – what I have called the drug-centred model – is our intuitive way of thinking about drugs that affect the brain. We are familiar with it when we think about the way that alcohol and other recreational drugs superimpose their effects onto our underlying thoughts and feelings, and most people understand the effects of tranquillising drugs like benzodiazepines in this way too. Yet, few people think about antidepressants like this.

How is it that the disease-centred model of drug action – the idea that drugs work by targeting underlying chemical imbalances or other brain abnormalities – has become the dominant way we understand drugs like antidepressants? How did this way of thinking eclipse the drug-centred model to such an extent that most people – professionals, academics and ordinary people alike – do not even consider that antidepressants are mind-changing drugs that inevitably alter the way we feel? How did we come to assume they work by acting on the mechanism of a hypothetical brain disease or abnormality?

We will see that the disease-centred model was embraced not because there was good scientific evidence to suggest it was correct, but because it fulfilled the ambitions of the psychiatric profession to be like other doctors and offer treatments that look like treatments in the rest of medicine. The success of this view is testimony to the power of the profession, backed by the mighty financial heft of the pharmaceutical industry, to set the parameters of our knowledge about psychiatric drugs.

History shows that the disease-centred model was not always the dominant view. Its evolution is also the history of the chemical imbalance theory of mental disorders and of antidepressants themselves. At least, it is the history of how we came to think of certain chemicals as being antidepressants. And it explains how we arrived at the worrying situation we now find ourselves in, in which millions of people are using chemicals whose effects we do not properly understand. It is also a story of how science can go hopelessly astray.

The evolution of ideas about drug action

Prior to the 1950s, drugs prescribed for mental health problems were implicitly understood according to a drug-centred model. Barbiturates, which were recognised as sedative drugs, were marketed for insomnia and anxiety and in the late 1930s, amphetamine was introduced. Amphetamine was understood to be a stimulant and was known to make people more alert, energetic and happy or euphoric. It was used as an appetite suppressant and also prescribed for fatigue and low mood.[1]

There was little reticence about prescribing mind-changing drugs at this time, and advertisements frankly depicted the sort of behavioural changes the drugs could produce. Advertisements for amphetamine depicted smartly dressed men and women, looking confident, alert and ready for action.[2] Adverts for barbiturates showed people being calmed and going off to sleep.[3]

Iproniazid, the drug that is usually referred to as the first antidepressant, was also initially described in a drug-centred way – in terms of how it alters mental activity and behaviour in general. Iproniazid was one of a group of drugs being used for tuberculosis, which was still a common disease in the mid-twentieth century. The old mental hospitals had special wards for people with the condition, and within these wards it was noticed that people who were taking the anti-tuberculous agents became lively and elated. They were said to be dancing in the wards, the story goes.[4]

The 1950s was a time of great excitement within psychiatry about the possibility of finding treatments for serious mental health problems. A new range of tranquillising drugs had been introduced for people diagnosed with schizophrenia, and there was a keen desire to find drugs that would help people with depression too. So, when the effects of the tuberculosis drugs were observed, some psychiatrists concluded they had found just what they were looking for, and they started to give these drugs to patients with depression.[5]

Early accounts of the effects of iproniazid make it plain that it was a stimulant-like substance, as well as being an antibiotic. Papers described its ability to increase energy, reduce fatigue and to produce overactivity, insomnia and occasionally paranoia, similar to amphetamine – and like amphetamine, it could make people euphoric.[6] The similarity was acknowledged at the time and iproniazid was described as a 'drug with stimulant properties'.[7]

Views about the nature of the new drugs being employed in psychiatry were changing rapidly, however. Although they were initially regarded as tranquillisers, the drugs introduced for the treatment of people diagnosed with schizophrenia in the 1950s and 1960s were soon imagined to be working, not through a general process of tranquillisation but by targeting the underlying disease mechanism. They gradually came to be known as 'antipsychotics', the term we still use, reflecting the fact that they were thought to target the psychotic symptoms of schizophrenia in a disease-centred manner.[8]

The same transformation occurred with iproniazid, which was increasingly positioned, not as a stimulant but as a specific drug for depression. Academic papers started devoting separate sections to its so-called 'therapeutic effects' and its 'side-effects' or 'toxic effects'. The therapeutic effects were said to consist of a vaguely defined 'psychological improvement' and this was now disconnected from the general stimulant profile of the drug, which was no longer described. Only in the small print of the 'side-effects' section was it mentioned that iproniazid led to 'overstimulation' and insomnia.[9] It was an exercise of smoke and mirrors. You describe the drug's effect on mood, you suggest this could reflect its action on the underlying mechanism of depression, you omit to mention its stimulant effects, which could equally explain its effects on mood, and hey presto, you have an antidepressant!

A leading American psychiatrist of the time, Nathan Kline, proposed that iproniazid and similar drugs were different from regular stimulants because they could selectively stimulate the mind without stimulating the body. He referred to them as 'psychic energisers'.[10] There was no evidence for this view, but it helped support the idea that there were drugs that could target psychological or emotional problems. It also enabled a line to be drawn between drugs for depression (the term antidepressants had not yet come into vogue) and amphetamine, which was starting to acquire an unsavoury reputation because of its popularity in the burgeoning recreational drug scene. Amphetamine was well recognised to induce general alterations to mental and physical functioning, and hence positioning it as a targeted medical treatment was challenging.

Imipramine and the concept of an 'antidepressant'

The Swiss psychiatrist Roland Kuhn was the first person to use the term 'antidepressant' in a way that caught on. Kuhn's training was influenced by psychoanalysis, popular in Switzerland in the early twentieth century, but when new physical treatments like ECT arrived in psychiatry, he became an advocate of biological approaches to mental disorders. In the late 1950s, he published two similar papers about a drug called imipramine, which he referred to as having 'markedly anti-depressive properties' and 'potent antidepressant action'.[11]

Imipramine is chemically similar to a drug called chlorpromazine, which was the first of the new tranquillising drugs introduced for people diagnosed with schizophrenia. Far from having stimulant properties, imipramine has sedative effects, like its tranquilliser relatives, although it is not as potent as these. In fact, Kuhn was initially given imipramine by the drug company Geigy to test in schizophrenia. Kuhn swapped the chlorpromazine his patients were taking for imipramine and the story that has arisen since is that imipramine didn't help the symptoms of schizophrenia but made patients elated. These effects inspired Kuhn to think it might be useful for depression.

However, imipramine does *not* make people elated, and what seems to have happened, according to the later reflections of Kuhn and Alan Broadhurst, a chemist from Geigy, is that imipramine was not as effective a tranquilliser as chlorpromazine. Therefore, patients taking imipramine became agitated and, in some cases, over-aroused or psychotic, most likely due to having had the tranquillising effects of their chlorpromazine withdrawn.[12]

Having observed that the drug failed in people with schizophrenia, Kuhn gave it to people with depression. He reported its effects in glowing terms, complete with claims of miraculous transformations and cures, reminiscent of early reports of Prozac, three decades later.

Even by the standards of the time, Kuhn's approach was lacking, however. Neither of his two early papers contained any figures or systematic comparisons, consisting instead of Kuhn's personal impressions and opinions, including unlikely claims that people who had been depressed for years were cured in a matter of days. He also alleged that people had coincidentally been cured of various physical ailments, including sexual problems and constipation, which is improbable since these are recognised side-effects of the drug. According to Kuhn, though, the drug had almost no side-effects. The fact that several patients collapsed during treatment was mentioned so briefly that it could easily have been missed.

Although Kuhn did not explicitly set out how he thought imipramine might work in these papers, he implied it worked by targeting the underlying biological mechanism of depression, or at least some types of depression. He stressed how, if the drug was stopped, 'the illness breaks out again',[13] suggesting that although the drug might not permanently cure the problem, it counteracted the faulty mechanisms producing the symptoms in a disease-centred manner. Nowhere did he describe the general alterations that imipramine produces, such as its sedative effects, or how these might impact on people's mood. Later, Kuhn declared more explicitly that imipramine had 'achieved a specific treatment of depressive states'.[14]

Despite the fact that Kuhn's papers on imipramine barely resembled scientific papers, and that Kuhn himself subsequently admitted his 'methods were entirely different from those that are nowadays applied in clinical research',[15] imipramine was quickly adopted, inaugurating the idea of the 'antidepressant'. Drug-makers were so confident of its benefits, they produced a generation of copycat drugs, which became known as the tricyclic antidepressants (due to their three-ring chemical structure). Some of these drugs are still prescribed today, particularly amitriptyline, which is used for depression, anxiety, insomnia and pain.

The fact that Kuhn's papers convinced people so readily demonstrates the appetite that existed within psychiatry for a drug that could be thought of as an antidepressant, and how little proof was needed that such a drug really existed. There were sceptics, however. Some were not convinced that the new drugs being touted as antidepressants did anything more specific than make people feel drugged in one way or another.

A group of British psychiatrists ran a trial comparing imipramine with a drug called Drinamyl (a mixture of amphetamine and a barbiturate, popularly known as the 'purple heart'). There was no difference, and they concluded that 'imipramine has no specific antidepressive action'.[16] American researchers compared imipramine with the tranquillising drug chlorpromazine. They also found no difference and concluded that there was no evidence for the existence of drugs that had specific antidepressant properties.[17]

Although both these groups comprised highly respected psychiatrists and researchers, they were swimming against the tide. The majority embraced the idea that drugs like iproniazid, imipramine and others that were introduced into the emerging antidepressant market had targeted effects on the biological basis of depression. In a conference held in 1959, one psychiatrist described how the new antidepressants had 'strong and clear-cut effects on pathological states and almost no effects on normals'.[18] No evidence was provided, and none existed, that they did not affect so-called 'normal' people. Others described their effects as 'curative',[19] and many repeated the claim that they were more specific than stimulants.[20]

What this brief historical sketch illustrates is that the idea that certain drugs have antidepressant properties came about not through a careful process of scientific selection, but because psychiatrists wanted it to be the case. They convinced themselves the drugs were effective long before there were proper clinical trials to test this supposition. We will come back to the evidence, or lack of evidence, from such trials later, but the point is that before they were even considered, the psychiatric community had decided they had a range of targeted and effective treatments for depression.

Changing ideas about depression

Before understanding the origins and development of the chemical imbalance theory, we need to understand what was happening to ideas about depression in the mid-twentieth century. Our modern idea of depression as a common medical condition did not formally exist in the first half of the twentieth century. Depression wasn't even seen as a single, distinctive condition.[21] At this time, people who went to see doctors with complaints of distress, anxiety or difficulty coping with life were said to have 'neurosis', the term popularised by Sigmund Freud. People whose neurosis was characterised by sadness or a loss of interest and pleasure in life might be said to have a 'depressive neurosis' or 'neurotic depression'. Drugs were frequently prescribed for 'neurotic' conditions, commonly barbiturates and other sedative drugs, despite the fact that they were understood to reflect people's emotional reactions to past and present life events and circumstances.

The relatively rare and severe condition known as 'melancholia' was regarded as a different situation from the more common 'neurosis'. There was not thought to be any 'specific form of therapy' for melancholia.[22] People usually got better of their own accord, and it was the job of psychiatrists and other professionals to nurture people's natural recovery.

In the 1930s, amphetamine started to be marketed by the drug company Smith, Kline & French for people with mild or neurotic depression. By the 1940s, it was being widely prescribed by GPs and psychiatrists and it was referred to as an 'antidepressant' in advertisements.[23]

In 1938, ECT was introduced into psychiatric hospitals. It was initially intended for the treatment of people diagnosed with schizophrenia, but it was given to people with all sorts of diagnoses, and psychiatrists started to think it was particularly useful for people with melancholia.

By the mid-twentieth century, therefore – before the first drugs that were generally accepted to be antidepressants came along – there was an evolving idea that there was a form of neurosis characterised by depressive symptoms and treatable with a drug, namely amphetamine. In parallel, ECT emerged as a treatment for melancholia or severe depression.[24]

For the next few decades, there was a debate about whether these two situations – neurotic depression and severe depression – were the same condition. Some leading psychiatrists argued they were categorically different and only severe depression had a biological basis. Others maintained depression was a single disorder with no fundamental distinction between severe and milder varieties.[25]

Drug companies marketing early antidepressants didn't want to restrict their market to severe depression, so they helped promote the idea of depression as a single condition that was common and amenable to medical treatment. In his book on the history of antidepressants, psychiatrist and historian David Healy reported how, in the early 1960s, Merck – the company that produced amitriptyline, the most successful of the tricyclic antidepressants – distributed 50,000 copies of a book by psychiatrist Frank Ayd called *Recognizing the Depressed Patient*.[26] Ayd's message was highly attractive to the pharmaceutical industry. It suggested that depression was much commoner than generally recognised and often went undiagnosed. Ayd estimated that one in ten of the general population needed psychiatric treatment of some sort, most commonly for depression.

This view of depression as a single entity was not cemented until the publication of the third edition of the *Diagnostic and*

Statistical Manual of Mental Disorders, psychiatry's diagnostic bible, in 1980, which finally killed off the increasingly fragile concept of neurosis.[27] But the idea that depression was common and required drug treatment was already taking root in the 1960s.

Noradrenaline and depression

So, before the chemical imbalance theory of depression was first articulated in the mid-1960s, psychiatrists increasingly saw depression as a medical ailment that originated in a biological process, and they had come to believe they had drugs to treat it that worked by targeting that process.

In the first half of the twentieth century, there was considerable interest in what is known rather curiously as the 'sympathetic nervous system'.[28] The sympathetic nervous system is the body's activation system: it keeps us awake and alert and readies us for action. Adrenaline and noradrenaline are the main chemical messengers in this system. Together, they have wide-ranging actions, but only noradrenaline is found in the brain.

Stimulant drugs, such as amphetamine and a related drug called ephedrine (commonly used as a decongestant, then and now), were recognised early on to stimulate the sympathetic nervous system in a similar way to adrenaline and noradrenaline.[29] Because they also elevated mood, early researchers hypothesised that depression was caused by decreased activity of the sympathetic nervous system, perhaps resulting from a deficiency of noradrenaline in the brain.[30]

Iproniazid fitted this theory. It was known to have stimulant effects,[31] and it was believed to enhance the effects of adrenaline and noradrenaline by inhibiting the enzyme that deactivates them.[32] This enzyme is known as monoamine oxidase, because noradrenaline and adrenaline are 'monoamines'. Iproniazid and later drugs developed to replicate its effects were subsequently called monoamine oxidase inhibitors (MAOIs).

Imipramine and the reuptake mechanism

The idea of imipramine improving mood was a puzzle, however, because it was not known to affect noradrenaline or the sympathetic nervous system. Most drugs that act on the brain affect most neurotransmitters in one way or another, though, so if you want to find such an action, you probably can.

In the 1950s, a young biochemist called Julius Axelrod was researching the effects of adrenaline and noradrenaline. Axelrod was not a psychiatrist, he had no particular interest in mental health, but he became the unlikely hero of the early antidepressant story. By attaching radioactive labels to the chemicals he was investigating, Axelrod was the first person to reveal the process of 'reuptake'. He showed how adrenaline and noradrenaline were absorbed back into the nerve cell body after they had played their part in transmitting nerve impulses in the synapse and were thereby inactivated.[33] This process is now known to occur with all neurotransmitter chemicals, including serotonin.

Shortly after this, Axelrod showed that drugs with diverse effects, including drugs with sedative properties like imipramine and chlorpromazine and the stimulants, amphetamine and cocaine, inhibited noradrenaline reuptake in various body tissues.[34] This was regarded as evidence that these drugs could bolster the actions of noradrenaline because by inhibiting the reuptake process, more noradrenaline would remain in the synapse (the gap between the nerve cells), where it was active. The peculiarity of substances with such contrasting effects on arousal having the same effects on the primary chemical involved in the arousal system didn't appear to raise any doubts.

At this stage, the inhibition of reuptake seemed to be an effect common to many different drugs and not just those considered to be antidepressants, but it hadn't yet been demonstrated to occur in the brain. Then in 1964, Axelrod and a colleague published the results of an experiment that compared imipramine with the tranquilliser chlorpromazine, and showed that imipramine, but not chlorpromazine, inhibited noradrenaline reuptake in brain tissue.[35] This was inferred to mean that imipramine, specifically, increased the activity of noradrenaline in the brain.

It seemed to provide the missing piece of the jigsaw because it enabled psychiatric researchers to claim that all antidepressants of the time increased brain noradrenaline, but other drugs didn't. It has been assumed ever since that inhibition of reuptake is the mechanism of the action of imipramine and other tricyclic antidepressants. Indeed, they are sometimes referred to as 'monoamine reuptake inhibitors' or MARIs.

Yet, the idea that tricyclic antidepressants would result in a net increase of noradrenaline activity is nonsensical. Noradrenaline is a stimulating substance, but imipramine is a sedating drug. Drowsiness is a well-recognised side-effect of imipramine and all tricyclic antidepressants, and studies with 'healthy volunteers' (people without a mental health problem) show these drugs make people tired and impair their mental abilities.[36]

Other evidence confirms that Axelrod's findings were either mistaken or were real but irrelevant. In fact, it has never been possible to demonstrate that tricyclic antidepressants increase noradrenaline activity as supposed, and most evidence suggests they decrease it, which would be consistent with their sedative effects.[37] Moreover, not all tricyclic antidepressants demonstrate reuptake inhibition when tested in experiments similar to Axelrod's.[38] If some of them do inhibit the reuptake mechanism, this may simply be swamped by their many other actions, since all tricyclic antidepressants have a wide spectrum of activity, influencing 'all neurotransmitters, many neuropeptides and most hormones'.[39]

In other words, it is unlikely that drugs like the tricyclic antidepressants increase noradrenaline, because they are sedative substances that reduce wakefulness and activity, and noradrenaline is part of the body's activating system. Axelrod's findings were a red herring.

This obvious contradiction didn't seem to occur to the psychiatric world, however. Psychiatrists of the time were desperate to have drugs they could call antidepressants and to create a theoretical mechanism of depression that could justify their use. They were happy to ignore facts that didn't concur with their needs and Axelrod's research looked, on the surface, as if it was just what was needed for everything to fall into place.

Freud and everyone else who thought depression was best explained as a reaction to misfortune and adversity were wrong. Depression was a biological condition, they thought; it was caused by specific abnormalities of specific brain chemicals and happily these turned out to be the target of a range of new wonder drugs: the antidepressants.

It is difficult to overstate the significance that was, and still is, attached to the supposed reuptake inhibiting properties of imipramine. Axelrod, who was awarded the Nobel Prize in 1970 for this work, among other things, is often remembered for having demonstrated the mechanism of action of the tricyclic antidepressants.[40] Yet, their reuptake properties were important more in imagination than in reality.

The first presentation of the chemical imbalance theory

Axelrod's findings were a key part of the case put forward by Joseph Schildkraut in his famous 1965 paper, which articulated the chemical imbalance theory of depression clearly for the first time. Schildkraut, a researcher based in New York, described the idea that 'some, if not all, depressions are associated with an absolute or relative deficiency of [...] norepinephrine [noradrenaline ...] in the brain'. The majority of the evidence he reviewed to support his hypothesis consisted of the effects of drugs – both those that he thought of as antidepressants and drugs that had been observed to produce depression.[41]

Schildkraut's main example of a substance that can cause depression was reserpine, a drug derived from an Indian plant called Rauwolfia. Reserpine was used as a treatment for high blood pressure in the 1950s and briefly as a tranquilliser for patients in mental hospitals. In common with other tranquillisers of this sort, reserpine can produce symptoms of physical and mental restriction similar to Parkinson's disease, and sometimes apathy and depression.[42] At the time Schildkraut was writing, many scientists thought reserpine exerted its effects by depleting the brain of noradrenaline.

Drugs that boosted noradrenaline activity, according to Schildkraut, included amphetamine, iproniazid and imipramine. He described the 'behavioural stimulation' produced by iproniazid and amphetamine, and suggested it was related to increased noradrenaline activity (which it probably is, among other mechanisms). He then went on to discuss how the 'riddle' of imipramine – that it had not been known to affect noradrenaline – had been solved by Axelrod's 'discovery' that it inhibits noradrenaline reuptake.[43] Axelrod's experiments allowed Schildkraut to conclude that drugs that were deemed to be antidepressants increased the activity of noradrenaline and drugs that produce depression reduced it.

He was wrong on both counts. Not all drugs that were thought to be antidepressants increase noradrenaline – it is unlikely that imipramine or other tricyclic antidepressants do so – and not all drugs that increase noradrenaline are regarded as antidepressants. Schildkraut himself didn't classify amphetamine, which increases noradrenaline activity, as an antidepressant, admitting that it had only 'variable results in the treatment of depression'.[44] As for drugs that produce depression, it is now agreed that reserpine produces its principal effects through its actions on dopamine, not noradrenaline – and its effects on emotions are not equivalent to regular instances of depression in any case.[45]

Schildkraut's paper illustrates again the sleight of hand by which select drugs were transformed into antidepressants. Although the paper started by describing the 'behavioural stimulation' caused by amphetamine and iproniazid, it ended up referring to the supposed antidepressant effects of iproniazid and imipramine. A theory that at first sight looked to be about the effects of noradrenaline on arousal, became one about mood. And this enabled drugs with contrasting effects on arousal – iproniazid and imipramine – to be inserted into the same schema without having to acknowledge the incongruity. No one even seemed to *notice* the incongruity. A story about antidepressants curing an underlying chemical problem was unfurling, and most of psychiatry was entranced by it.

What took place over the course of the 1950s and '60s was a revolution in views about the nature of drugs prescribed for psychological problems and what they might be doing. A crude and often implicit drug-centred model of drug action that existed up until that time – the idea that drugs cause general changes in arousal, emotion and mental activity – was supplanted by the disease-centred model – the idea that drugs target underlying disease or symptom mechanisms. This transformation did not occur because there was evidence to support the truth of the disease-centred view. It came about because psychiatrists *wanted* the disease-centred model to be true, and that coloured the way they interpreted what they were seeing when they gave their patients the new drugs. The disease-centred model was established so quickly and so comprehensively that people soon forgot there was any other way to think about psychiatric drugs.

By the time Axelrod was doing his work on reuptake, most researchers already overlooked the fact that the drugs they were using were mind-altering substances that changed people's usual feelings and behaviour. No one thought it was important to explore the typical changes produced by imipramine, for example, to guide them in interpreting the laboratory findings. Therefore, no one questioned the contradictory idea that a sedating drug might increase noradrenaline activity.

This can be seen as the point at which the scientific community lost interest in the actual effects of the drugs it let loose on patients. This is the situation we have inherited.

6

Serotonin Arrives on the Scene

Serotonin is part of the same family of chemicals as noradrenaline, which are collectively known as monoamines. Therefore, serotonin was always loosely associated with emerging ideas about the chemical basis of depression. In the 1960s, the focus was mainly on noradrenaline, partly because the functions of noradrenaline had been more clearly identified by then than those of serotonin, which even now remain largely mysterious.

There was considerable interest in serotonin in the mid-twentieth century, across many areas of medical research. The first person to isolate the chemical was an Italian scientist, Vittorio Erspamer, in the 1930s, who came across high concentrations of the chemical in the cells of the gut.[1] Later, American scientists detected its presence during their research on the chemical basis of blood-vessel constriction.[2] They called it serotonin because it derived from the serum or blood. By 1951, it had been artificially synthesised in small quantities and in 1953 it was found to be present in the brain.[3]

Following this, research was conducted into the role of serotonin in high blood pressure and migraine, among other areas. Interest in the role of serotonin in mental activity was partly stimulated by the discovery of LSD because there are similarities between the chemical structure of LSD and that of serotonin. Animal experiments showed that LSD opposed the constricting action of serotonin on the uterus and blood vessels,[4] although it was also proposed that LSD mimicked the actions of serotonin.[5]

In the mid-1950s, two sets of researchers, one based in the UK and one in the USA, separately proposed the first chemical imbalance theory of a mental disorder involving serotonin, but it related to schizophrenia rather than depression. They both suggested schizophrenia was caused by a 'lack of serotonin'.[6]

Ideas about serotonin and depression

Later in the 1950s, when interest in the biochemistry of depression was mounting, several researchers started to consider links between serotonin and depression. In 1959, two British psychiatrists speculated that iproniazid might produce its purported effects on depression through increasing the availability of serotonin.[7] At the same time, an American group, headed by a biochemist called Bernard Brodie, proposed that the effects of reserpine, including the depression it induced, were mediated by its actions on serotonin. Brodie and his colleagues never fully developed their ideas, but they were inclining towards the idea that depression was caused by *high* levels of serotonin, because their experiments suggested that serotonin produced some sedative effects, similar to reserpine.[8]

In the USA, interest among depression researchers switched to noradrenaline, but Brodie's findings were influential with two

European researchers: Arvid Carlsson from Sweden, who worked in Brodie's lab for six months in 1955, and Alec Coppen from the UK.[9] In 1963, Coppen published a small experiment involving twenty-five people with depression. They were all given an early antidepressant (tranylcypromine, a similar drug to iproniazid) and, alongside it, half of them were given large doses of tryptophan, the amino acid from which serotonin is made. The study seemed to show that those who took tryptophan improved more than the those who did not.[10]

Coppen and others went on to conduct further studies with tryptophan that did not confirm these effects;[11] nevertheless, Coppen remained convinced that serotonin played a role in depression. He started testing the urine of his patients for levels of serotonin and its break-down products and looking at serotonin levels in the brains of people who had recently died from suicide. He reported on these and other early experiments in two papers, published in 1967 and 1968, in which he reviewed the state of the evidence for a link between depression and brain chemicals in general, and focusing on serotonin in particular.[12]

Coppen's 1967 paper could be a manifesto for the chemical imbalance theory of depression and for the disease-centred theory of antidepressant action. It was also the first paper to make a strong case for the role of serotonin. Coppen opened by acknowledging that some might find the idea of depression as a biochemical disorder 'provocative', but then went on to say, 'In my view, the weight of evidence, although it is by no means conclusive, suggests that biochemical changes are most important' in the causation of depression and other mood problems. It followed from this, he explained, that treating the disorder involves targeting the underlying abnormality: 'A biochemical aetiology implies that there are certain biochemical changes in the brain which need to be restored to normal before the patient's clinical condition will improve.'[13]

Coppen assumed that the drugs that were by then considered to be 'antidepressants' *must* act via a disease-centred mechanism. They 'exert their therapeutic effect by altering the biochemical abnormalities that are responsible for the illness,' he declared.[14] He did not consider other possibilities. He was not interested in the way the various substances he described might alter general mental and physical functions, or how these alterations might interact with people's underlying moods and feelings (as a drug-centred model would encourage).

Like Schildkraut's paper, much of Coppen's was devoted to the way that various drugs were thought to modify mood, including antidepressants and reserpine. Coppen cited the effects of reserpine as evidence for a biochemical basis for depression, but Coppen thought reserpine's effects were mediated through serotonin rather than noradrenaline (both were wrong). Coppen cited the work of Brodie and colleagues, but, in contrast to them, he interpreted it as showing that low serotonin activity was associated with depression. Coppen also described his initial study of tryptophan as evidence for the role of serotonin, and although he acknowledged the unconvincing findings of other studies, he concluded that serotonin 'may be an important monoamine in reducing depression'.[15]

However, after twenty-seven pages describing the latest findings on the biochemistry of depression, Coppen had to admit that despite all the experiments and enthusiasm no one really knew what was going on in the brain when someone was depressed. In fact, he suggested, 'In spite of all the numerous investigation and very exciting leads that are now opening up, we are perhaps only in a slightly better position than Sanctorius of Padua' 300 years ago.[16]

Yet, he remained supremely confident that brain chemistry held the key to understanding depression. In his 1968 paper, he concluded that although we need 'more information about the function of the amines in the central nervous system, [...] it is clear that they have a prominent role in the etiology of depression'.[17] Coppen embodied the spirit of therapeutic fervour that was starting to capture the psychiatric world at this point.

Arvid Carlsson, a pharmacologist, is another key figure in the development of the serotonin story and in the evolution of modern serotonin-targeting antidepressants. By the 1960s, Carlsson was already famous for his discovery that dopamine acted as a brain chemical neurotransmitter, and that dopamine deficiency was the chemical basis of Parkinson's disease.[18] Although it was Carlsson's own experiments that showed that reserpine acted mainly by reducing brain dopamine activity, rather than through serotonin or noradrenaline, Carlsson started to believe that some of the early antidepressants might be exerting their effects via the serotonin system. By this time, some of the tricyclic antidepressants (the class of antidepressants that includes imipramine), had been shown to block the reuptake of serotonin as well as noradrenaline; although, as we saw, the relevance of this effect is questionable.

Carlsson later described how he was influenced by the impressions of a Swiss psychiatrist called Paul Kielholz, who proposed that different tricyclic antidepressant drugs had different effects. Kielholz published a paper in 1968 containing tables and graphs that categorised tricyclic antidepressants – there were now at least seven of these on the market – into those with a 'sedating and anxiolytic component' and those with an 'activating component' or 'stimulating' effects.[19] The idea that any tricyclic antidepressant has 'activating' or 'stimulating' effects is hard to understand, seeing as they are chemically similar and all have a strongly sedative profile, but Carlsson liked the idea that the different agents might have different applications.

Then it was found that tricyclic antidepressants differed somewhat in their effects on serotonin and noradrenaline reuptake. Although the relevance of this to their actual effects had not been clarified, Carlsson speculated that some tricyclic antidepressants might primarily restore 'drive' through their effects on noradrenaline, which was known to be involved in the body's arousal system, and that others might specifically affect mood, via their effects on serotonin.[20]

The first SSRI

These thoughts inspired Carlsson to approach various pharmaceutical companies to persuade them to develop drugs that had more selective effects on the serotonin system. He collaborated with scientists from the Swedish company Astra to produce the drug generally regarded as the first SSRI: zimelidine. The patent was obtained in 1971, and Astra then undertook clinical trials, which reported in 1981. The drug was released in Europe under its trade name Zelmid in 1982, but it didn't last long because it was found to cause a potentially dangerous hypersensitivity reaction and a serious neurological condition called Guillain–Barré syndrome. It was withdrawn from the market in 1983, before it ever reached the USA.[21]

Before it was withdrawn, however, Zelmid had been given to more than 200,000 patients in Europe. This was an impressive reach for a relatively small drug company and for a drug that was only licensed for severe depression. It was even more remarkable given that Zelmid had been tested on a relatively small number of patients prior to its release: identifying and recruiting people with severe depression had been difficult and there was controversy about the optimal dose.

Scientists, including Carlsson, recommended a graduated dose regime, whereas the company wanted a uniform single dose to make prescription and administration easier. Astra prevailed, and despite the fact the drug was only approved for severe depression, it launched a vigorous marketing campaign aimed at GPs. By blurring the difference between severe and less-severe depression, Astra demonstrated the sizeable and largely untapped market for an antidepressant drug, along with the benefits of a simple dosing strategy and aggressive promotion. The rest of the pharmaceutical industry took note, and the brief 'success' of Zelmid was one of the sources of inspiration for the production and release of the more familiar serotonin-based antidepressants a few years later.[22]

The story of Zelmid also illustrates that, two decades after thalidomide, there was still scant concern for the safety of new drugs, at least in Europe. Zelmid was approved on the basis of trials that were far too small to detect rare, adverse effects, and too short to identify the consequences of long-term treatment.

The beginnings of Prozac

Long before Zelmid was released, scientists at Eli Lilly, an American firm, heard about Carlsson's ideas and also started working on producing a drug that targeted the serotonin system. In 1974, David Wong and his team at Lilly published the first report of experiments involving a drug they had just synthesised, which they referred to as 110140. This was fluoxetine, later marketed as Prozac. The paper reported how the new drug was a 'highly selective inhibitor of serotonin uptake [meaning reuptake]' into the nerve cell terminals in tissue preparations made from rat brains.[23]

The paper didn't make a big splash at the time, and the authors were uncertain of the implications of their research. They suggested their new drug might be useful in clarifying the functions of the serotonin system, and that it might find a use as a 'therapeutic agent', most likely in depression and possibly in a subgroup of people with depression who 'are deficient in serotoninergic function and would be helped more by a drug that acts selectively on 5HT [serotonin] than by currently available drugs'.[24] There were few hints of the Prozac phenomenon that was to come.

Science going astray

By the 1970s, the idea that depression could be the manifest result of an imbalance of brain chemicals was firmly established. It was inspiring the development of new drugs along with an extensive research effort to clarify the role of the various chemicals that were proposed to be involved. Drugs known as antidepressants were, from their very beginnings, believed to work by rectifying this presumed brain chemical abnormality.

Coppen's writings illustrate how, for many psychiatrists and researchers, the disease-centred model of drug action – the idea that drugs target an underlying disease mechanism – had already eclipsed the drug-centred model – that drug-induced alterations are superimposed on underlying problems. This ensured that any curiosity people might previously have had about the general alterations their new drugs produced was snuffed out. Drug-induced changes to arousal or wakefulness, and behaviour and mental activity were only considered, if they were considered at all, as extraneous effects (side-effects) that were a nuisance and an obstacle to the perceived restorative or therapeutic properties of the drugs. No one thought to ask how being artificially stimulated or sedated might affect people who were depressed, or how the therapeutic effects the drugs were supposed to have could be distinguished from such effects. For the same reasons, little attention was paid to the potential dangers of giving people brain-modifying chemicals.

To some extent, it was a different era. Scientists regularly tried drugs out on themselves, the ethics of human studies were rudimentary, and, despite thalidomide, there was still relatively little concern about the potential harms and dangers of prescribed medicines. The question of the duration of treatment was rarely discussed, so once started, people were often left on medication indefinitely and there was almost no interest in the possibility that psychiatric drugs might lead to physical dependence and withdrawal symptoms.

The scientists and clinicians working on antidepressants believed they were researching a 'cure' for depression. They believed that depression was a chemical problem and the drugs they had to treat it with were able to restore normal brain function. Understandably, therefore, they focused on the benefits they thought the drugs could produce and regarded other drug-induced effects merely as incidental irritations.

In some ways, we are in the same situation today because the people who do most of the research and write most of the papers still believe in the disease-centred model of antidepressant action. They believe antidepressants are targeting the underlying biological mechanisms of depression. Although they are surely more alert to the dangers and harms of drugs than people working in the 1950s and 1960s, there remains an underlying assumption that taking a drug like an antidepressant must be beneficial because it is rectifying an otherwise intractable biological defect.

The point is that long before Prozac and the other SSRIs arrived, the scene was already set. Scientists and psychiatrists believed that at least a significant proportion of people with depression had a chemical disorder that could be treated with drugs. Yet, the serotonin and noradrenaline theories of depression – often collectively referred to as the monoamine theory – were riddled with inconsistencies right from the start.

Reserpine, which was thought to induce depression, produces its effects primarily by depleting dopamine, rather than through its actions on noradrenaline or serotonin. In any case, reserpine was shown to *improve* symptoms of depression in several randomised trials, rather than making it worse (which reflects the fact that numerous substances not generally classified as antidepressants have marginal effects on depression that are similar to antidepressants).[25] The significance of the reuptake mechanism of tricyclic antidepressants is unclear and experiments using the molecular building blocks (precursors) of serotonin and noradrenaline, such as the trials of tryptophan conducted by Coppen and others, do not consistently demonstrate beneficial effects in depression.

None of this deterred the researchers committed to the idea that depression is fundamentally a biological condition. They set off to conduct a boundless number of experiments on all aspects of the noradrenaline and serotonin systems to try to demonstrate a link with depression. Results were inconsistent – some were positive, and these were highlighted and discussed, some were negative, and these were quietly forgotten. The theory was irrefutable because when negative results accumulated in one area, using one technique, people just left it behind and started looking at another area or started using another technique. We are still in this position today.

The history of the 'monoamine theory' of depression illustrates how easily science can go astray, especially when it is trying to address complex areas of human life, such as emotions and behaviour, that cannot simply be transposed into biological events. A great scientist like Carlsson, whose work on dopamine and Parkinson's disease was undoubtedly a seminal achievement, was beguiled by simple ideas and, as he expressed later in life, by the 'beautiful picture' in Kielholz's article. Carlsson subsequently admitted that his suggestion that noradrenaline was involved in activation and serotonin in mood 'may not be true after all'.[26]

Yet, he and others had been so enamoured with the disease-centred model of drug action and caught up in studying the action of drugs on particular brain chemicals and receptors, they overlooked the question of how drugs affect our biology and behaviour more generally, and what they do to the human being as a whole. In a comprehensive review published in 1987, David Healy suggested the chemical imbalance theory of depression owed its success, in its early years, to having just the 'right measure of simplicity and ambiguity'.[27] It provided a simple message for patients and the media, and although it sounded like it had a clear and definite meaning, it could be interpreted in different ways to fit diverse and conflicting findings. Moreover, the increasing amount of research that was being carried out made it look as if the science was progressing, even when it wasn't.

Early research on the chemical imbalance theory of depression

In the 1980s, the National Institute for Mental Health (NIMH), a US body that funds research, set up a programme designed to resolve some of the outstanding issues in what it called the 'psychobiology' of depression, but was essentially the biology of depression. From perusing the publications that stemmed from the programme, it seems its leaders were already committed to the idea that depression has a biochemical basis, involving the monoamines, serotonin and noradrenaline.

Their main objectives were to clarify which chemical was involved in which type of depression and how the two chemicals might relate to the actions of different antidepressants. Nevertheless, they also tested the validity of the monoamine hypothesis itself by comparing measures of noradrenaline and serotonin in people with depression and people without. They routinely measured the breakdown product of serotonin in the cerebro-spinal fluid (the most direct way serotonin could be measured at the time and, arguably, today), for example; and in a paper describing the project's aims and rationale, they explicitly hypothesised that 'levels for depressed patients as a group will be lower than those found in comparison subjects'.[28] No data from these comparisons between people with and without depression were ever published, however, which seems highly suggestive that no differences were found. Instead, the researchers reported various confusing findings about the response to antidepressants by people with different subtypes of depression, but even these showed no clear relationship with measures of brain chemicals.[29]

The monoamine theory that depression is caused by an insufficiency of noradrenaline or serotonin has inspired decades of research devoted to chasing the chemical origin of depression, all of which represents billions of dollars of wasted time and effort. It has led to the development of drugs targeted at particular chemical pathways, whose impact on the normal functioning of the body and brain have not been properly investigated. Almost no research was conducted, or at least published, on how the drugs that came to be known as antidepressants affect basic biological functions such as wakefulness, arousal, sensations, sexual activity or sleep, let alone how they impact on more complex human attributes, including thinking abilities, emotions and behaviour.

In 1987, just before the arrival of Prozac, David Healy concluded that the monoamine theory of depression was a hypothesis 'in search of evidence'. He thought the lack of confirmation from the NIMH research programme would finally kill the theory off, but it proved far too useful to be abandoned so easily.[30]

7

The 'Age of Depression'

So, while it had always been flaky, by the late 1980s the monoamine hypothesis – the overarching chemical imbalance theory of depression – should have been dead in the water. Yet, it managed to survive long enough to be revitalised by the pharmaceutical industry a few years later in the interests of marketing the new generation of blockbuster drugs: the SSRIs. In the process, the theory was transformed from an unsubstantiated supposition into what was perceived as a scientific truth, and this was what persuaded subsequent generations to flock to their doctors to get pills for depression.

On a cold, grey day in February 2023, I spent an afternoon at the Royal College of Psychiatrists' headquarters in London looking through documents in the college archive. I went with Mark Horowitz, who was looking for information for an upcoming BBC *Panorama* documentary about antidepressants. We felt like spies who had miraculously managed to get access to classified information in the heart of an enemy organisation. I was particularly interested in materials relating to the Defeat Depression Campaign, a campaign launched in the early 1990s to 'raise awareness' of depression. Raising awareness meant encouraging people to see depression as a medical condition and to seek treatment for it. I was curious about the role this campaign and others like it had played in changing people's ideas about the nature of depression and how to respond to it.

The demise of the age of anxiety

I'll get to what I unearthed later, but, first, the key to what happened in the 1990s was the fate of the benzodiazepines and the market for anxiety treatments. Benzodiazepines, such as Librium and Valium, were introduced in the 1960s as an advance on the previous generation of tranquillisers – the barbiturates and barbiturate-like substances that had dominated the market for decades. The problem with barbiturates is that they are extremely toxic in overdose (they are responsible for high-profile deaths, including those of Marilyn Monroe and Jimi Hendrix) and they are associated with a dangerous withdrawal reaction.

The people who consumed barbiturates in the first half of the twentieth century, and later benzodiazepines, were largely women, mainly in middle age, who were unhappy, worried, overwhelmed, unfulfilled or stifled by their lives. Advertisements told doctors they could help women who were 'emotionally overworked, overwrought ... and probably overwhelmed'[1] to cope with 'environmental pressure',[2] 'emotional distress'[3] and feelings of 'inadequacy and isolation'.[4]

Because of their sedative and calming effects, barbiturates and benzodiazepines were principally promoted as treatments for anxiety. Advertisements told doctors the answer to the problems that filled their waiting rooms[5] was an 'anxiety-allaying agent which has a prompt and predictable calming action'.[6] By relieving 'anxiety, tension, agitation and irritability', the drugs could strengthen people's ability to cope with their 'day-to-day problems'.[7] Doctors passed this message onto their patients and in this way people were encouraged to understand their difficulties as consisting of anxiety or 'nerves' – a state that was easily and safely (so they were told) alleviated by one of these 'well-tolerated' drugs.[8]

This carefully constructed 'age of anxiety', as author Andrea Tone called it, helped create the first blockbuster pharmaceuticals.[9] Miltown, a barbiturate-like substance, became the most popular prescription drug in the USA in the 1950s. It was a cultural phenomenon, a bit like Prozac, featuring in cartoons in the *New Yorker* and on greetings cards, and by the late 1950s it was estimated that one in twenty Americans had used it.

Then Librium, the first benzodiazepine, came onto the market in 1960, followed by Valium in 1963, and these quickly succeeded Miltown to best-selling status. Between 1968 and 1981, Valium was the most widely prescribed drug in the Western world[10] and by 1971, around 10 per cent of women in the USA were using a benzodiazepine 'regularly'.[11] Between them, Valium and Librium helped their maker, the Swiss drug company Hoffmann La Roche, become one of the largest and richest pharmaceutical companies in history (and, incidentally, enriched the Sackler family, the owners of Purdue Pharma, the originators of the US opioid crisis. Arthur Sackler owned and ran the company that conducted the advertising campaign for Valium).[12]

Benzodiazepines were initially marketed as a safe and non-addictive alternative to barbiturates. They were indeed safer, but non-addictive they were not. Withdrawal reactions characterised by agitation, insomnia and occasionally epileptic fits were noted following the abrupt discontinuation of high-dose Librium as early as 1961.[13] From the late 1960s, there were reports of people experiencing withdrawal symptoms when they stopped taking more moderate doses.[14]

For many years, no one took much notice, but then there was a dawning realisation that these widely used drugs were, in fact, addictive substances and that millions of people had become unwitting 'addicts'.

It is important to clarify the meaning of the terms 'addiction' and 'dependence' here, which I will use interchangeably as they are used in ordinary speech. Official definitions of these terms have been the cause of much confusion, and this confusion has enabled the fact that antidepressants cause significant withdrawal reactions to be denied or played down. The problem is that it had long been assumed that only drugs that make people feel good, or 'high', can cause addiction or dependence. Therefore, both terms have commonly been associated with the sort of compulsive or drug-seeking behaviour people engage in when they enjoy the effects of a drug. For example, the *International Classification of Diseases* (*ICD*) defines 'dependence' as including 'a strong desire to take the drug' and 'difficulties in controlling its use', but not necessarily the occurrence of physical withdrawal symptoms.[15]

It is now clear, however, that most drugs that affect the brain, if used repeatedly, induce biological changes that give rise to withdrawal symptoms when the drug is stopped (although some doctors remain unaware of the fact). In other words, people become physically dependent on them. This is not related to whether the drug has enjoyable effects. Furthermore, physical dependence is not restricted to drugs that affect the brain, nor to drugs that are used for pain, anxiety or other mental health problems. Steroid withdrawal is a well-recognised phenomenon and cessation of some blood-pressure medications can also cause a withdrawal reaction.[16]

Barbiturates and benzodiazepines, unlike antidepressants, are generally pleasurable to take, so they were commonly diverted onto the recreational drug scene in the 1960s. This allowed it to be claimed that addiction or dependence were problems of addicts and junkies, and not one that involved 'normal' law-abiding people. Drug companies and medical textbooks argued that addiction to benzodiazepines only afflicted people who used the drugs in excessive quantities and had dependence-prone personalities to begin with.[17] In other words, they blamed the patients.

It was only when prominent figures in the USA, such as First Lady Betty Ford, went public about their benzodiazepine addiction in the late 1970s that the problem started to be taken seriously. This prompted a US Senatorial Committee hearing, held in 1979, led by Senator Edward Kennedy. Studies had already shown that people could become dependent at normally prescribed doses by then, but the president of Hoffmann La Roche told the hearing such dependence was 'extremely rare'. Other witnesses, including several doctors who had become dependent on Valium, testified otherwise.[18]

In the UK, a prime-time national television programme, *That's Life*, was devoted to the subject on two separate occasions, in 1983 and 1985, featuring people who reported excruciating withdrawal symptoms after discontinuing benzodiazepines. Following the first programme, the producers received so many letters they commissioned their own MORI poll. This estimated that a colossal 23 per cent of the British population were taking benzodiazepines.[19]

By this time, the level of benzodiazepine use was becoming a major cause of concern in itself. In fact, back in the 1970s, British doctors had written in the *British Medical Journal* and the *Lancet* of a 'psychotropic drug juggernaut' that was leading to the 'total tranquillisation' of the British people.[20] The drugs were being prescribed quite inappropriately, they suggested, for the mollification of people experiencing everyday worries and real material hardships.[21] The fact that women made up the majority of consumers also prompted a feminist backlash, with scholars describing the drugs as a means of social control, which kept women in their place by suppressing their complaints and stifling their protests.[22]

By the middle of the 1980s, tranquillisers had acquired a thoroughly bad reputation, and no drug marketed for anxiety could escape the stigma. It was accepted that benzodiazepines were addictive and that they had been widely used as a social pacifier to numb people to the troubles of life. A drug called buspirone, which was brought out around this time and marketed as a non-addictive tranquilliser, failed to establish a good customer base because people simply no longer believed that a tranquilliser could be non-addictive.[23] The pharmaceutical industry, accustomed to enticing doctors to medicate away their patients' reactions to the stresses of life with a mild degree of inebriation, had to change tack.

The 'age of depression'

The launch of Prozac in 1987 inaugurated what American sociologist Allan Horwitz dubbed a new 'age of depression'.[24] Horwitz suggested that psychiatrists had, in fact, long preferred depression to anxiety for a number of reasons, including that the existence of the monoamine theory suggested it might have a neurochemical basis. In addition to this, the fact that some people were temporarily shocked out of their depression by ECT seemed to suggest it was physical in nature and the episodic character of depression also made it look more like a treatable condition.

Anxiety, on the other hand, was tainted by its association with psychoanalysis, which had the idea of neurosis at its core.[25] From the 1970s onwards, psychoanalysis, previously central to psychiatry, at least in the USA, started to become an embarrassment to the profession. Philosopher Karl Popper referred to it as a 'pseudo-science' and others suggested it was more akin to religion than science.[26] The concept of 'neurosis' was duly expunged from the psychiatric lexicon with the publication of the third edition of the *Diagnostic and Statistical Manual of Mental Disorders* (*DSM* III) in 1980, and as the profession endeavoured to salvage its scientific reputation, it was more than willing to embrace depression as its central concern.

By 1987, professional organisations, such as the US National institute of Mental Health (NIMH), were already funding research on depression (including the 'psychobiology' programme), but only after the introduction of Prozac did they start to reach out to the public. The NIMH launched Depression Awareness, Recognition and Treatment in 1988, a campaign designed to inform the public that depressive disorders are 'common, serious and treatable'.[27] I couldn't find out for certain whether this campaign was supported by Eli Lilly, makers of Prozac, but its timing, a year after Prozac was brought to market, suggests there would have been collaboration with the drug-maker.

Prozac was a runaway success. It showed the fastest growth of any psychiatric drug in history, with sales increasing rapidly from the outset. It was named 'the product of the year' by *Fortune* magazine in 1990[28] and, by 1994, it was the second-best-selling drug in the USA and the entire world (after the anti-ulcer drug Zantac).[29]

Prozac became a cultural as well as a medical phenomenon. In the early 1990s, it featured on the front covers of several leading magazines, including *Newsweek*, *Time* and *New York*; it was the subject of numerous television talk shows and books about it became best sellers. *Prozac Nation*, a book by Elizabeth Wurtzel that described the author's chaotic and troubled young adulthood supposedly relieved, at least for a while, by Prozac, was made into a film.[30]

Magazine articles featured grateful patients who felt their lives had been miraculously transformed by the drug and clinicians who were apparently amazed by its effects. The 1990 *Newsweek* cover story, for example, told the story of 'Susan A', who suffered bouts of depression and bulimia, misused drugs and alcohol, and had tried to kill herself. Within a month of starting Prozac, she reported she felt '1,000 per cent'. She had started a job and her marriage was 'five times better'. 'Ellen M' was an editor, who had taken a variety of different antidepressants since the age of 11, none to much effect. Finally, she tried Prozac and felt 'normal' at last. A pharmacist told the magazine his customers told him they had 'never felt better'.[31]

Although it was only officially licensed for depression at first, almost immediately Prozac was being prescribed for a whole gamut of other psychological conditions, such as anxiety, eating disorders, obsessional behaviour and addiction. Soon it was suggested it could also make people 'better than well'[32] – that, as well as curing medical disorders, it could transform people who did not have a formal diagnosis into more confident, assertive and successful versions of themselves.

Like Valium before it, Prozac was primarily consumed by women, but rather than the bored and frustrated housewife of the Valium era, Prozac was presented as the drug of the professional working woman, including the archetypal 1990s 'supermom'. Advertisements stoked this stereotype with images of women at work and captions such as 'for both restful nights *and* productive days'.[33]

Peter Kramer's famous book, *Listening to Prozac,* opened with the story of Tess, a middle-aged woman who, despite a successful career, lacked confidence and self-esteem and had spent her life lurching from one abusive relationship to another. After starting Prozac, she became more confident, she enjoyed dating a variety of men and started to find her work more satisfying. Kramer concluded that Prozac had transformed her personality from a shy, timid, self-effacing person who lived for others, to someone who was confident, outgoing and asserted her own needs. With echoes of dystopian science fiction, he suggested Prozac was the first of a new generation of sophisticated chemicals that would enable doctors to 'sculpt the patient's personality trait by trait'.[34]

A subsequent *Newsweek* article from 1994 described how people with no history of psychological problems were benefitting from taking Prozac. Helen, a successful public relations executive, was not depressed but sometimes had difficulty prioritising and focusing at work. She took Prozac to 'give herself an edge'. 'Now that she's on the antidepressant,' the article read, 'she not only handles job pressures more gracefully but sports a more buoyant personality.'

Prozac was also credited with making people more content and less combative or argumentative.[35] Susan, who featured in the 1990 *Newsweek* article, described how on Prozac she finally 'liked Mom and Dad' and was well liked at work. A *New Yorker* cartoon from 1993, entitled 'If they had Prozac in the 19th century', depicted Karl Marx with a speech bubble declaring, 'Sure, capitalism can work out its kinks'.[36]

Yet, it was emphasised, Prozac was not like Valium or street drugs. A *New York Times* article from 1993, which described the fascination with Prozac as indicative of a 'legal drug culture', nevertheless stressed that people taking Prozac were 'not talking about getting high, or escaping'. They were 'talking about not feeling depressed anymore, or feeling better able to cope or, in some instances, simply feeling more like themselves'.[37]

The ability of Prozac and similar antidepressants to numb or blunt emotions suggests that what Kramer was observing may have been, along with some creative interpretation, the consequence of a Prozac-induced reduction in people's emotional sensitivity. However, the similarity between stories from the early days of Prozac and those described by Roland Kuhn in relation to imipramine suggests the miraculous transformations reported were largely a function of the hype accompanying the introduction of a new medication.

Most of Kramer's patients had already tried the tricyclic antidepressants, hailed as miraculous a generation earlier, and failed to improve on them or failed to improve for long. We don't know what happened to his patients in the long run, but Elizabeth Wurtzel certainly wasn't cured by Prozac. Although she described feeling better for a short time after starting it, before long she was experiencing renewed fits of depression and taking regular overdoses again. In the book's epilogue, she admitted, 'The secret I sometimes think that only I know is that Prozac really isn't that great.'[38] Enthusiasm can engender a powerful placebo effect, but the effect wears off as the drug loses its novelty.

The chemical imbalance

In his book on the history of 'happy pills', historian David Herzberg describes how, from the start, it was Prozac's targeted effects on the serotonin system that were credited for its supposed ability to cure depression and modify inconvenient aspects of temperament. Prozac was described as if it was a piece of precision engineering that could accurately tweak bits of the brain responsible for unwanted emotions and character traits, leaving the rest more or less untouched. 'Instead of using a shotgun,' said a Professor of Psychiatry in 1990, 'you're using a bullet.'[39]

Serotonin itself became a 'minor celebrity', as it was increasingly believed to constitute the chemical basis of happiness and success. By the late 1990s, an article in *Time* magazine opened by asking, 'Could a single brain chemical hold the key to happiness, high social status and a nice, flat stomach?'[40] The *Guardian* newspaper wondered whether the British had become a 'low-serotonin people'.[41] As David Healy pointed out, the psychoanalytical 'psychobabble' of the ID and ego, popular in the 1970s and 1880s, gave way to an equally opaque 'biobabble' of neurochemical imbalances, receptors and the mysterious and essentially meaningless term 'dysregulation'.[42]

The pharmaceutical industry ensured the message about serotonin being the basis of depression and antidepressant action saturated the minds of prescribers and their patients alike. In his book *Blaming the Brain*, Elliot Valenstein, of the University of Michigan, reproduced some of the advertising copy released in the early days of Prozac and the other SSRIs.[43] Even before the official legalisation of direct-to-consumer advertising in the USA in 1997, pharmaceutical companies had access to the public in various ways. In 1996, for example, a consortium of American drug companies inserted a booklet called 'New Hope for depression and other mental illnesses' into copies of major magazines including *Time*, *Newsweek* and *Reader's Digest*. The booklet told readers, 'Mental illnesses are medical illnesses just like diabetes, high blood pressure or heart disease'. It went on to present depression as having been demonstrated to be caused by abnormalities of brain chemicals:

> Today scientists know that many people suffering from mental illness have imbalances in the way their brain's metabolise certain chemicals called neurotransmitters. Too much or too little of these chemicals may result in depression, anxiety, or other emotional or physical disorders.[44]

Doctors were also used as conduits and provided with materials designed to be passed on to their patients. Eli Lilly produced a sheet of this sort, sometime during the 1990s, which told people that 'serotonin, an important chemical found in the brain, is linked to depression'. It featured two pictures of the same woman: one with her looking sad, accompanied by the caption, 'Serotonin in short supply', and one with her looking happy, with the caption, 'Serotonin in good supply'.[45]

When the FDA lifted restrictions on direct-to-consumer advertising in the USA, it opened the floodgates to a deluge of advertisements on television, billboards and in newspapers and magazines. Much of this told people that depression was a physical illness produced by a shortage or imbalance of serotonin or other brain chemicals.

An advertisement placed in *Cosmopolitan* magazine in 1997, for example, told readers, 'When you're clinically depressed, one thing that can happen is that the level of serotonin (a chemical in your body) may drop [...] To help bring your serotonin levels closer to normal, the medicine doctors now prescribe most often is Prozac.'[46] The famous television 'blob' advert I described in Chapter 2 was released in 2001 and featured an animation of the antidepressant Zoloft (sertraline) replenishing the alleged shortage of serotonin molecules in the synapse.[47]

Disease awareness campaigns

As if the pharmaceutical industry was not doing well enough on its own, the medical profession was happy to lend a helping hand. The Defeat Depression Campaign was conducted by the Royal College of Psychiatrists and the Royal College of General Practitioners between 1992 and 1996, although it was predominantly run by the former. I remember the campaign well and I visited the archive because I wanted to see what I could learn from unpublished documents and whether I could confirm my suspicions that it received funding from the pharmaceutical industry. This was not disclosed in any of the numerous leaflets produced by the campaign, but I felt sure I had seen it reported somewhere.

In the archive I found a copy of a letter from 1997 written by the then President of the Royal College of Psychiatrists, Robert Kendell, to Charles Medawar, a health campaigner. Medawar had written to the college to complain that the Defeat Depression Campaign had ignored the dependence-forming nature of antidepressants, and he enquired whether the campaign had accepted donations from pharmaceutical companies. In his reply, Kendell stated that 28 per cent of the funding of the campaign had come from the industry.[48] However, I came across another document that presented a breakdown of the campaign's funding and this suggested the contribution was 44 per cent, plus an unknown amount from Eli Lilly for the production and distribution of some leaflets.[49]

Whether it was 28 per cent or 44 per cent, the Royal College of Psychiatrists never acknowledged the drug company sponsorship publicly. None of the other documents I reviewed mentioned it, except for one version of a report on the campaign. However, another version of the same report omitted this particular section.[50] It looked as if the college had tried to avoid recording its links with the pharmaceutical industry as far as it could.

In his reply to Medawar, Kendell stressed how the college had only accepted money on the basis that the industry would have no influence on the content of the campaign, and it is true the campaign never recommended individual drugs. However, the importance of company sponsorship is illustrated by the fact that a meeting to discuss the future of the campaign in 1996 was held at Eli Lilly's headquarters in London.[51]

The function of the Defeat Depression Campaign was to persuade the population that depression is a common medical condition that requires medical treatment. An illustrated booklet published for the campaign, called *Down with Gloom*, claimed that between a third and half of people will be afflicted by depression at some time in their lives, and that at any one time, one in seven or eight people is currently depressed.[52] Other campaign materials claimed that only half the people who suffered from depression were diagnosed or treated. In some documents, people with depression were depicted as an iceberg, with the tip above the water representing the small proportion of people who were supposed to be receiving appropriate treatment.[53] The conclusion was that GPs needed educating in the recognition and treatment of depression, and the public needed encouragement to identify themselves as having a medical problem.[54] 'Making depression a more legitimate reason for visiting the GP' was a campaign priority.[55]

In order to achieve this, the campaign set out to overturn people's previous views about depression, views that were rooted in centuries of commonsense. To prepare for the campaign, in 1991 the Royal Colleges conducted focus groups and commissioned a MORI poll to find out what people thought were the causes of depression, and what their attitudes were to taking medication for depression. Focus-group participants felt that everyone gets depressed at some point in their lives and identified the causes of depression as being 'bereavement, moving house, isolation, marriage breakdown, having a baby, illness, and redundancy'.[56] They didn't mention a chemical imbalance or anything else about the brain. In the poll, although 73 per cent of people agreed with the statement that 'depression is a medical condition', only 33 per cent thought depression could be caused by 'biological changes in the brain', compared with almost 80 per cent who though it could be caused by unemployment, bereavement and other life events.[57]

In other words, people generally held the view of depression I outlined in Chapter 3: a meaningful emotional reaction to adversity. The Royal College of Psychiatrists, on the other hand, concluded that 'the confusion between the social origins of depression and the medical nature of depression needs to be addressed' – in other words, people's sense that depression is a normal reaction to challenging life events and losses needed to be overwritten with the idea that it is a medical condition that arises from medical – that is, biological – causes.[58]

Both doctors and patients also needed persuading that antidepressant treatment was effective, simple and safe. Hence the campaign also set out to wear down people's natural and sensible cautiousness about using drugs that modify emotions. 'There is a strange resistance to taking drugs for depression,' the

Down with Gloom booklet commented.[59] In the 1991 poll, only 16 per cent of respondents thought people with depression should be offered an antidepressant and less than half of them (46 per cent) thought antidepressants were effective for depression. In contrast, 90 per cent thought people with depression should be offered counselling and 85 per cent of people thought counselling was effective.[60] *Down with Gloom* concluded, 'Clearly, then, the public needs far more education and persuasion in the taking of antidepressants when they are needed.'[61]

A major theme of the Defeat Depression Campaign and much early promotional material was that antidepressants did not cause addiction or dependence. The 1991 survey found that 78 per cent of the British public thought antidepressants were addictive. The leaders of the campaign thought people had incorrectly extrapolated from their knowledge about benzodiazepines to conclude that antidepressants were also addictive.[62] They worried that this would reduce people's willingness to take antidepressants and so they advised doctors to tell their patients 'the facts that antidepressants are not habit-forming or addictive'.[63] The *Down with Gloom* pamphlet told readers, almost hysterically, 'It needs, apparently, to be shouted again and again from the housetops: ANTIDEPRESSANTS ARE NOT ADDICTIVE.'[64]

The campaign was particularly concerned about the fact that people only took antidepressants for a short time, and it urged doctors to encourage their patients to take them for at least four to six months *after* they started to feel better. Campaign literature estimated that most people took their antidepressants for less than three weeks, and hence this recommendation alone stood to increase the use of these drugs by a vast amount. The leaders of the campaign speculated that 'patients may believe that the drugs are addictive so naturally they do not wish to take them for a long time'.[65]

When the campaign said antidepressants were not 'addictive', however, it didn't mean they were easy to stop, although this was not explained to the campaign's audience. In his response to Medawar's challenge that antidepressants cause dependence just like benzodiazepines, Royal College of Psychiatrists President Robert Kendall admitted that antidepressants might cause withdrawal symptoms. However, he argued that because they lack the appealing qualities that lead to compulsive and harmful use, they do not cause 'dependence'. He cited the International Classification of Disease's definition that equates dependence with drug misuse rather than the propensity of a drug to cause withdrawal effects. Withdrawal symptoms, Kendall suggested, were of no great concern and should be regarded simply as 'an adverse effect that should be weighed in the balance with other adverse effects against the drug's benefit'.[66]

It turns out Kendall was wrong, and the public was right to suspect that getting off antidepressants was not a trivial affair and the longer you took them, the more problematic it became. Looking back, it is tragic to see that ordinary people had a better sense of the dangers of antidepressants than members of the profession, who were supposed to be the experts, and even more tragic that this sense was drummed out of people so they would become willing recipients of the latest pharmaceutical money-spinners.

Although the Defeat Depression Campaign clearly positioned depression as a medical problem and antidepressants as a targeted medical treatment, it did not explicitly claim that depression was due to a chemical imbalance. US organisations were not so reticent. The National Alliance for Research on Schizophrenia and Depression (now the Brain and Behavior Research Foundation) placed large advertisements in national newspapers, which claimed that 'recent research has taught us that depression is often biological, caused by a chemical imbalance in the brain'.[67] A pamphlet produced by this organisation, entitled 'Conquering Depression', which was funded by

Wyeth-Ayerst, makers of the hugely successful antidepressant Effexor (venlafaxine), told people, 'Scientists believe that major depression is caused by an imbalance of neurotransmitters – natural chemicals that allow brain cells to communicate with one another'.[68]

In the UK, an organisation called Neurolink, funded by Wyeth-Ayerst, produced a guide for GPs in the early 2000s, entitled 'Depression: A Guide to its Recognition and Management in General Practice'. The guide told recipients, 'Depressed people have reduced levels of serotonin and noradrenaline. Drugs which increase the levels of these neurotransmitters can restore the balance and improve mood.' It also instructed doctors, 'Depression should be treated regardless of whether the cause is an understandable reaction to life events or circumstances'.[69] Among the experts working for Neurolink (and therefore indirectly for Wyeth) who had endorsed the guide was psychiatrist David Nutt. Nutt was an enthusiastic promoter of antidepressants prior to his conversion to psychedelics and is also famed for losing his job as a government advisor after suggesting that taking Ecstasy was no more harmful than riding a horse.[70]

Use of antidepressants

The Defeat Depression Campaign itself had only modest success by its own standards. A poll conducted in 1997, a year after the end of the campaign, revealed that 43 per cent of people now agreed depression could be caused by 'biological changes in the brain' (up from 33 per cent in 1991), but the proportion of people who endorsed antidepressant treatment for someone with depression was still only 24 per cent (it was 16 per cent in 1991).[71]

However, the combination of pharmaceutical marketing and professional authority eventually proved an irresistible mix. In the UK, the number of prescriptions issued for antidepressants rose by 235 per cent between 1992 and 2002.[72] In the USA, prescriptions rose to a staggering 1,550 per cent between 1988 and 2002, from 2 million to 33 million.[73]

International organisations were swept up by the propaganda, too, helping to establish a worldwide antidepressant market. In 1996, the World Health Organization proclaimed depression to be the second-leading cause of disability on the planet after cardiovascular disorder[74] and by 2017 it was said to be the number one cause.[75] No one questioned how so many people had developed a new or previously rare disease at the same time as the world's population was richer and healthier than ever before.[76]

The marketing of Prozac and the antidepressants that followed was a trailblazer in selling a disease along with a drug claimed to treat it. Numerous 'disease awareness' campaigns followed the example of the early depression campaigns, persuading people to view situations such as premenstrual tension, baldness, shyness and sexual difficulties as diseases in need of medical treatment, creating a myriad of new markets for new drugs.[77]

In the aftermath of the revelation that benzodiazepines were highly addictive substances like their predecessors, the barbiturates, the depression awareness campaigns reassured people that antidepressants were not zombifying tranquillisers and would not get you hooked. They were drugs that precisely targeted underlying chemical defects or imperfections. They treated real medical conditions and might even make you a more productive and successful person by tweaking the chemical framework of your personality.

The popularity of the deadly barbiturates in the middle of the twentieth century, as well as the widespread and frequently lethal use of opium in the nineteenth century, demonstrates the human appetite for a chemical solution to the troubles of life. In a meeting I attended to discuss how to reduce antidepressant prescribing in the UK, a GP protested that doctors simply *must* have a pill to give to patients in distress, and at least modern antidepressants didn't kill people like the drugs of the past.[78]

Yet, although the deluge of marketing that Prozac unleashed may have found a willing ear in some respects, it also had to overcome people's equally ingrained suspicions of using chemicals to adjust one's emotions and personality – suspicions that had been reinforced by the benzodiazepine affair. As David Healy commented back in 2004, we need to 'contemplate the possibility that the Era of Depression we have recently been living through in the West has stemmed primarily from the need of pharmaceutical companies to market compounds such as Prozac, Zoloft and Paxil'.[79] It is not an exaggeration to say that the pharmaceutical industry made us depressed.

Part 3

The Science

8

Reviewing the Evidence on the Serotonin Theory of Depression

Now that we understand the origins of the theory that depression is caused by a deficit of serotonin or serotonin activity, it is time to take a closer look at the modern evidence for the theory.

When I set out to review the evidence, I knew it would be a mammoth task. It would require a team of people to sift through a massive volume of research papers, pick out the relevant ones and summarise what they revealed. In 2019, I managed to gather a team together. It included Mark Horowitz, who was working with me on a government-funded study of antipsychotic drugs at the time, and several researchers with expertise in conducting systematic reviews. We wrote the protocol for the review and then divided up the different areas of research between the members of the team. Before I come to what we found, however, I need to provide a realistic picture of what we know and what we don't know about the biological functions of serotonin.

Evidence on the functions of serotonin

Serotonin is a chemical found in various parts of the body, including the brain. Actually, most of it is located in the gut and in blood cells known as platelets. Only about 8 per cent is found in the brain, where it is produced by structures known as the raphe nuclei. From there, it is distributed to other parts of the brain, where it acts as a neurotransmitter.

So, what do we know about the sort of behaviours and feelings that are influenced by serotonin-related transmission in the brain? Returning to the metaphor of the *Mona Lisa* from Chapter 3, in one sense this is like asking how the chemical structure of the paint affects the meaning of the picture. We might wonder how relevant this is, but regardless, there have been hundreds, if not thousands, of studies that have attempted to identify the effects of various brain chemicals on emotions, intelligence, learning and behaviour.

Despite the volume of this research, there is little evidence of any links. How the brain works, in general, is incredibly complex, involving numerous interrelated systems, and we lack clear knowledge even about something as basic as how the brain keeps us awake.[1] You wouldn't know this, however, from reports in the press that regularly describe how the 'neurochemistry of love' or anger or aggression has just been identified,[2] or how serotonin produces 'a sense of well-being and happiness'.[3]

The scientific literature is also misleading and frequently overstates its findings. A typical paper tells us, 'Serotonin regulates mood, behaviour, appetite, and energy expenditure'.[4] So, what is the evidence that serotonin is involved in any of these things? Many of these claims are based on studies using drugs that manipulate the serotonin system, but this research is problematic because most drugs have effects on a variety of brain chemicals, and brain-chemical systems are also deeply interconnected.

Appetite is frequently said to be regulated by serotonin, for example, but the principal evidence for this assertion comes from research on the appetite-suppressant drug fenfluramine. Fenfluramine was used as a drug for weight loss until it was pulled from the market in 1997, due to the discovery that it could damage the heart valves.[5] Since it was thought to act by increasing serotonin activity, it has been concluded that serotonin reduces appetite. However, it turns out that fenfluramine wasn't a very good appetite suppressant – in fact, it was usually prescribed in combination with the stimulant drug phentermine (in a preparation known as fen-phen) – and what's more, it's not clear that it works by affecting serotonin anyway. Fenfluramine is derived from the stimulant drug amphetamine, and we know that amphetamine, which also suppresses appetite, exerts its effects principally through increasing the activity of noradrenaline and dopamine.[6] There is no compelling evidence, therefore, that serotonin plays a specific role in appetite regulation.

Evidence on sexual function is stronger, although, again, much of this also comes from the effects of drugs that are not likely to be entirely specific to the serotonin system. Broadly, animal studies show that drugs designed to increase the action of serotonin, such as SSRIs, reduce sexual activity, and drugs that inhibit serotonin increase sexual activity.[7] Injecting serotonin into parts of the brain that are linked with sexual behaviour reduces sexual activity and deliberately damaging parts that produce or are rich in serotonin, such as the raphe nucleus, increases sexual activity.[8]

Studies with humans indicate that SSRIs reduce genital sensitivity and delay orgasm, effects that are consistent and potent enough that SSRIs have been trialled as treatments for premature ejaculation.[9] No one knows the precise mechanisms that underpin SSRIs' impact on sexual function; many other drugs, including other types of antidepressants, which predominantly affect other chemical systems, impair sexual function too. Overall, however, the evidence suggests serotonin inhibits normal sexual function in various ways.

Serotonin is frequently claimed to be involved in learning, intelligence and motivation. A typical review of the extensive animal research in this area, written by three scientists from Cambridge University, claimed that evidence indicates 'a role for serotonin in modulating context-dependence parameters of action selection, affect, and social cognition; and concurrently supporting learning mechanisms, which promote adaptability and behavioural flexibility'.[10] This might sound plausible, but reading the paper closely reveals it is actually a tortuous attempt to salvage something out of research that finds nothing.

The paper reported that one animal experiment or another had demonstrated serotonin is associated with increased 'waiting behaviour' (animals wait longer for a reward), 'fleeing behaviour' (animals are quicker to flee from a threat), 'persistence' (animals are slower to flee from a threat), inhibitory behaviour (animals become less active) and locomotion (animals become more active). In other words, experiments produced highly inconsistent results. The authors admitted the literature they surveyed was replete with 'failures of replication' and 'contradictory effects in similar paradigms'[11] and described the findings as 'difficult to interpret'.[12] They acknowledged that the overall functions of serotonin 'remained elusive', and even though they made a valiant effort to explain away the inconsistencies, their findings indicate that manipulating the serotonin system results in no obvious pattern of effects on intelligence, learning or motivation.

No doubt serotonin is involved in many of our biological functions. It is found all over the brain, so this wouldn't be surprising. The authors of one scientific review concluded that 'serotonin modulates virtually all human behavioural processes' and, they go on, 'indeed, it is difficult to find a human behaviour that is not regulated by serotonin'.[13]

All this means, however, is that serotonin is present in the brain and, as such, is involved in most of what the brain does. It is equivalent to saying that paint is involved in a painting! And although you are unlikely to encounter a neuroscientist with an interest in serotonin who will admit the parlous state of our knowledge, it appears that, apart from its likely inhibitory effect on sexual function and sexual desire, we have no clear idea about serotonin's specific role in bodily functions, behaviour or mental activity.

How evidence is misinterpreted

Before I move on to the details of our review, I want to consider how it is that tentative or ambiguous scientific findings like these become accepted scientific 'knowledge', which sometimes get transformed into headline-grabbing 'breakthroughs'.

First, most experiments involve doing an array of tests, and researchers have a tendency to highlight the tests that produce positive or interesting results and ignore the rest. But, if you do enough tests, some will come up positive due to random fluctuations in our biological states, even when there is no real difference.

Second, much of the research on serotonin and depression involves studies that compare people with depression to people without depression. The latter are often referred to as 'healthy controls' or 'healthy volunteers' and they are meant to be similar to the participants with depression, except in not being or having been depressed. But they are often different in important ways: volunteers are likely to be physically fitter and healthier than the people with depression, for example, which may affect the serotonin system; they are less likely to be taking medicines, such as painkillers, which are known to influence serotonin; and of course, they are generally not taking antidepressants.

This is particularly relevant because in most of these studies, participants with depression are taking or have taken antidepressants, and evidence from animal and human studies suggests that antidepressants (and not just SSRIs) affect the serotonin system, both while they are being taken and after they are stopped.[14] Therefore, studies that involve a comparison between people with depression and 'healthy volunteers' may detect coincidental differences in the serotonin system, which are nothing to do with depression but are caused by things that are linked to depression, including the use of antidepressants.

Third, there is the issue of causation and correlation. If abnormalities in the serotonin system or anything else were to be found in people with depression, it doesn't necessarily imply they are the cause of depression. They might be the way the brain reacts when someone is in a low mood. In other words, they might be the physiological and biochemical *result* of feeling depressed, not its cause.

Typically, what happens is a small study is published claiming to find evidence of a relationship between serotonin and depression. Everyone gets excited, the media report that research has shown a connection, and the public are left with the impression that an important scientific advance has been made. When larger studies are conducted that fail to replicate the positive finding, they are either not published, as is likely to have occurred with the National Institute of Mental Health 'psychobiology of depression' studies of the 1980s, or they are published but ignored. Gradually, it becomes apparent that the research is leading nowhere, at which point the researchers give up and move on to a new area. But no one admits, at least not publicly and maybe not even to themselves, that the research failed to find evidence of the links it set out to study. So, the idea that there is evidence to support the original theory continues to circulate and is never publicly refuted. This is how long-defunct theories persist.

Serotonin and depression

The idea that serotonin is involved in mood derives primarily from research investigating whether serotonin is implicated in depression. This is what my team and I set out to look at in our review of the evidence for the serotonin theory of depression. Specifically, we aimed to evaluate the claim that low levels or reduced activity of serotonin causes depression.

Good-quality reviews need to be conducted systematically, using established principles and transparent methods. Since there is so much research on serotonin, we elected to conduct what is referred to as an 'umbrella' review. An umbrella review is a review of reviews – it is designed to provide an overview of all the systematic reviews, meta-analyses (a meta-analysis is an analysis based on a combination of different studies) and large-scale studies in a particular area. Because we were looking at research in several different areas, our review was effectively a series of mini-umbrella reviews.

We focused on the main areas of research on serotonin and depression, which have investigated concentrations of serotonin and its breakdown products (metabolites) in blood and brain fluid, serotonin receptors, the serotonin transporter protein and the gene for the serotonin transporter. Genetic studies have also tested whether there is an interaction between the serotonin transporter gene and adverse life events, which we also looked at. We also examined experiments using a technique called tryptophan depletion, which aimed to test whether lowering serotonin levels in the brain can induce depression in people who are not already depressed.

So, what did we find? You can see details of the research we included in our review in Table 1, but the results can be summarised quite easily. Except for the genetic studies, the research consisted of small studies that either showed no link between serotonin and depression or yielded inconsistent results. Moreover, few of them accounted for the likely impact of antidepressants. The recent genetic studies were very large, high-quality studies, and they were convincingly negative.

We were not the first to suggest the serotonin theory of depression has not been proven by research; so, overall, the results were as we expected. However, we had not been aware of quite how weak and confusing the evidence was. There were some surprising findings, too, particularly indications of how antidepressants affect serotonin. I won't describe all the research we examined because it involves a lot of technical details and you can read the paper if you want to,[15] but I'll give you a flavour of what we found.

Studies of the serotonin breakdown product in brain fluid

Because you can't stick needles into people's brains, it is generally agreed that, at present, the most direct measure we have of serotonin in the brain is the concentration of the main breakdown product of serotonin in the cerebrospinal fluid that surrounds the brain. Serotonin is an unstable molecule, however, so researchers prefer to measure its main breakdown product (known as 5HIAA), which is more stable. The cerebrospinal fluid can be sampled by doing a lumbar puncture, but this is an invasive procedure that carries risks of infection and injury, so, for this reason, studies of this sort are not common or large, but several have been done.

We identified two previous systematic reviews of studies of the concentration of the serotonin breakdown product in cerebrospinal fluid. The two reviews looked at nineteen separate studies between them. Neither of these reviews found any overall difference in the level of the breakdown product in people with depression compared to people without depression. So, the most direct method we currently have of assessing brain levels of serotonin suggests there is no difference between people with depression and people without depression.

Tryptophan-depletion studies

The area of research that is most often cited to support the serotonin theory of depression consists of a curious set of experiments known as tryptophan-depletion studies.[16] These are intended to reduce brain serotonin by depleting the supply of serotonin's parent molecule: tryptophan. Tryptophan is a naturally occurring amino acid (amino acids are the building blocks of the proteins that make up our bodies) and it is usually acquired through food, including milk, tuna, chicken and chocolate.[17]

The method of tryptophan depletion employed in recent times involves giving people a drink containing a mixture of common amino acids that specifically lacks tryptophan. The drink reduces the amount of tryptophan that crosses into the brain and it is assumed that this slows down the synthesis of serotonin in the brain. Within hours of having the drink, it can be shown that concentrations of tryptophan in the blood and brain reduce markedly. Whether the technique reduces serotonin levels in the brain has not been definitively demonstrated, but experts think it is likely it does, at least to some extent.[18]

The principal aim of tryptophan-depletion studies is to see if the technique can induce depression or lower mood in healthy volunteers who are not depressed to begin with. Numerous such studies have been conducted. The last review we could find was published in 2007, so in order to get a snapshot of more recent research, we also looked at the ten most recent studies of tryptophan depletion published at the time we did our review (Table 2).

The 2007 review has been highly influential. It was conducted by a group of researchers led by Professor Eric Ruhé from the Netherlands, and it surveyed thirty-two studies involving 'healthy volunteers' and nineteen studies involving people who had a history of depression.[19] Studies involving volunteers mostly showed that the tryptophan-depleted drink had no effect on people's mood compared to a control drink, including the higher quality, more robust two-group studies (studies that compare the effects of the experimental and control drinks in two separate groups of people as opposed to studies that compare the effects of the drinks sequentially in a single group).

None of the ten more recent studies we sampled detected any effect of the tryptophan-depletion technique on mood in healthy volunteers, either. Hence, the evidence does not suggest that reducing brain serotonin by tryptophan depletion induces depression in people who are not depressed to begin with.

In contrast, a number of the studies in the 2007 review that involved people with a history of depression showed that the tryptophan-depleted drink did appear to lower mood compared to the control drink. However, results of the individual studies were inconsistent, and the total number of people involved was small, suggesting the effects may have been a chance finding rather than a real effect. Moreover, it looked as if some studies had been double counted, which would suggest numbers were even smaller. Most participants had used or were using anti-depressants, which may also have modified the effects of the tryptophan-depletion procedure.

In our sample of more recent studies, two involved people with a history of depression and both found no effects of tryptophan depletion. In a supreme example of spin, it was claimed in one of them that tryptophan depletion did have an effect. What it actually showed, however, was that the control group experienced a slight improvement in mood for some reason, producing a difference between the real drink and the sham drink (the improvement was tiny and most likely a random and irrelevant fluctuation).[20]

So, tryptophan-depletion studies do not support the serotonin theory of depression. The experiments clearly show the technique does not provoke depression in volunteers. Some older studies suggested tryptophan depletion may lower mood in people with a previous history of depression, but results were variable and not confirmed in recent studies.

Studies of serotonin receptors and the serotonin transporter

We were surprised to find that some of the research we examined indicated that, if anything, there might be increased serotonin in people with depression. Studies of one of the serotonin receptors (the 5HT1a receptor), which mainly inhibits the action of serotonin, found evidence of reduced levels of this receptor in some brain areas. If this is a real finding, it suggests that serotonin activity is higher, not lower, in people with depression, because the receptor reduces the activity of serotonin. Findings varied across different brain areas, however, and the number of participants was small, so the results may well be random findings. The use of antidepressants was also not accounted for in the studies, yet antidepressants have been shown to modify serotonin receptors.[81] Hence, the results are most likely to be explained by chance or the effects of antidepressants.

Research on the serotonin transporter revealed a similar picture. Higher concentrations of the transporter would be expected to lower serotonin activity by removing serotonin from the nerve synapse, where it is active. Lower levels would be expected to increase serotonin activity. SSRIs inhibit this transporter, remember, which is how they are thought to increase serotonin activity. But some of the studies we looked at detected *lower* levels of the serotonin transporter in some brain areas in people with depression, implying *higher* serotonin activity. Increased levels of the transporter, which would be associated with lower levels of serotonin, were only detected in a single brain area in one poor-quality study. Overall, however, like the serotonin receptor, research on the serotonin transporter was inconsistent and the results most likely explained by chance or by the use of antidepressants. In most studies, people with depression were using or had used antidepressants.

Genetic studies

The genetic studies explored the effects of the gene for the serotonin transporter protein. It turns out that some people have a shortened version of this gene, which is thought to be less efficient and to result in reduced production of the serotonin transporter. In 1996, a study involving 1,024 people from different countries in Europe was published, which reported that people with depression were more likely to have the short version of the serotonin transporter gene than the normal version, compared with people without depression.[22] This study sparked a frenzy of interest and dozens of studies followed.

Results were disappointingly inconsistent, but, in 2003, a group of researchers based in London reported that people with the short version of the gene were more likely to have depression, but only if they also had a history of being exposed to 'life stress'.[23] This research was influential and led to a further proliferation of studies, with numerous research groups setting out to see if they could replicate the link between the gene, depression and adverse life experiences. As the studies mounted, more and more systematic reviews and meta-analyses were conducted. We looked at the five most recent analyses of data in this area.

Results of the genetic studies were conclusive. Two definitive, high-quality studies (Border et al., 2019, and Culverhouse et al., 2018, in Table 1),[24] both of which involved data from tens of thousands of people, found no evidence that having the short version of the serotonin transporter gene was associated with depression and no evidence of an interaction with stressful life events, a history of trauma, childhood abuse or any other measures of stress. The largest of these included data from over 100,000 people, and both of them incorporated much of the data from earlier reviews and studies.

The genetic studies clearly illustrate the pattern of research I described at the beginning of this chapter. Some of the earlier studies we looked at, especially those that looked at gene-stress interactions, reported positive findings, demonstrating how it is possible for data to give the impression that a real effect exists even when it doesn't. In fact, when we remember that evidence of the effect of the serotonin transporter gene was first reported in 1996, we can see that false-positive or misleading findings were accepted for more than two decades before bigger and better studies revealed the real situation. Genetic research is well suited to conducting large studies because of the massive banks of genetic samples that have been built up. Such big studies are more difficult in other research areas; therefore, it is likely that false-positive results get propagated for even longer.

As we were putting our results together, we noticed how the genetic studies also demonstrate the powerful link between negative life events and depression. Although studies that explored the gene-stress interaction found no effect of the gene, they all identified a strong relationship between depression and experiences of stress, adversity and abuse.

Antidepressants and serotonin

One unexpected result of our review was that some of the research we examined suggested the long-term use of antidepressants might *reduce*, not increase, serotonin levels.[25] One of the studies we included, for example, was a meta-analysis of blood levels of serotonin, which was based on data from three large studies involving a total of 2,469 post-menopausal women.[26] [27] The analysis showed that women who were using antidepressants for any indication (not just depression) had lower levels of serotonin in the blood than women who were not taking antidepressants. In contrast, women with depression who were not taking antidepressants did not have lower levels of serotonin than women without depression.

This is an important study because it was relatively large and it was not conducted by people with a particular interest in serotonin or antidepressants. The authors tested a number of chemicals and didn't even remark on the serotonin findings, they just presented the data.

Research on the serotonin breakdown product also highlighted evidence that people taking antidepressants had lower levels compared to people who were not taking antidepressants.[28] Moreover, it turns out there is animal research showing that prolonged administration of SSRIs, in particular, reduces the amount of serotonin in the brain and the serotonin breakdown product in brain fluid.[29] Therefore, despite the theory that SSRIs boost serotonin, there is evidence that they may, in fact, decrease the amount of serotonin in the blood and the brain, at least when they are used for a sustained period.

Possibly SSRIs increase serotonin initially and then the body reacts to this increase by trying to bring the serotonin concentration down again but overshoots and reduces it too much. This overshooting phenomenon has been found to happen with some other drugs. Opioids, for example, suppress pain sensitivity initially but can result in an increase in pain sensitivity when used on a long-term basis, which is thought to reflect the body overcompensating for the effects of the drug.[30]

Overall, we have little idea how SSRIs or any other type of antidepressant interact with the serotonin system, including whether they produce a net increase or decrease in serotonin activity.[31] There are some indications, however, that in the long run at least, they reduce it.

Conclusions

The research we surveyed in our review had been conducted over thirty years across several continents. The genetic studies were large, analysing data from tens of thousands of people, but studies in other areas tended to be small. A grand total of 5,843 participants were involved across all the individual, non-genetic studies. For comparison, studies of statins for heart disease prevention include hundreds of thousands of people.[32]

The research indicates there is little evidence to support the serotonin theory of depression – that is, the idea that depression is caused by low levels or low activity of serotonin in the brain. Studies of serotonin in the blood, its breakdown product in brain fluid, the inhibitory serotonin receptor and the serotonin transporter are either negative or unreliable. The few that suggest some abnormality of serotonin suggest it is higher, not lower, in people with depression, but these are likely to be the result of random fluctuations or antidepressant-induced effects. Reducing brain serotonin using the tryptophan-depletion method does not provoke depression in healthy volunteers and evidence from people with depression is not compelling.

Studies of the gene for the serotonin transporter are, overall, decisively negative. Besides, excluding the genetic studies, none of the research we looked at was designed to detect whether deviations in the serotonin system preceded the onset of depression. Therefore, even if the research we examined did suggest an abnormality of serotonin, none of it could show that this was a cause of depression, rather than simply a correlation of being in a depressed state.

No sensible scientist would accept this sort of evidence as establishing anything. At most, it provides a stimulus to further research.

Of course, other ways of looking at serotonin can be developed, and more studies can be done, and this will allow people to make new claims that there is a serotonin deficiency in people with depression. But the body of research I have described is the principal research on which the serotonin theory of depression stands or falls at present. And it definitely falls.

9

What Antidepressant Research Really Shows

Overwhelmingly, the most common response to our serotonin paper was that it doesn't matter because 'antidepressants work'. In the online magazine *The Conversation*, two UK-based psychiatrists wrote an article entitled 'Depression: low serotonin may not be the cause – but antidepressants still work' and an Australian psychiatrist published one called 'The chemical imbalance theory of depression is dead, but that doesn't mean antidepressants don't work'. Both pieces made the same argument: it's not important that we don't understand *how* antidepressants work, only that they do.[1]

So, before I cover the reactions to our paper and what they reveal about how public ideas about depression and its treatment are shaped and maintained, it is time to take a detailed look at the evidence for whether antidepressants actually help people. This involves presenting some dry facts about drug trials and how they are conducted and interpreted, but it is essential that people understand exactly what the much-repeated claim that 'antidepressants work' is based on. The issues are not difficult to grasp, so bear with me and hopefully the effort will be worthwhile. When you have read the next few chapters, you will be more informed than most doctors.

I hope it is already clear that how antidepressants exert the effects they do matters a lot, but whether they work is also doubtful. When I was training as a psychiatrist, I saw many people with depression who were starting out on antidepressants. Some got better, some didn't. Other psychiatrists and many patients thought the antidepressants were helpful, but I just couldn't see this. When people improved, usually the things that had made them depressed in the first place had resolved or improved – they had got a new job or recovered from a break-up, for example. I realised people can interpret the same situation in different ways. Many people are inclined to believe treatment is beneficial and they attribute improvements to treatment when there might be other explanations.

This is why we do drug trials. It is why we need to compare drugs like antidepressants to a placebo – that is, a 'dummy' tablet. We know that our moods go up and down naturally; we know moods reflect our circumstances; and we know that being seen by a professional – being listened to and sympathised with – all enhance people's chances of improvement.[2] Taking a pill we think *might* be effective can also make us feel better. Therefore, we need to know whether taking an antidepressant is more effective than not taking one, and, if it is, whether the effects are due to a specific pharmacological effect of the drug or whether they are down to people's beliefs about the benefits of the drug – what we call the placebo effect.

Most drug trials are what are called 'randomised-controlled trials'. This means people who enrol are assigned at random to take the active drug or the placebo. The randomness of the process ensures that there are no systematic differences between people allocated to the different sorts of tablets (the drug and the placebo tablets) that could influence the outcome of the trial.

When I was a junior doctor, I worked on a drug trial testing whether a particular drug (naltrexone) was helpful for people with alcohol problems. I was employed by an NHS hospital in London, but the trial was organised by a clinical research organisation (a company that conducts drug trials), which had been hired by the drug's maker – the pharmaceutical company DuPont. My job consisted of identifying patients who might be eligible for the trial, signing them up if they were willing, and then conducting medical examinations and taking blood for tests. My overriding memory is the inconvenience of having to lug round a large machine to spin the blood samples before I sent them off to the laboratory.

The experience gave me an invaluable insight into how trials work on the ground. I learned, for example, that most people who sign up for a trial want to get the real drug, not the placebo. Many of the people I recruited were desperate and would try anything that might help them stay sober. They were also intensely curious about the identity of their tablets and tried to guess whether they were taking the active drug or the placebo. We'll come to why this is important shortly.

Results of antidepressant trials

Many hundreds of trials have been conducted that involve comparing an antidepressant with a dummy tablet or placebo. Most have been run by pharmaceutical companies and typically last around six to eight weeks. The main thing that is measured is the level of symptoms people experience, which is assessed using questionnaires that ask people questions about their feelings and other symptoms of depression, anxiety or whatever condition is being treated.

So, what do these trials show? Because there are so many of them, the results of individual trials are commonly combined using the technique of meta-analysis. In depression, meta-analyses indicate that, overall, people assigned to take an antidepressant show slightly more improvement during the course of the trial than people assigned to take a placebo. The difference is 'statistically significant', meaning it is not just a chance finding,[3] but it is small.

The most commonly used depression questionnaire was designed by a psychiatrist called Max Hamilton back in the 1960s and is called the Hamilton Depression Rating Scale.[4] The usual version has seventeen questions and a maximum score of 52 points. Meta-analyses show that the average difference on this scale between people randomised to take an antidepressant and those randomised to take a placebo is 2 points or less.

A meta-analysis published in 2022, for example, which was based on data from antidepressant trials submitted to the US drug regulator, the FDA, found an average difference of 1.8 points.[5] A large and influential meta-analysis published in 2018, by a team based at the University of Oxford, revealed an overall difference of 2 points (although this was not how the results were presented).[6]

The relevance of antidepressant-placebo differences

So, the next question is, what does this mean? Is a two-point difference between an antidepressant and a placebo a relevant and helpful difference, and does it reflect a pharmacological effect, or might it be due to something else? On the face of it, a 2-point difference on a 52-point scale doesn't sound like much, but what does the evidence suggest?

Measuring depression is not a simple task, of course. It is not like taking someone's blood pressure or measuring the amount of sugar in the blood. Depression-rating scales consist of questions about a number of manifestations or symptoms of depression. The Hamilton Depression Rating Scale, like other depression scales, is an arbitrary collection of some of these. It doesn't include a question on loss of pleasure in life, which is often considered a cardinal indication of depression, and it contains several questions about physical symptoms, such as gastrointestinal symptoms and menstrual disturbances, which might have nothing to do with a person's mood.

The way the items are rated is also questionable. Take the depressed mood item presented here, for example:

DEPRESSED MOOD (sadness, hopeless, helpless, worthless)

- **0 Absent**
- **1 These feeling states indicated only on questioning**
- **2 These feeling states spontaneously reported verbally**
- **3 Communicates feeling states non-verbally, i.e. through facial expression, posture, voice and tendency to weep**
- **4 Patient reports virtually only these feeling states in his/her spontaneous verbal and non-verbal communication**

You are considered to be more depressed if you spontaneously tell the person doing the assessment you are depressed (score of 2) than if you only admit to it after being questioned (score of 1). People taking both antidepressants and placebos in clinical trials usually score between 1 and 2 at the end of their treatment, so this is a critical distinction.[7] But people have different styles of communication, and no one has established that telling someone about your mood directly indicates you are more severely depressed than if you are more reserved. We might expect that sometimes, at least, it would be the opposite.

It is also not necessarily true that people who show their feelings non-verbally, by crying for example (and would score 3), are more affected than people who don't (and would score 1 or 2).

Some people have suggested the Hamilton Depression Rating Scale isn't a very good scale, which is true, and that other scales might reveal larger antidepressant effects – they don't. The other most commonly used scale is the Montgomery–Åsberg Depression Rating Scale (known as the MADRS), named after the two psychiatrists who developed it.[8] Trials using this scale find modest differences between antidepressants and placebo that are roughly equivalent to the 2-point difference on the Hamilton Depression Scale.[9]

The problem is, there is no objective way of identifying or measuring depression; therefore, we don't know whether these scales are really measuring what they say they are measuring. When it comes down to it, we can't be confident that someone who scores 20 points on a depression scale is more depressed than someone who scores 10 points, and it certainly makes no sense to say they are precisely twice as depressed.

Given this, you could be forgiven for thinking that antidepressant trials are complete nonsense – and I would say this is not far from the truth. But putting aside more fundamental concerns about the whole enterprise of measuring depression, what evidence do we have about what a 2-point difference in Hamilton Depression Scale scores might mean? Most efforts to establish this suggest it doesn't represent a helpful or even noticeable difference.

One way you can evaluate the meaning of depression scores is to compare them to scores on a widely used rating scale called the Clinical Global Impressions Scale, which assesses how people are doing overall.[10] This scale requires a researcher to classify people into one of seven categories: 'very much improved', 'much improved', 'mildly improved', 'no change', 'minimally worse', 'much worse' or 'very much worse'.

A group of researchers from Germany, led by the respected and prolific Stefan Leucht, analysed data from a trial in which people were rated using the Hamilton Depression Scale and the Clinical Global Impressions Scale at the same time. Their analysis revealed that a change of 3 points or less on the Hamilton Depression Scale equated to the 'no change' category on the Clinical Global Impressions Scale. A change of 7 or 8 points equated to a rating of 'mildly improved'.[11] In other words, a difference of 2 points does not even register as a difference on the Clinical Global Impressions Scale and a difference of 7–8 points would be needed to indicate that antidepressants had even a 'mild' advantage over a placebo.

Various other methods have been proposed to establish the size of a meaningful difference in Hamilton Depression Scale scores. None of the methods are perfect, by any means, because of the difficulty of measuring something like a mood, but they also indicate that a difference of 2 points would not qualify.[12] So, antidepressants trials show that antidepressants are not meaningfully different from a placebo.

The amplified placebo effect

There is another major problem with interpreting antidepressant trials, however, which suggests the small difference between antidepressants and placebo may not even be a pharmacological effect at all. It may be an 'amplified' placebo effect.

When I was a junior psychiatrist wondering why my colleagues thought antidepressants were so effective, I asked Geoff, one of the more senior doctors on my team, what he thought. Geoff was a supportive mentor. He always had good advice on how to manage situations in which people were suicidal, acutely psychotic or heavily intoxicated – the daily challenges of my work on the night shift in a busy accident and emergency department in London. Geoff said he thought antidepressants were 'active' placebos, and he referred me to a paper published in 1982 in the *British Journal of Psychiatry*. Reading the paper was a lightbulb moment for me. Everything fell into place. Now I understood why antidepressants might look a little bit better than a placebo in a clinical trial but had no convincing effect in the real world.

The paper Geoff signposted me to was called 'Side effects and placebo amplification' and was written by a psychiatrist called Richard Thomson.[13] Thomson pointed out how placebo-controlled trials do not necessarily eliminate the placebo effect. This is because antidepressants are active drugs and, therefore, the experience of taking them is different from the experience of taking an inert substance, such as chalk or lactose – the usual constituents of placebo tablets. Antidepressants have recognisable side-effects, such as nausea and drowsiness, and they are psychoactive drugs that change people's feelings and sensations in more- or less-subtle ways. Based on these effects, it is likely that at least some people taking part in antidepressant trials will be able to figure out whether they are taking the antidepressant or the placebo. The staff working on trials may also be able to guess who is taking the antidepressant and who is on the placebo by the profile of side-effects that participants report.

The point of running a randomised placebo-controlled trial is that none of the people involved, neither the participants nor the researchers, know who is getting the real drug and who is not. They are meant to be 'blind' to the nature of the tablets. This is what is known as the 'double-blind' design. But if people can guess what they are taking, or if the researchers can guess who is taking what, then the study is not double-blind.

In this situation, the results may be influenced by people's common belief that the drug will be effective. Those who guess they are taking the real thing will be more optimistic and hopeful and this may improve their mood in itself. Conversely, those who suspect they are on the placebo may feel disappointed and dejected, which will make their mood worse. Researchers often have the same expectations, and they might rate people they suspect to be taking the real drug as doing better than those they think are taking the placebo.

Therefore, when a trial is not properly double-blind, and participants and researchers can guess who received the drug and who received the placebo, all or part of the effects of the drug may be due to an 'amplified' placebo effect. This is a combination of the ordinary placebo effect, which is the consequence of taking some sort of tablet, amplified by the extra boost people derive from the side-effects and other effects that suggest to people they are getting the real drug. In this context, the drug acts like a placebo with special powers.

This problem was recognised back in the early days of psychiatric drug research in the 1960s. To try to address it, several trials were set up that compared an antidepressant with an 'active' placebo, which is a drug that produces some of the same side-effects as the antidepressant being tested, without being thought to be an antidepressant. Thomson described seven such studies conducted in the 1960s and 1970s, which used the drug atropine as an active placebo in trials of various tricyclic antidepressants that were being used at the time. Atropine mimics some, though not all, of the side-effects of tricyclic antidepressants, particularly a dry mouth.

Thomson found these trials were less likely to detect an effect of antidepressants compared to trials using regular, inactive placebos. The paper made such a strong impression on me that as soon as I managed to obtain a post where I could do my own research, I updated Thomson's review and confirmed that there is little, if any, difference between antidepressants and an active placebo.[14]

Since the 1970s, no one has paid much attention to this problem and there have been no further antidepressant trials using an active placebo. Yet, a recent study clearly demonstrates the power of people's beliefs about medication. Psychologists in Sweden enrolled forty-seven people who had been diagnosed with social anxiety disorder and gave them all the SSRI escitalopram, which is thought to be an effective treatment for anxiety.

Only half the participants were told the drug was escitalopram, however. The other half were told they were receiving a placebo. After nine weeks of treatment, the people who were told they were receiving the drug had a 51 per cent reduction in their social anxiety symptoms and those who were told they were being given the placebo only showed a 26 per cent reduction, a large and statistically significant (non-random) difference.[15]

A clinical trial that compared the effects of the SSRI sertraline, St John's Wort (a plant extract, also known as hypericum, which is occasionally used as an antidepressant) and a placebo in people with depression also shows the influence of people's belief about what they are taking.[16] As the left-hand columns in Figure 2 show, the results of this trial revealed minimal differences (1 point or less on the Hamilton Depression Rating Scale) between the treatments in the degree of improvement in people's depression scores, and these differences were not statistically significant (they could have occurred by chance).

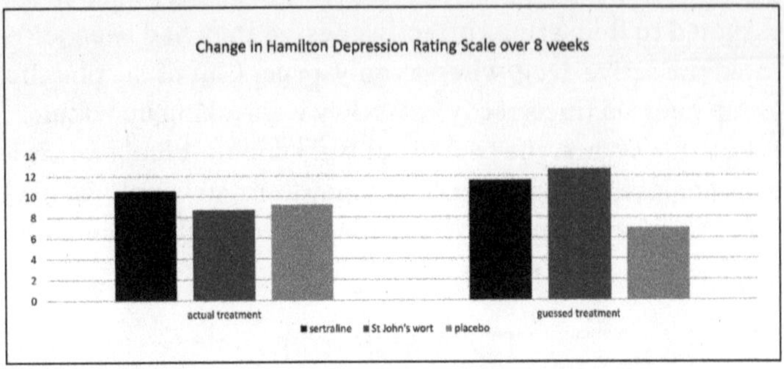

Effects of guesses on depression symptoms in a randomised trial of sertraline vs St John's Wort vs placebo (derived from data in Chen et al., 2011).

The columns on the right-hand side, however, show that when the data were analysed according to what people *guessed* they were taking, rather than what they were *actually* taking, there was a more substantial and statistically significant difference. People who guessed they were taking sertraline improved by 5 points more than people who guessed they were taking the placebo, and the difference between those who guessed they were taking St John's Wort and those who guessed they were taking the placebo was almost 6 points.

Participants in this trial didn't guess what they were taking more accurately than would be predicted by chance, maybe because the trial involved two different active drugs, making guessing quite complicated. Therefore, people's guesses didn't influence the ultimate results of the trial, which was negative. It clearly demonstrates, however, that whether people think they are taking a real antidepressant or a placebo has a significant influence on their mood, regardless of what they are actually taking.

In contrast, in most trials in which people are asked to guess the identity of their tablets, they do guess better than chance.[17] In a trial of fluoxetine (Prozac) and placebo for the treatment of people with alcohol problems, for example, 80 per cent of those assigned to fluoxetine correctly guessed they had been allocated the active drug, whereas only 45 per cent of the placebo group guessed (incorrectly) that they were taking fluoxetine.[18] When this occurs, the trial is not truly double-blind and, as a consequence, the antidepressant may exert an 'amplified placebo effect', which makes it look more effective than it really is.

The TADS study

Data from another study illustrate how this can happen. The Treatment for Adolescents with Depression Study, known as

TADS, was conducted in the early 2000s in the USA and has been influential in producing a consensus that fluoxetine is an effective antidepressant for children and young people. The study had a complex design that involved comparing fluoxetine with a placebo, with some participants also having cognitive behavioural therapy and one group only having the therapy. The main paper, published in 2004, reported that adolescents treated with a combination of fluoxetine and cognitive behavioural therapy showed the greatest improvement in their depression scores, followed by those taking fluoxetine alone, followed by those assigned to a placebo or cognitive behavioural therapy alone.[19]

Years later, Professor Jon Jureidini of the University of Adelaide, Australia, obtained the data from the trial and led a group of researchers, including myself, in looking at the effects of people's guesses about the identity of their tablets, which had not been reported previously. Like the study of sertraline and St John's Wort, we found that what the adolescents guessed they were taking when they were asked six weeks into the study strongly predicted their mood ratings at the end of the study, six weeks later (the double-blind part of the trial lasted twelve weeks in all). But unlike in the previous study, everyone involved in the TADS trial – including the adolescent participants, their parents, their doctors and the researchers – could guess the identity of the tablets slightly better than expected. Instead of being correct 50 per cent of the time, as would be predicted by chance, they were correct between 60 and 62 per cent of the time.

Our analysis was unique in that we were able to use statistical techniques to explore how people's guesses interacted with the effects of the drug. This showed that when we accounted for the effects of people's guesses, the actual nature of the medication (whether it was fluoxetine or placebo) had no impact on depression scores. However, when we removed the effect of guessing from the analysis, the apparent effect of the medication increased, and people assigned to fluoxetine showed a marginal statistical advantage over those allocated to the placebo.[20]

So, we showed that if you don't account for the effects of people's guesses when you conduct an antidepressant trial, you can end up with a spuriously positive result – the drug appears to be more effective than the placebo, when it isn't. This is the amplified placebo effect. If the TADS trial had involved an antidepressant with more noticeable effects than fluoxetine (which has relatively few side-effects), people's guesses might have been more accurate. In that case, the difference between the antidepressant and the placebo would likely have looked larger.

While most advocates of antidepressants ignore the issue of amplified placebo effects, some have suggested it is not relevant because people's guesses may be based on the benefits they get from the drug, rather than on its side-effects.[21] However, the TADS study showed that guesses could not be due to a therapeutic effect of the drug because there was none.

Effects of other substances in depression

Now we can see why it is relevant that people who enrol in randomised trials want to get the active drug and are highly invested in working out what sort of tablet they have been allocated to, as I observed in the alcohol treatment trial I was involved in long ago. People's beliefs about the likely effectiveness of a drug influence their ultimate outcome substantially, and if they can guess whether or not they are taking the real drug, those beliefs can influence the results of the trial.

This explanation for antidepressants' effects makes sense of some curious facts about antidepressants. It explains why they are such a disparate collection of chemicals, with little in common except that they affect the brain in some way, and why numerous substances that are not normally thought of as antidepressants have been found to produce similar effects to antidepressants on symptoms of depression. These include benzodiazepines, stimulants, amphetamine, methylphenidate (Ritalin), opioids, buspirone (the 1980s anti-anxiety drug), many antipsychotics (including chlorpromazine) and 'purple hearts', as found by researchers back in the 1960s.[22]

It also makes sense of the most contradictory finding of all: a drug that has the opposite effect of the SSRIs, a serotonin reuptake *enhancer*, has been licensed and is used as an antidepressant. It is called tianeptine, and it is prescribed in some European and South American countries. Like other antidepressants, tianeptine has gone through clinical trials and been shown to be marginally better than a placebo.[23] What all these chemicals have in common is that they produce noticeable physical and mental changes or side-effects. So, the fact that they all produce much the same effect in depression suggests they are working through an amplified placebo effect.

Anxiety

Research on anxiety is similar to research on depression. There are fewer trials but, overall, they reveal that antidepressants improve anxiety symptoms a little better than a placebo. In a recent meta-analysis of trials involving people with general anxiety, antidepressants outperformed placebo by only 2–3 points on an anxiety symptom scale that has a maximum score of 56.[24] In obsessive compulsive disorder, usually classified as an anxiety disorder, antidepressants show an advantage of 3 points on a 40-point scale.[25][26]

There is no comparable research on the meaning of these differences in anxiety or obsessive compulsive disorder, but they don't look impressive. Moreover, people with anxiety are just as likely to be able to guess the identity of their tablets as people with depression, and to be influenced by positive expectations of treatment, as we saw in the experiment with people with social anxiety disorder. So, the evidence for the effects of antidepressants in anxiety are the same as for depression. Placebo-controlled trials reveal small differences that are unlikely to be relevant and may represent amplified placebo effects.

Antidepressant development

At this point, you might be wondering how particular drugs are selected as antidepressants, given what I have said about their variability. Surely, you might suppose, there is a scientific process of drug development that identifies drugs with antidepressant action on a rational basis?

I thought this was the case, too, until I started doing research for my first book. During my investigations, I came across a scientific review of antidepressant effects in 'animal models' of depression.[27] 'Animal models' are used to test drugs for antidepressant effects and involve inducing depression-like states in animals, such as rats and mice. The best known is called the Forced Swim Test, which involves making the animals swim in a tank they can't get out of and measuring how long it takes them to give up trying (sounds cruel, I know). Drugs that keep them swimming for longer are interpreted as having antidepressant properties.

I had assumed that antidepressants are identified using these models, and then tested in humans and brought to market. This is what is claimed by people who do these studies.[28] But it turns out animal model experiments are highly unreliable: tests done in different laboratories' yield different results. Antidepressants don't always show the predicted effects and drugs that are not considered antidepressants, such as amphetamine, often show what are referred to as 'false-positive' effects (because they are not deemed to be antidepressants, they are not meant to show positive effects). Yet, given the stimulant properties of amphetamine, it is not surprising that it keeps animals swimming for longer.

Putting aside the obvious problem that animal models of complex human emotions are flawed to begin with, this suggests there is no systematic scientific process behind the identification of drugs that are deemed to be antidepressants. As you may have realised already, what gets branded as an antidepressant is determined instead by a combination of the latest vogue in neurotransmitter theory and what drug companies think will sell best at a particular time.

Other outcomes

I have described how antidepressants have small and irrelevant effects on symptoms of depression, but what do we know about how they affect people's actual lives? Do they help people to manage their day-to-day responsibilities better and enable them to enjoy their social relationships and leisure activities? There is little evidence on these questions for the simple reason that clinical trials focus primarily on depression symptoms. Sometimes, what is called 'quality of life' is measured using questionnaires, but these overlap considerably with depression questionnaires; their results are not consistently reported and they are also susceptible to amplified placebo effects, just like depression questionnaires. There is almost no data from clinical trials on such important things as whether antidepressants help people get back to work, how productive people are, how reliant they are on health services, or how people's intimate relationships, social lives and recreational activities are affected by treatment.

Conclusions

Recommendations for the use of antidepressants by authorities such as NICE (the National Institute for Health and Care Excellence) are based on the placebo-controlled trials I have described.[29] These trials set out to measure depression as if it were high blood pressure, disregarding the obvious fact that human emotions are not readily amenable to being quantified. They last a mere few weeks in most cases, and rarely provide objective data on how people are managing their lives. It is doubtful that antidepressant trials tell us much at all, therefore, but if we accept these trials on their own terms, they reveal that antidepressants are barely better than a placebo, and the small difference detected is likely to be accounted for by amplified placebo effects.

All this begs the question: how has this meagre evidence been transformed into the much-trumpeted idea that 'antidepressants work'?

10

Spinning Straw into Gold: How We Came to Believe that Antidepressants are Effective

We have known for a long time that antidepressants are not very different from a placebo. Irving Kirsch, a world leader in the field of placebo research, led a team that showed this back in 2002. They conducted a widely publicised meta-analysis of antidepressant trials from which they concluded the pharmacological effects of antidepressants, as opposed to their placebo effects, are 'clinically negligible'.[1]

So, how is it we have been led to believe that antidepressants are effective and useful? And what about other evidence on antidepressants, such as whether they help people over the long term, and how they fare in the real world? What does this suggest?

Ignoring inconvenient facts is one of the tactics employed to massage the evidence. Even though the amplified placebo effect has been discussed periodically in the scientific literature since Thomson's paper in 1982, few trials require people to guess what they have been assigned to take or consider the possibility that amplified placebo effects might account for the results. A recent review of 295 antidepressant trials, for example, found that only 5 per cent reported participants' guesses of what they were taking.[2]

Non-publication

Another strategy is the non-publication of negative studies – that is, studies that find antidepressants to be no different or worse than a placebo. This is referred to as 'publication bias'. Drug companies or researchers can decide not to publish negative trials, so trials that make it into the scientific literature are more likely to show positive antidepressant effects. In 2008, Eric Turner, former reviewer of drugs for the US FDA, and his team showed that 49 per cent of the antidepressant trials submitted to the US regulator were negative, but almost all of these had either never been published or had been published in such a way as to suggest they were positive.[3]

There is also no obligation to submit studies to the regulators either, and it has been suggested that there are hundreds of negative antidepressant trials for which there is no public record.[4] Pfizer documents released during legal proceedings demonstrate how several early trials of its SSRI sertraline (Lustral or Zoloft) were negative. Memos record company discussions about how to manage this situation, which was causing European regulators to refuse to grant the drug a licence. But Pfizer just kept on doing trials until some of them brought in the required result.[5]

The manipulation of data in published papers was laid bare by the now notorious Study 329. Study 329 was a randomised trial conducted by GlaxoSmithKline, comparing their SSRI paroxetine with the old tricyclic antidepressant imipramine and a placebo in adolescents. It was initially published in 2001 and the lead author on the publication was a professor at Brown University Medical

School in New York, although it later transpired that the article had been written by a 'ghost writer' employed by the company.[6]

The article claimed that paroxetine was more effective than a placebo, with generally mild side-effects, and the trial formed the basis of a marketing campaign that declared paroxetine had 'REMARKABLE safety and efficacy'.[7] But papers released after publication, including company emails, revealed how GlaxoSmithKline researchers had adjusted the data, replacing the originally designated primary outcome measure, which showed a negative result, with one that was positive.[8]

They also underestimated paroxetine's side-effects. The study was eventually reanalysed according to the original protocol by a group of independent researchers, including David Healy and Jon Jureidini, and published in the *British Medical Journal*. This revealed there were no differences between paroxetine and the placebo for any of the primary or secondary outcomes that had been specified in the original protocol, and serious side-effects, including suicidal thoughts and suicide attempts, had not been reported.[9]

The response-rate illusion

Reputable researchers can also present evidence in misleading ways. The 2018 meta-analysis conducted by the University of Oxford team, for example, which was widely proclaimed to confirm that 'The drugs do work: antidepressants are effective', used a method that inflates the apparent difference between antidepressants and placebos.[10]

The published paper did not present the depression symptom scores collected during the studies that the analysis was based on. Instead, it reported the likelihood of showing a 'response' to an antidepressant compared to a placebo. Each antidepressant was considered individually, and for the old antidepressant, amitriptyline, which showed the greatest advantage over placebo, the chance (technically the odds)[11] of showing a response to the drug was about twice that of the placebo (for example, if 30 per cent of people taking the placebo showed a response, 60 per cent taking the antidepressant would show a response). For sertraline the chance was 1.7 times that of placebo, and for other antidepressants it varied from 1.4 to 1.9 times. Presenting the data in this way gives the impression that treatment for depression has a binary outcome – either you get better or you don't – and taking an antidepressant can double or almost double your chances, which sounds pretty good.

Recovering from depression is not like this, however. There is no natural distinction between showing a response and not showing a response. People improve to different degrees. The 'response' that is reported in trials and in this meta-analysis is an artificial figure constructed by categorising the data from depression questionnaires using an arbitrary cut-off point. The trouble with this is that people with similar scores can end up in different categories and if a lot of scores are close to the cut-off, this can end up making a small difference seem larger than it is.[12]

Statisticians repeatedly advise not to categorise data from scales in this way,[13] but this is what the researchers did. They could have chosen to look at overall depression scores instead, but they didn't. It was only when a group from Denmark analysed the data that this figure was revealed.

Among the trials included in the meta-analysis that had used the Hamilton Depression Rating Scale (the most commonly used scale), the average difference in scores between people assigned to an antidepressant and people assigned to a placebo was, like other meta-analyses, a tiny 2 points.[14] In other words, by categorising people into 'responders' and 'non-responders', the Oxford team had transformed a 2-point difference in depression symptoms scores into the more impressive but deceptive statistic that you are twice as likely to respond if you take an antidepressant compared to a placebo.

This technique of dividing data into artificial categories, alongside the selective publication of positive results and the overlooking of likely amplified placebo effects, is how the small and inconsequential difference between antidepressants and placebo has come to be perceived as evidence for the effectiveness of antidepressants. When challenged, most psychiatrists admit the difference is small, though they don't often say this in public. When they do admit it, they frequently argue that, nonetheless, some people experience a worthwhile effect, even if many don't. It is commonly claimed, for example, that antidepressants are particularly effective for people with more severe depression.

Do antidepressants work for severe depression?

In fact, there is little evidence that antidepressants have substantially greater effects in people with more severe depression. Several meta-analyses have explored whether people who have more severe depression show a greater relative improvement with an antidepressant (versus placebo) than people with less severe depression. Some show this, some don't.[15] In the ones that do, the difference between antidepressants and placebo among people with severe depression is still small. In the large analysis of FDA data published in 2022, for example, the 5 per cent of people who had the most severe symptoms only showed a difference of 2.5 points.[16] This is still below all estimates of a meaningful effect and easily accounted for by amplified placebo effects (recalling that the difference produced by people's beliefs about what they were taking was 5 points or more in the trial of St John's Wort and sertraline).[17]

What about people with really severe depression, including the 'melancholic' depression I described in Chapter 3? As it happens, antidepressants have not been shown to be helpful in this situation. A seminal study, funded by the Medical Research Council, was conducted in the 1960s with people who had been admitted to hospital with severe depression. It consisted of a randomised trial comparing the effects of two early antidepressants – imipramine and phenelzine – with a placebo and ECT. Although it is sometimes reported as showing that imipramine worked but phenelzine did not (because imipramine had slightly larger effects), in fact, neither of the antidepressants appeared to work. Neither were superior to the placebo in the main outcome of the trial, which was the percentage of people who showed a 'substantial improvement' after four weeks, and there was no difference in symptom scores. People who received ECT, on the other hand, did better than those on a placebo.[18] Other studies from this era did not find that antidepressants were more effective in very severe depression than in milder 'neurotic' or 'reactive' depression.[19]

As an aside, ECT is not a targeted treatment either. ECT can sometimes temporarily lift the mood of someone with severe depression, but not because it reverses an underlying biological deficit – at least, there is no evidence that it does this. As I explained in my book, *The Myth of the Chemical Cure*, ECT causes a sudden and dramatic alteration to the brain's normal state that commonly results in changes to mental capacities, including memory loss. Occasionally, it produces an artificial state of euphoria, similar to that which can occur after a brain injury. These effects can temporarily override feelings of depression, but they wear off within a few weeks and the depression returns. Some memory deficit can be permanent, but there is no evidence that ECT produces a lasting improvement in mood.[20]

Depression that occurs in the course of the condition known as manic depression or bipolar disorder is often thought of as more severe than other instances of depression; yet, two large, modern meta-analyses suggest that antidepressants are no more effective than a placebo in people with this condition.[21]

Antidepressants are also frequently claimed by their proponents to 'save lives' by reducing people's chances of committing suicide. Yet, antidepressants have never been shown to reduce suicide. It is difficult to prove anything about suicide because it is so rare, but there is no evidence from randomised trials that antidepressants modify rates of actual suicide. In fact, as we will see in the next chapter, they slightly increase the rates of suicide attempts and suicidal thoughts in trials involving young people.

Therapist Lucy Cavendish, writing in *The Guardian*, expressed the common belief that if people don't get better with a non-medication-based intervention, such as having therapy or taking more exercise, they must *need* an antidepressant and that antidepressants *must* be helpful in this situation.[22] But just because other things don't work, doesn't mean antidepressants do work.

Many people assume that antidepressants undoubtedly work for people with severe depression, so it is important to stress that this has not been demonstrated. People who are more deeply depressed do not respond to antidepressants in a more convincing way than people who have a milder condition. And there is no evidence that antidepressants save lives.

Long-term use of antidepressants

Another significant limitation of antidepressant research is that studies last for relatively short periods compared to the time people often take these drugs for in real life. Of the 522 trials included in the Oxford team's 2018 meta-analysis, 75 per cent lasted for eight weeks or less and only 2 per cent of them lasted longer than three months.[23] Yet we know many people take antidepressants for years.

The studies that are used to justify long-term treatment with antidepressants are a different set of studies, sometimes referred to as 'relapse-prevention' studies. These studies involve people who are already taking an antidepressant, who are then randomly assigned either to continue their antidepressant or to be switched to a placebo. A summary of such studies published in 2003 reported that 40 per cent of people had a relapse of their depression after being switched to a placebo, compared to only 18 per cent of those who continued on their antidepressant.[24]

There are two major problems with these studies. First, like 'response', the meaning of 'relapse' in a condition like depression is unclear. Feelings of depression fluctuate, and people will have different views about what constitutes a relapse. The definitions used in trials vary and, as with 'response', many use arbitrary criteria that have not been shown to correlate with anything in real life.

Second, antidepressants produce withdrawal symptoms, including changes in mood, sleep and concentration. It has been shown that these can mimic relapse in people who are switched from taking antidepressants to placebo, especially because the antidepressants are usually stopped abruptly, which is likely to provoke particularly intense withdrawal symptoms.[25] The occurrence of withdrawal symptoms may also lead to a genuine decline in mood, since if people are not aware they are experiencing withdrawal, they may become frightened they are about to relapse. In this situation, people's negative expectations may become a self-fulfilling prophecy – the opposite scenario to the amplified placebo effect. The fact that the issue of withdrawal has been ignored in relapse-prevention studies until recently means most of them are worse than useless for providing evidence on the benefits of continued antidepressant treatment.

A study published in 2021, known as the ANTLER study (ANTidepressants to prevent reLapse in dEpRession) and run by colleagues of mine at University College London, was designed to minimise the effects of antidepressant withdrawal.[26] ANTLER was a good study in many ways. It was a placebo controlled discontinuation trial, and, to minimise withdrawal symptoms, people assigned to the placebo group had their antidepressants reduced gradually over a period of two months before they were fully transferred to placebo tablets. Participants were asked about withdrawal symptoms as well as being given the usual depression scales and other measures to complete; relapse was defined as a reported period of low mood lasting at least two weeks, rather than a cut-off on a depression scale.

The problem is that we now know that reducing antidepressants over two months is not necessarily long enough to prevent withdrawal symptoms, particularly in people who have been taking antidepressants for several years.[27] Seventy per cent of the participants in the ANTLER study had used antidepressants for more than three years prior to entering the study.

The ANTLER trial reported that 56 per cent of people who were allocated to stop their antidepressant and switch to a placebo relapsed within a year, compared to 39 per cent of those who were randomised to continue their antidepressant. This is a smaller difference than is found in most previous trials, suggesting the gradual lowering of antidepressants may have helped reduce the impact of withdrawal symptoms. However, there was evidence that withdrawal symptoms still occurred, including nervousness, crying, insomnia, fatigue and poor concentration, and these may have been mistaken for relapse. This is especially likely since several symptoms that were considered indicative of relapse, including 'restlessness' and loss of concentration, are recognised withdrawal symptoms.

The researchers who conducted ANTLER acknowledged it showed some people could stop antidepressants successfully, but they also concluded that 'for many patients, long-term treatment is appropriate'.[28] However, scientific letters sent to the *New England Journal of Medicine*, in which the trial was published, highlighted the problem of withdrawal effects potentially explaining relapse, and that the trial was not reliably double-blind: most people randomised to antidepressant discontinuation had been able to work out what they had been assigned to.[29]

There are no studies that compare the effects of starting out on an antidepressant and taking it for several years, as many do in practice, with taking a placebo. But the studies that are meant to justify long-term use cannot do so because the occurrence of withdrawal symptoms means that stopping an antidepressant is not the same as never having taken one. It follows that there is no robust evidence for the benefits or harms of using antidepressants for more than a few months. As Allen Frances, leading US psychiatrist and editor of the fourth edition of the *DSM*, acknowledged to a Cable News Network (CNN) newscaster, 'We're doing a kind of public health experiment on hundreds of millions of people around the world without really understanding the long-term effects.'[30]

In real life

Placebo-controlled trials are important, but they are highly artificial situations. Many trials advertise for patients and, as a consequence, the people who take part are not necessarily the same people who seek help from services. Moreover, participants in trials are monitored closely, they receive attention from enthusiastic young researchers and they feel they are doing something worthwhile, so the results are not likely to be the same as the results of routine treatment in a busy clinic. For these reasons, it is worth looking at what other evidence tells us about the effects of antidepressants, especially in relation to long-term treatment. It does not look promising.

The STAR-D Study (Sequenced Treatment Alternatives to Relieve Depression) was a US Government-funded study that enrolled over 4,000 people and is the largest study of depression treatment ever conducted. Its aim was to evaluate the effects of gold-standard treatment with regular patients in regular services. No placebo was employed.

People who enrolled were all treated with the SSRI citalopram for twelve weeks to begin with. Those who didn't improve sufficiently were then randomly allocated to several different treatment variations, including switching to other antidepressants, CBT and various combinations of antidepressants with each other and with other drugs. It was designed to reflect the way depression is treated in the real world – in that when someone doesn't get better, they are usually offered another treatment and then another, and so on. The study lasted a year and participants received continuing care throughout that time with the aim of helping people not just to get better, but to stay better.

The main results of the study were published in 2006 and the headline was that 67 per cent of people 'recovered' from depression after receiving between one and four of the treatment options.[31] But the results always looked fishy because the analysis was not based on the Hamilton Depression Scale, which had been specified as the main outcome measure in the study protocol. Instead, the researchers used a questionnaire they designed themselves, which was originally intended to monitor how people were doing in the clinic. They also arrived at the figure of 67 per cent by including patients who were technically ineligible for the study because they met the criteria for recovery before they even started, and by ignoring people who dropped out early on, even though such people were meant to be classified as not getting better.[32]

Ed Pigott is a practising psychologist from Rhode Island, USA, who, by his own account, became 'immediately obsessed' with the STAR-D trial when it was published because of its 'apparent biases'.[33] In 2010, Ed and some colleagues published an article showing how abysmal the results actually were. They highlighted that when no assumptions were made about people who dropped out, only 46 per cent of the 4,041 people who started the study got better at some point, using the researchers' questionnaire. However, most of these people relapsed or dropped out later, and only 108 people, a paltry 2.7 per cent of the original sample, stayed well and remained in the study at the final follow-up a year later.[34]

In 2023, Pigott teamed up with some more researchers, including Irving Kirsch, to produce a comprehensive reanalysis of the STAR-D data according to the original protocol (using the Hamilton Depression Rating Scale to define recovery). This revealed an even worse result, with only 35 per cent of people recovering at some point during the year the study lasted.[35]

This is a remarkably poor result, given that most people with depression eventually get better on their own. One study of people referred to mental health services, for example, found that 85 per cent of people who did not receive initial treatment for a depressive episode recovered in the following year.[36] A community survey found that 86 per cent of people who were not treated for depression had recovered by the time they were next assessed two years later.[37]

The STAR-D study offered people free, 'state of the art', high-quality and continuing care; yet only just over a third got better, and 90 per cent of those subsequently relapsed or dropped out.[38] The results raise the question of whether standard medical treatment for depression might *hinder* recovery, rather than promote it.

Some other evidence suggests this may, in fact, be the case. A fifty-year study of 591 people conducted in Zurich, Switzerland, between 1978 and 2008, found depressed people who took antidepressants had more severe depression at subsequent follow-ups than depressed people who didn't take them. This result was obtained after the nature and severity of people's original symptoms were taken into account – that is, it wasn't just that people who took antidepressants were more depressed to begin with.[39]

So not only are antidepressants more or less indistinguishable from a placebo in short-term clinical trials, in the real world, it looks like taking antidepressants might be worse than doing nothing.

Why do people think antidepressants work?

Despite the research evidence, many people feel they have been helped by taking antidepressants. When *The Guardian* asked readers to write in about their experiences in 2013, more than 3,000 people responded and the majority felt antidepressants had been beneficial. Lou said of her time taking antidepressants, 'I finally felt like myself again; although it's a cliché, I genuinely felt like a cloud had been lifted.' Andrew spent years taking two different antidepressants that didn't make any difference, but then eventually he started on one that he felt had helped him. 'I wish I didn't have to take them [antidepressants],' he said, 'but I know they stop me spiralling into a low.'[40]

How is it possible that people hold these beliefs if antidepressants don't really work? It comes down to two things: the power of the placebo effect and the fact that depression is a fluctuating condition and most people will improve with time.

The placebo effect particularly influences people's subjective ratings of how they are (and researchers' ratings of how their participants are doing). This is illustrated by a cleverly designed randomised trial for people with asthma. The study found that people treated with either a standard asthma drug or two placebo interventions rated their breathing as substantially more improved (between 45 and 50 per cent) than people who had no treatment (who only rated it as 21 per cent improved). When the researchers measured people's breathing objectively using a spirometer, however, they found that only people on the active drug had improved. The placebos made no difference to people's breathing, but people *felt* better for them.[41]

Depression is a special case because an inherent part of the placebo effect is hope. So, not only is the outcome subjective (people's evaluation of their feelings or symptoms), but since hopelessness, despondency and pessimism are part and parcel of depression, anything that restores hope is likely to prove a powerful antidepressant – at least temporarily. This is what the studies that demonstrate the amplified placebo effect suggest.

I asked Mark whether he experienced a placebo effect when he started antidepressants and he said he wasn't sure. The antidepressants made him feel slightly 'spaced out', which was 'unsettling', but he kept taking them because he felt he should. He thought, they 'are probably good for me' and because they made him feel a bit strange, he concluded they were 'definitely doing something'.

Despite his uncertainty, he encouraged his friends to take antidepressants and he defended them against critics. When a GP suggested he stop them because he seemed to be doing well, he told her that if he was doing well, it was because he was taking his medication. Someone who had met Mark at this time would have concluded that he felt antidepressants had helped him, even if, deep down, he was uncertain.

The fact that people's moods go up and down naturally and in response to life events can also lead people to think that taking a tablet has had an effect when it hasn't. People often go to the doctor when they are at their lowest point or when they hit a crisis. Visiting the doctor in itself can be a wake-up call that something needs to change, and can help motivate people to work out what that is and what to do about it. The fact that antidepressants are commonly perceived to take two weeks or more to work is most likely down to the fact that in a few weeks, many life crises have resolved and people have naturally started to feel better.[42]

People who are depressed and anxious are in a vulnerable state; when the doctor tells them they have a chemical imbalance and there is a pill to put that right, they are predisposed to feel relief and gratitude. When they start taking the tablets and experience side-effects that indicate they are taking a real drug, they will feel encouraged that they have found something to help them.

What's wrong with the placebo effect?

You might think it doesn't matter if antidepressants are only acting as placebos. If they give people hope and help them improve, surely that's a good thing, even if it has nothing to do with their pharmacological effects? But antidepressants are not sugar pills. They are real drugs that produce side-effects and physical complications. We will come to these shortly, but there is a downside to the placebo effect itself, too.

Joe Tudor, who we will meet again later, is a young man who became depressed in his early twenties. When he was given an antidepressant, he initially 'felt a bit of a bounce' from taking something he thought was going to help him. But when the distress crept back again, he felt worse than ever. The treatment had failed, so he thought there must be something wrong with him. He was worried he would be in this state forever. He thought his life was over.

Let me give you another typical scenario.[43] A young woman is struggling during her first year of university. She has always been anxious and has found it difficult to make friends. She starts to drink too much; she becomes socially withdrawn and she neglects her studies. Towards the end of the year, she realises she needs help and approaches the student health service. The person she sees recommends she start an antidepressant, but she doesn't want to. She has counselling and she manages to reign in her drinking. She pays more attention to her work and finds some like-minded friends. Gradually, she gains confidence, she feels better about herself, her anxiety lessens and her mood lifts.

If this young woman had accepted the antidepressants she was offered, her improvement would have coincided with taking them, and she would probably find it difficult to resist the idea that they had played a necessary part in her recovery. In this situation, she might not have appreciated the importance of the measures she took to change her lifestyle. Even if she was sceptical of drug treatment, she would live with a nagging suspicion that she had needed the antidepressants to get better. This might have undermined her confidence in her own abilities to manage her feelings and take charge of her life, making her more susceptible to becoming depressed in the future.

These negative effects of taking a drug that people have been persuaded will fix their broken brains may explain the pitiful results of the STAR-D study and the other evidence that people who take antidepressants have worse outcomes in the long run than people who don't. Drugs like antidepressants, which most likely act as placebos, may make people feel better initially but, in the end, they are likely to erode people's self-assurance and leave them in a worse state than they were in to begin with (quite apart from the physical complications they may suffer).

Emotional numbing

Alongside placebo and amplified placebo effects, there is the possibility that antidepressants improve people's depression scores by numbing their emotions, as I alluded to in Chapter 4. I will describe evidence that most antidepressants reduce the intensity of emotions of all varieties, including sadness and anxiety, but also happiness, in the next chapter. Logically, it seems to make sense that drugs that dampen emotions would reduce the intensity of depression and lead to lower scores on scales like the Hamilton Depression Scale. We will see how some people seem to appreciate this effect, whereas others don't like it. Yet, the clinical trial data suggests it is unlikely this effect translates into a meaningful benefit for people overall.

Moreover, whether the small effects of antidepressants are attributable to amplified placebo effects, emotional numbing or a combination of these, there is no evidence that they are rectifying an underlying chemical imbalance or any other aberrant biological process. In other words, they are not doing what people have been told they are doing.

Why are we still using antidepressants?

What are we to make of the fact that antidepressants, among the most commonly used drugs of modern times, have not been convincingly shown to be beneficial, either in the short term or the long term? Sertraline, for example, is now the most widely prescribed antidepressant in the UK, despite the fact that Pfizer struggled to get it licensed because the early trials showed it was no better than a placebo. Many renowned figures, including Irving Kirsch, have been pointing out for decades that the evidence tells us that antidepressants do not have worthwhile effects.[44] So, how is it possible that doctors, policy-makers, the media and the public have carried on as if they do?

We will come to some of the explanations for this situation later, including that the psychiatric profession does not want to admit that its most commonly prescribed treatment is a fancy placebo. Politicians and policy-makers also want to believe in antidepressants to avoid the formidable task of constructing a political solution to the widespread misery and discontent that seems to characterise modern society.

Doctors sometimes complain they feel under pressure from patients to prescribe antidepressants.[45] It is not surprising that people want to believe there is a quick and simple solution to personal and social problems, but we should also remember how the pharmaceutical industry and the medical profession have coached people for years into believing that antidepressants are safe and effective and that they correct an underlying chemical imbalance. If people have come to expect a pill for every ill, this is exactly what they have been told to do.

We cannot be complacent about this situation. Taking a drug that has not been established to have beneficial effects is rarely the best thing to do. In the following chapters we will look at evidence that antidepressants can significantly impair people's physical health and well-being. Hope can be beneficial, but false hope is harmful.

11

How Antidepressants Affect Feelings and Sex

In this chapter and the next I want to focus on what are commonly referred to as 'side-effects' of antidepressants. Many people feel these are just something they have to put up with, which is partly because the term 'side-effects' is misleading; it implies the effects are incidental and secondary to the drugs' disease-targeting effects. But we have seen that antidepressants have not been shown to have disease-targeting effects. Hence, the side-effects I will describe are not strictly 'side-effects', they are the 'expected effects' of taking a substance that changes the body's, including the brain's, normal chemical composition and interferes with its natural functions.

Modern antidepressants are not as dangerously toxic as barbiturates or the older tricyclic antidepressants, but their side-effects are not trivial – they can significantly impact people's quality of life – and, disturbingly, they don't always go away when people stop their antidepressants. Antidepressants change people's state of mind, and these effects are relevant to the way they might affect our moods.

We need to know what these changes consist of to evaluate antidepressants according to the drug-centred model I described earlier (the idea that drug-induced, 'mind-altering' effects are superimposed on underlying emotional problems) and to work out whether their effects might be useful – and also what harm they might do us.

Emotional effects

In Chapter 4, I described how antidepressants commonly make people feel a bit 'woozy' or foggy and how they alter people's usual emotional experience. Most psychoactive drugs affect our emotions. Alcohol and drugs with similar effects, such as benzodiazepines, can make us more emotional, but they also make our emotions cruder, less refined, less in tune with what we are reacting to. The 'antipsychotic' drugs used to treat people diagnosed with schizophrenia or psychotic episodes dramatically suppress people's emotions and people taking them sometimes talk of having no feelings left at all.[1] Opiates like heroin and morphine (and synthetic opioids such as OxyContin or fentanyl) produce a more pleasurable state of emotional indifference.

Although their effects are more subtle than those of antipsychotics or opiates, many antidepressants also dial down the intensity of emotions. This has taken time to be recognised because doctors have been reluctant to acknowledge that antidepressants have general psychoactive (brain- and mind-altering) effects, rather than targeted actions.

Back in the 2000s, I was also unsure about the emotion-blunting effects of antidepressants, but I was keen to investigate the changes wrought by antidepressants further. So, when a promising student called Lucy Goldsmith approached me with funding to do a summer project, I suggested we do this. Lucy and I analysed several hundred reports about two commonly used antidepressants – fluoxetine (Prozac) and venlafaxine (Efexor) – on an online website set up for patients to record experiences with all types of medication. The results quashed any doubts I might have had.

People frequently described a numbing or blunting of emotions while taking both of these antidepressants. They reported being less in touch with their feelings, being unable to cry, feeling uncaring or unmotivated, and some felt they were no longer themselves. One person described feeling 'less creative, less motivated, and it seems less me'. Another said they felt 'distanced from life'. One described themselves as 'uncaring and emotionally flat most of the time'. We also found the emotional effects were linked with sexual dysfunction.[2]

In 2009, a group of researchers from Oxford University, including the well-known biological psychiatrist Guy Goodwin, described these effects in more detail in a paper published in the *British Journal of Psychiatry*.[3] People interviewed for this research described their emotions as being 'flattened', 'dulled', 'blocked' and 'toned down'.[4] They reported their ability to experience positive emotions such as joy, excitement, enthusiasm and happiness was diminished, as well as the intensity of negative feelings, such as sadness, anger, irritability and anxiety. They felt less love or affection for family members and friends, and their interest in life had diminished.

Some described feeling detached from their emotions and from their previous cares and concerns – a feeling of being 'in limbo' or 'disconnected' from the world. Many reported apathy and reduced motivation, even though their depression had improved. Some felt they no longer cared about anything, and described a reckless disregard for themselves and their responsibilities.[5] This last effect was described vividly in another study, conducted by British psychologist John Read and colleagues, in which a former antidepressant user explained, 'I had no perception of danger around me and I often had near misses with cars and in the kitchen (e.g. with cutting food and switching off appliances)'.[6]

Some researchers have characterised the effects of antidepressants as consisting of 'loss of motivation, anergy [lack of energy], and lack of curiosity'.[7] Read and his team suggested that antidepressants could lead to 'a sort of "closing down", a withdrawal from the emotional and interpersonal world'.[8]

Some of the participants in the Oxford research felt the blunting effect had been useful initially, when they were acutely distressed, but when they started to feel better they became concerned about their lack of emotions. They recognised the drug was blocking them from reacting appropriately to bad news, sad situations, or to enjoyable or rewarding events. However, others welcomed feeling more emotionally detached from life and were happy to continue this experience (echoing Peter Kramer's stories of the personality transformations produced by Prozac). All the participants clearly identified the emotional effects to be a consequence of their antidepressant treatment, rather than as arising from their depression or underlying mood.

By the 2010s, therefore, emotional numbing was recognised as a typical consequence of taking antidepressants, but it wasn't yet clear how common it was. In 2014, John Read published a survey of the effects of antidepressants in a sample of almost 2,000 people from New Zealand, where he was living at the time. In response to questions about their emotions, 60 per cent of people described experiencing numbing of emotions and 42 per cent had noticed a reduction in positive feelings. Half of the respondents (52 per cent) said they didn't feel like themselves any more and 39 per cent said that they cared less about other people.[9] In another study published in 2017 by the Oxford team, 47 per cent of people who responded to an online survey reported 'significant emotional blunting'.[10]

People who respond to surveys are mostly long-term users, so these figures do not necessarily apply to people who have used antidepressants for short periods; nevertheless, they suggest the emotional numbness induced by antidepressants is a common experience. Still, there was the possibility that people were mistaking the causes of their numbed emotions: people might think the effect was to do with their antidepressants, when really it was part of their depression.

It is true that some people with depression feel emotionally numb, and the Oxford group showed a correlation between emotional numbing and depression symptoms in their 2017 survey. However, the survey also showed that numbing is more severe among those with depression who are taking antidepressants compared to those who are not, even after accounting for the severity of people's depressive symptoms.

Some people describe how the emotional numbing produced by antidepressants is a distinctive state that feels different from their normal emotions. A participant in the Oxford research likened the experience to having 'chemical feelings'. Moreover, the connection between loss of emotions and loss of sexual feelings, which has now been documented by several research groups, is compelling evidence that these are complementary aspects of a single pharmacological effect.[11]

The issue of how antidepressants affect normal emotions and whether they cause emotional blunting could be resolved by conducting a study with people who do not have depression. 'Healthy volunteers' could be randomised to take an antidepressant or a placebo tablet for a few weeks and asked to rate the intensity of a range of emotions.

No one has conducted such a study, as far as I am aware, but a group of academics from the University of Copenhagen provided less direct evidence that antidepressants reduce emotional responsiveness in volunteers. In this study, published in 2023, sixty-six healthy volunteers were randomised to take either the SSRI escitalopram or a placebo for three weeks. At the end of this period, they were given a series of psychological tasks to perform.

One of these was the Probabilistic Reversal Learning task, which is designed to test how responsive people are to positive feedback. The study found that people taking escitalopram were less sensitive to positive feedback than people taking the placebo, suggesting they had lower motivation or cared less. People who took the antidepressant were more likely to experience sexual dysfunction than those on the placebo, as expected, but there were no differences in people's mood or levels of anxiety or anger.[12]

So, even though we are still waiting for the definitive study of volunteers, few people now deny that antidepressants blunt emotions. A thorough review of the subject published in 2023 by a team including Professor David Baldwin, a leading UK antidepressant researcher and advocate of the drugs, concluded that 'antidepressant-induced apathy' (used as a synonym for emotional blunting) is a significant problem that deserves 'careful clinical attention'. The review noted how these effects have been recorded in people with a variety of diagnoses and are present after people get better from their original problem. It considered how the effects could explain the actions of antidepressants, citing my work on the drug-centred model. It also highlighted how many people taking antidepressants might not recognise the emotional changes they were experiencing, implying the effects may be even more common than current data suggest.[13]

Denial and minimisation

Following the publication of our serotonin paper, I started to describe the emotional blunting produced by antidepressants on air and in the popular press, and I discussed how this might impact on people with depression and other emotional problems. I pointed out how it might make people feel less intensely distressed in the short term, and how some people might welcome the emotional anaesthesia. But I also stressed that, ultimately, it could be detrimental to people's chances of recovery by preventing them from addressing the causes of their suffering and learning other ways to manage their feelings.

Despite the general acknowledgement of antidepressant-induced emotional blunting, I expect my discussing the effect in public made some psychiatrists uncomfortable. Perhaps this is because it undermines the idea that antidepressants are targeted medical treatments that act in a disease-centred way. It also highlights how antidepressants are doing something unnatural to our brains and our emotions, which sounds worrying.

So, following the publication of our review, several psychiatrists weighed in to play down the significance of the emotion-numbing effects of antidepressants. In September 2022, Ronald Pies and another leading American psychiatrist, George Dawson, published a blog entitled 'Antidepressants Do Not Work by Numbing Emotions'. Thirteen years earlier, Pies had acknowledged that antidepressants 'may leave some individuals feeling somewhat "flat" emotionally. They may also complain that their sexual energy or drive is reduced, or that their thinking seems a little "fuzzy" or slowed down.'[14] In the 2022 blog, Dawson and Pies didn't quite contradict Pies' previous statement, but they did argue that 'it should not be assumed that the patient's antidepressant is necessarily *the cause* of the patient's complaint [of emotional numbing]'.[15] They suggested the cause is often depression itself and antidepressant-induced numbing has been overstated and cannot account for the effects of antidepressants.

I agree with Dawson and Pies that it is difficult to say that emotional blunting accounts for the beneficial effects of antidepressants because, as we have seen, the beneficial effects are minimal and likely to be attributable to amplified placebo effects. Yet the emotional effects of antidepressants, which few people now completely deny, can hardly be irrelevant to the way they influence people's emotional state.

Agitation, suicidal behaviour and aggression

Somewhat paradoxically, as well as numbing emotions, some antidepressants, particularly the SSRIs, occasionally provoke feelings of agitation or tension and, very rarely, these manifest in suicidal impulses or aggression. How these effects relate to emotional blunting is not clear and, although some have suggested that blunting may reduce inhibitions or emotional regulation,[16] we don't really know. Yet again, these effects underline how little we really understand about antidepressants.

The connection between antidepressants and suicidal behaviour has been hotly debated since the early 1990s. Some commentators contend the risk has been exaggerated and warnings about it may have led to more suicides by deterring people from seeking what is assumed to be effective treatment.[17]

David Healy has been at the forefront of exposing these hazards of antidepressants. Based on observations of his own patients and emerging reports from elsewhere, as early as 1991 Healy started to suspect that SSRIs, in particular, could induce an unusual state of 'mental turmoil'.[18] Even at that time, there was evidence to suggest this state could occasionally occur in people with no history of nervous complaints and could induce people to become uncharacteristically suicidal or violent.[19] Healy became further convinced when he conducted a study of the SSRI sertraline and another antidepressant in volunteers from the staff of his local hospital: two of the twenty people involved became suicidal shortly after taking sertraline.[20]

Healy campaigned for years to highlight these issues and, in 2002, he persuaded the BBC's investigative *Panorama* programme to cover the story. The programme focused on paroxetine (also known as Seroxat or Paxil) and described two high-profile tragedies: one a suicide and one a murder, both committed by people taking paroxetine.[21] Following the programme, the drug's makers, GlaxoSmithKline, had a series of meetings with the UK medicines regulator, the Medicines and Healthcare Products Regulatory Agency (MHRA), who demanded that the company present its data on adverse events occurring in the course of its clinical trials.

When the company finally produced the data, it revealed that paroxetine was associated with a slight increase in suicide attempts and suicidal ideas in trials involving children and adolescents. Among those assigned to paroxetine, 3.4 per cent showed signs of suicidal behaviour or thinking, compared to 1.2 per cent of those assigned to a placebo.[22] The data led the UK regulator and then the FDA in the USA to issue warnings about the potential for paroxetine to provoke suicidal thoughts and behaviour in children and adolescents; a warning that was extended to all antidepressants following the results of an analysis commissioned by the FDA.[23]

Suicide and suicide attempts are thankfully rare events, so they are uncommon in clinical trials, especially as such trials usually exclude people who are feeling suicidal to begin with. However, several subsequent meta-analyses have confirmed an increase in suicidal behaviour, such as suicide attempts, in children or young people taking antidepressants, compared to those taking a placebo.[24]

One of these analyses was conducted by a group of Danish researchers who obtained unpublished clinical trial reports on seven antidepressants. Their analysis showed that children and young people taking antidepressants were more than twice as likely to exhibit suicidal tendencies than those taking a placebo and were more likely to be aggressive. Moreover, they found many of the incidences of suicidal behaviour and aggression recorded in the reports had not been included in the published versions of the trials.[25]

The issue of the relationship between antidepressants and violence has also been the subject of controversy. Several non-randomised studies show that young people who take antidepressants are more likely to commit acts of violence than those who are not taking them.[26] However, these don't prove that antidepressants cause aggression, because young people who are troubled to begin with are more likely to be prescribed antidepressants. The Danish meta-analysis is the only evidence based on randomised trials, which are not subject to this limitation, and it suggests that aggressive behaviour may be slightly increased among young people taking antidepressants.[27]

Overall, it seems that Healy's initial inclinations were right and occasionally antidepressants, particularly SSRIs, can provoke violent and suicidal behaviour. Why this should occur mainly or exclusively in children and younger people is not clear, although we know that the immature brain is more susceptible to drugs.[28] SSRIs may also have a somewhat different profile of effects in children and young people as compared to adults: the former are more susceptible to the drug-induced agitation that is thought to be related to suicidal and aggressive impulses, whereas adults are more strongly affected by sedation and apathy.[29]

Antidepressants and sex

It is well recognised that most antidepressants disrupt normal sexual function, with SSRIs being the worst offenders due to the inhibitory role of serotonin in our sexual biology. Antidepressants can reduce sexual desire, decrease sexual excitement, delay and reduce the intensity of orgasm, and produce erectile problems and delayed ejaculation. As we saw in Chapter 8, SSRIs consistently reduce sexual activity in animal studies and their effects are reliable enough that they are prescribed to sex offenders to reduce their sexual drive,[30] as well as being trialled for premature ejaculation.

Although the prevalence of sexual dysfunction is difficult to study because of people's natural reticence, Healy, who is also a leading researcher on the sexual side-effects of prescription drugs, thinks some impairment of sexual pleasure and performance is a near-universal effect with SSRIs. He suggests reduced genital sensation can occur within thirty minutes of taking the first dose, and delayed and weakened orgasm can occur soon after, whereas loss of libido takes longer to develop. He describes a dramatic example of a woman taking an SSRI whose genitals were so numb she could brush them with a hairbrush without feeling anything.[31]

Post-antidepressant sexual dysfunction

One of the most worrying complications of taking antidepressants is that the sexual side effects can persist after the antidepressant is stopped. Although still not widely recognised, persistent sexual dysfunction was first reported to the regulators in 1991, according to Healy.[32]

In 2005, an internet forum was set up called SSRIsex, on which many people described sexual problems that endured after they had stopped their antidepressant. In 2008, researchers from the University of Pittsburgh interviewed members of this forum and published some typical stories. These included that of a 44-year-old man who described loss of libido, numbing of his genitals, reduced intensity of orgasm and difficulty sustaining an erection four years after stopping the SSRI citalopram, which he had taken for eighteen months, and a 28-year-old man suffering with persistent loss of libido, genital numbing and loss of pleasure during orgasm after he ended two years of treatment with an SSRI.[33]

In a letter to a sexual health journal published in 2009, two doctors working in a sexual health clinic in Belfast described how they were seeing more and more patients with persistent sexual dysfunction following treatment with antidepressants, consisting particularly of 'lost sensation and arousal'. They commented on how the condition impinged on people's 'quality-of-life and relationships'.[34]

Since that time, there have been increasing reports of antidepressant-related persistent sexual dysfunction, often referred to as post-SSRI sexual dysfunction (PSSD) because SSRIs appear to be the most frequent culprits. It is also associated with SNRIs (Serotonin and Noradrenaline Reuptake Inhibitors), however, and possibly with some tricyclic antidepressants too (possibly those that have more significant effects on the serotonin system).[35] Usually, it occurs in people who have used antidepressants for months or years, but it is also reported by a few people who have only used antidepressants for a few weeks or even a few days. Characteristic symptoms include numbness or reduced sensitivity of the genitals, reduced sex drive, erectile dysfunction or issues with vaginal lubrication and delayed and weak orgasm.[36]

In 2019, in response to a request and petition led by David Healy, the European Medicines Agency recognised the condition and required companies that produce SSRIs and SNRIs to list persistent sexual dysfunction after stopping the drug as a side-effect in their official 'product information'.[37]

Like emotional numbing, sexual problems can occur during depression, so they are not always attributable to antidepressants. However, numbness of the genitals, which is a common and typical complaint among those with antidepressant-associated sexual dysfunction, is not a symptom of depression.

Animal research is also persuasive. Two studies showed that adolescent rats treated with various SSRIs, including fluoxetine (Prozac), were subsequently less sexually active than rats who did not have SSRI treatment.[38] Another showed that newborn rats who were given the SSRI citalopram showed deficits in sexual activity when they matured into adults.[39] A systematic review of fourteen animal studies showed persistently reduced sexual activity and ejaculation in rats previously treated with SSRIs compared to rats that had been given a placebo.[40]

The fact that persistent sexual dysfunction can occur after treatment with some other drugs, including the hair-restoring treatment finasteride and the acne drug Roaccutane, suggests that sexual functioning is vulnerable to various chemical substances. The mechanisms that underpin such effects may vary according to the drug involved.[41]

It is notoriously difficult to estimate the prevalence of sexual problems, because people are too embarrassed to report them. Israeli researchers estimated that post-SSRI sexual dysfunction might affect 1 in 200 men in particular, based on the number of cases identified among men attending a local erectile dysfunction clinic. However, a survey of young people conducted in Canada found that 13 per cent of those who had taken antidepressants reported persistent genital numbness, compared with only 1 per cent of those who had taken and stopped other prescribed medicines, suggesting it could be a common problem.[42]

On social media, people describe the persistence of emotional numbing as well as sexual dysfunction following the discontinuation of antidepressants. For many, the two experiences are intrinsically linked. Another group of Israeli doctors with experience of treating people with persistent sexual dysfunction suggested there was 'a degree of non-specific emotional malfunctioning' in most people they saw with antidepressant-induced sexual dysfunction, characterised by reduced enjoyment, apathy and blunting of emotional sensitivity.[43]

Our emotions and our sexual desire and enjoyment are fundamental parts of human life. Losing them can feel like losing one's identity. Roy, now aged 38, describes his story on the Post-SSRI Sexual Dysfunction (PSSD) Network website. Almost immediately after starting the SSRI citalopram, when he was only 22, he experienced sexual side-effects including 'genital numbness, a nearly complete loss of libido, and pleasureless orgasms'. A little later, he noticed his emotions had been dialled down. He wrote:

> The emotional numbness has also had a profound effect on my life. I can no longer feel a whole range of emotions that I used to experience. I can't feel excited to go on holiday, to spend time with a friend, or to do a hobby; and I can't feel sad, feel romantic feelings, or empathise with others in the same way as before. I also can't enjoy music like I used to, as my emotions are too numb to enjoy the emotional effects.[44]

Another victim of this effect is Dr Audrey Bahrick, a psychologist at the University of Iowa and one of the authors of the 2008 paper on the stories from the SSRIsex forum. Audrey had started taking Prozac when she was 37, she told the *New York Times,* when she was interviewed for an article on post-SSRI sexual dysfunction in 2023, and immediately 'her clitoris and vagina felt numb. "It was like there was a glove over them – a very, very muffled sensation".'[45] At first, she thought it was an 'acceptable temporary' side-effect, but two years later, when she met someone she wanted to have a relationship with, she stopped the drug, expecting the numbness to resolve. It didn't. The relationship broke down because of her lack of interest in sex, and although she remained hopeful the problem would get better if she ate well and stayed healthy, it persisted. Audrey was interviewed for the BBC *Panorama* programme, broadcast in 2023, about antidepressants and she told the filmmakers, 'I continued to hope for months and then years.' She paused, 'It's been twenty-seven years.'[46]

Audrey wanted to publish papers on the condition to help people in her situation. 'It was a long, lonely journey,' she said of the time before she linked up with other sufferers on the internet, and one of the hardest things was not being believed. The last scene in the *Panorama* documentary is of Audrey in the garden with her dog. 'You asked what I think my life might have been like if this hadn't happened,' she replied to the programme-maker. 'It's a really painful question. It's left an indelible mark on my life.' Her composure and resignation make the statement even more affecting, but Audrey was also pleased that, at last, her condition was being given some attention. 'I have been waiting for you to show up for fifteen years,' she told the crew.[47]

There is no known cure for antidepressant-induced persistent sexual dysfunction, and we don't know how long it lasts. Anecdotally, it appears to improve over time in some people, but in others, like Audrey, it can last for many years. Not surprisingly, it can lead to desperation and despair. Roy described living with it as a 'form of prolonged mental torture'.[48]

Doctors' reactions

Despite increasing coverage of the condition in the medical literature and the press,[49] many doctors are either unaware of it or reluctant to believe it is a genuine, drug-induced condition. There has been a common assumption that drugs can only impact the body while they are being ingested and a slowness to appreciate they may have enduring effects.

In 2019, Healy and colleagues published a paper about the experiences people had when they reported their post-antidepressant sexual dysfunction to their doctor or psychiatrist. One person reported how a psychiatrist had 'dismissed PSSD as impossible and suggested that I was asexual and traumatised'. Another psychiatrist 'could not engage with the notion of SSRI's having a long-term impact, instead pretending not to hear me or move onto another topic of conversation. This was a surreal experience.' Another was told he was 'talking absolute rubbish' and his sexual symptoms were the result of his 'psychological constructs'.[50]

US psychiatrist Anita Clayton, who has conducted research on the sexual side-effects of SSRIs in the past, has also denied that post-antidepressant sexual dysfunction exists. She told the *New York Times* for its 2023 piece, 'I think it's depression recurring. Until proven otherwise, that's what it is.'[51] But generally, when a potential complication of this gravity is highlighted, we should assume it's the drug until proven otherwise. George Dawson, though not denying the possible existence of the condition outright, accused those who highlight the disorder as having an 'ideological bias'.[52]

Mostly though, medical professionals have just taken no notice of the mounting evidence of post-antidepressant sexual dysfunction. If they took it seriously, there would, at least, be widely circulated warnings about it. There would be guidelines about how to discuss the issue with patients before starting an antidepressant, and how to recall people already taking one to discuss their options. No such warnings or edicts have been issued.

Even if it is rare, people taking antidepressants are now so numerous that persistent sexual dysfunction is likely to affect significant numbers and, for those affected, it can be devastating. Everyone taking or contemplating taking antidepressants needs to be warned about this potential complication, especially young people who risk losing years of sexual pleasure and intimacy.

Antidepressants, it transpires, can diminish core parts of the human experience. In rare, but not exceptional, cases they deprive people of some of the most important and potentially fulfilling aspects of human life and stifle people's social and emotional development. Roy's sexual side-effects persisted throughout his young adult life. 'I also feel that I didn't develop properly as a young person in many different ways because of PSSD and emotional numbness,' he wrote.

When the *New York Times* covered the story, Yassie Pirani, a counsellor in Vancouver, told the newspaper, 'People put on these drugs at a young age may just never know who they might otherwise be if they hadn't been on this drug.' People who take antidepressants need to know they are gambling with their sex lives and their emotional health, possibly for years to come.

Antidepressants, fertility and pregnancy

The effects of antidepressants on reproductive functions also need to be more widely publicised. The following information may be shocking to women who took antidepressants during pregnancy without knowing all the facts and is not meant to make anyone feel guilty about their choices. It is meant to ensure women are better informed in the future.

Research indicates that antidepressants can have numerous adverse effects on pregnancy. Women who take antidepressants are more likely to suffer a miscarriage, a haemorrhage, pre-eclampsia (a dangerous condition involving high blood pressure in late pregnancy), a premature birth, a small baby and a stillbirth compared with those who don't take them.[53] These effects are also found in animal studies using rats, mice and sheep, which confirms they are not simply due to the adverse circumstances that are associated with being depressed and taking antidepressants, although these may play a part.[54]

After birth, 30 per cent of babies born to mothers taking antidepressants suffer a withdrawal syndrome, in which they are jittery and have breathing and feeding problems.[55] It can be serious, and one study found that 13 per cent of babies exposed to antidepressants during pregnancy needed resuscitation in the delivery room compared to 4 per cent of babies who were not exposed.[56]

Many studies show that the babies of women who took antidepressants during pregnancy are more likely to have a birth defect compared to babies of women who didn't take antidepressants, including defects of the heart, kidney, nervous system, digestive tract, abdomen, muscles and bones.[57] There is ongoing debate about whether this is due to antidepressants, specifically, or whether it reflects the circumstances or behaviour (such as smoking) of women who take antidepressants, but several high-quality studies suggest that antidepressants play a role.[58]

The children of women who have taken antidepressants are also more likely to have language difficulties and behaviour problems, and to be given a diagnosis of autism or ADHD. Again, however, other influences such as genetics, social circumstances and parental behaviour are likely to account for some of this effect.[59] Animal studies are inconsistent, but some find behavioural changes in the offspring of antidepressant-treated mothers, including reduced social and exploratory activity.[60]

Exposing the developing brain to a foreign chemical substance is always taking a chance. Serotonin plays a central role in the growth and organisation of the baby's brain and nervous system[61] and we don't know how drugs that modify that system, such as antidepressants, might affect these processes. If antidepressants were a life-saving treatment, their risks might be an acceptable price to pay, but, as I've argued above, they are not.

Increasing numbers of women of child-bearing age are using antidepressants. In 2018, women in the UK were prescribed antidepressants at some point in 13.4 per cent of pregnancies, which was up from 3.2 per cent in 1996.[62] Adam Urato, a US-based maternal-foetal medicine specialist, has called this situation a 'public health emergency' and reflected that 'never before in human history have we chemically altered developing babies like this, especially the developing fetal brain'.[63]

The medical establishment is in denial about this situation, as it is about antidepressants' emotional and sexual side-effects. Following a FDA panel convened in 2025 to hear evidence about antidepressants and pregnancy, medical organisations voiced their outrage that the panel had included critics of the drugs, such as Adam Urato, David Healy and myself.[64] Medical publications rushed to reassure women that 'SSRIs are safe' or 'confer minimal risk'.[65] They claimed that depression, not antidepressants, causes the complications in women taking antidepressants, and that not treating women is what puts them at risk. This has not been demonstrated, however, partly because studies of the effects of depression in pregnancy mostly fail to account for the effects of antidepressants.[66]

Antidepressants have negative effects on male fertility as well as on pregnancy. Studies in animals and humans show SSRIs reduce the concentration and quality of sperm cells, and increase damage to the genetic material or DNA they contain.[67] In 2012, a warning about 'sperm impairment' was added to the label of several SSRIs.[68]

Antidepressants may also influence fertility through their effects on sexual desire and performance. No doubt, many factors are at play in the falling rates of sexual activity that are apparent in high-income countries (the amount of time people spend on screens, pornography, anxiety),[69] but it's not implausible that the widespread use of drugs that inhibit sexual function could be playing a part.

Overall, evidence suggests antidepressants are profoundly disrupting some of our most basic drives and biological functions. With millions of people taking these drugs on a long-term basis, we have to consider how they might be changing us. What is the widespread and poorly understood chemical manipulation of our emotions, our sexuality and our reproductive health doing to us and to our society?

12

Dependence and Withdrawal Effects of Antidepressants

In the previous chapter, I described common ways in which antidepressants alter our mental and emotional states and their effects on sexual functioning. In this chapter, I describe the issue of dependence and withdrawal effects. We will see that, like sexual dysfunction, withdrawal effects can be protracted and can persist long after people have stopped taking their antidepressant.

David Healy coined the term 'legacy effect' for an effect that persists after a drug has been stopped.[1] A well-recognised legacy effect is a neurological complication of taking antipsychotic drugs called 'tardive dyskinesia', which consists of involuntary movements and some degree of general mental impairment.[2] It usually starts during long-term treatment and often persists after the drug is stopped, although it generally improves gradually over the course of time.[3]

Persistent sexual dysfunction and protracted withdrawal states caused by antidepressants can also be viewed as legacy effects. Their occurrence suggests antidepressants disrupt the brain and nervous system in a way that can take a long time to revert to normal.

Withdrawal effects

Antidepressants do not generally make people euphoric, like recreational drugs. In fact, they often make people feel mildly below par, but as I explained earlier, this doesn't mean they can't cause dependence. Dependence occurs because the body changes its biological structure and activity in response to the ongoing ingestion of a drug. When the drug is stopped, these changes lead to withdrawal effects.

Dr Tom Stockmann, who was part of the serotonin review team, started working with me when he was a junior psychiatrist in 2015. During one of our supervision sessions, he disclosed he had been taking an antidepressant and was trying to come off it. Even though he had only been taking the drug for eighteen months, it was proving to be a difficult process.

Tom had been prescribed the SNRI duloxetine (Cymbalta), which is similar to the more widely prescribed venlafaxine (Efexor), both of which are recognised to cause particularly severe withdrawal symptoms. Getting off duloxetine and venlafaxine is difficult, in part because they don't come in small doses, so Tom was having to break open the capsules and measure out a slowly decreasing number of the tiny beads of the drug contained inside. This was the only way he could reduce the drug at a slow enough pace to keep the withdrawal symptoms just about tolerable. If he went too fast, he became light-headed, had trouble concentrating and experienced excruciating vertigo and 'brain zaps' (a feeling like electricity being passed through the brain).

It took Tom about a year to get off the drug altogether. 'I had no idea how hard it would be,' he said in an interview with the *New York Times* in 2018. But it was worth it because Tom was fortunate not to suffer persistent effects. After he stopped, his emotions, which had been stifled when he was on the drug, returned. 'There was a really significant moment,' he recalled in the same interview, 'I was walking down near my house, past a forest, and I suddenly realized I could feel the full range of emotions again. The birds were louder, the colors more vivid – I was happy.'[4]

As part of a series of articles on withdrawal, published in 2018, the *New York Times* invited readers to describe their experiences of coming off antidepressants. Almost 9,000 people replied. They reported dizziness, nausea, fatigue, flu-like symptoms, anxiety, panic attacks, crying a lot, fogginess and the weird but characteristic 'brain zaps' Tom had experienced, which are also described by people withdrawing from benzodiazepines.[5]

It was still unclear how common such problems were, though, so James Davies, a respected academic and author,[6] and psychologist John Read conducted a review of the literature on antidepressant withdrawal to see what the evidence indicated. They were motivated by the fact that antidepressant withdrawal was portrayed in most official sources as trivial and short-lived. The American Psychiatry Association's 2010 clinical guideline suggested that withdrawal reactions 'typically resolve without specific treatment over 1–2 weeks', for example.[7] The 2009 NICE guideline advised that withdrawal 'symptoms are usually mild and self-limiting over about 1 week', although it did add that they 'can be severe, particularly if the drug is stopped abruptly'.[8] In the 2020 edition of the *New Oxford Textbook of Psychiatry*, antidepressant withdrawal is listed in a table, but not described at all in the text itself.[9]

Davies and Read identified fourteen studies that had explored the prevalence, severity and duration of antidepressant withdrawal symptoms, including surveys and randomised trials. The proportion of people experiencing withdrawal symptoms varied between 27 per cent and 86 per cent across these studies, likely reflecting the different designs of the studies, the fact that some antidepressants are more likely to induce withdrawal symptoms than others and that people had been taking antidepressants for varying lengths of time before withdrawal. The average proportion was 56 per cent, and almost half of these people (46 per cent) – a quarter of the total – reported that the withdrawal effects had been 'severe'. Several studies recorded instances of withdrawal symptoms lasting for weeks, months and sometimes years.[10]

Davies and Read's review, which was published in a journal called *Addictive Behaviours*, was widely publicised and influential in changing the conversation about withdrawal. Still, it was limited by the nature of the studies on which it was based. The surveys it included, for example, had been put out online for anyone to respond to, and therefore potentially recruited people who had had particularly bad experiences with antidepressants or antidepressant withdrawal (although the majority of people who answered the surveys believed their antidepressant helped them).[11] So, just before the Covid pandemic, Dr Horowitz and I set up a survey of people attending a local NHS psychological therapy service. Our aim was to explore withdrawal experiences among a more typical group of antidepressant users.

We recruited 310 people who had taken an antidepressant and stopped or tried to stop it at some point. Almost 80 per cent reported experiencing withdrawal symptoms of some sort. For many people these were mild, but almost half the sample (49 per cent) reported having had moderate or severe withdrawal symptoms (15 per cent had severe symptoms). Most tellingly, however, 38 per cent of people had tried to stop their antidepressants but couldn't.

We also found that, on average, withdrawal became more severe the longer someone had used antidepressants. Four out of five people who had used an antidepressant for more than two years had been unable to stop when they tried. Although withdrawal symptoms lasted a few weeks for most people, 10 per cent indicated they lasted longer than a year.[12]

Antidepressant withdrawal effects had been described back in the 1950s, as it turns out,[13] but, as we saw earlier, the promotional and professional campaigns of the 1990s and 2000s went to lengths to erase this knowledge from the collective memory. Even after it became widely accepted that the SSRI paroxetine (Paxil or Seroxat) caused significant and severe withdrawal effects (partly due to coverage by the BBC's 2002 *Panorama* programme) and although the use of paroxetine plummeted after this,[14] the belief continued that for most antidepressants, withdrawal effects were minimal.

Along with Davies and Read's review, our findings suggest this impression is wrong. Our survey was subject to the usual limitations of surveys, such as that people may attribute symptoms to withdrawal that are not, in fact, related to it, and those who took the survey may have had particularly bad experiences. Yet it appears that severe and prolonged withdrawal symptoms are relatively common, especially among people who use antidepressants long term, and may result in many people being trapped on medication they don't want to take.

Protracted antidepressant withdrawal

Adele Framer is someone who discovered some of the dire consequences of antidepressant withdrawal for herself. Adele grew up in New York State in the 1960s, and she told me she had had a difficult childhood because her mother preferred to play bridge and have affairs than look after her children, while her father was too dejected to compensate. Despite this, she went to college, graduated with a bachelor's degree, moved to San Francisco and went to work in the expanding information technology sector. In the

1990s, she was prescribed Prozac by a gynaecologist for premenstrual difficulties. Prozac had just hit the streets and Adele, like millions of others, was persuaded to try it.

Prozac brought its typical sexual dysfunction, but no other significant adverse effects, and she stopped it after a couple of years without too much difficulty. A few years later, working for a failing dotcom, she was given paroxetine (Paxil or Seroxat) for social anxiety. She took this drug faithfully for the next two years, but became increasingly numbed by it, both emotionally and sexually. So, in 2004, she decided to stop it and weaned off it over a period of a few weeks.

This was the start of a hellish experience that lasted for several years. At first, she felt elated and she was hyperactive, along with more typical withdrawal symptoms, such as brain zaps and depersonalisation (a feeling of being disconnected from your body). As time went by, these subsided and new symptoms appeared – particularly insomnia, an inability to concentrate, disorientation and sharp, short spells of panic and deep despair. These came and went in a pattern people now describe as 'windows and waves'. She struggled to concentrate and to work; having a social or personal life was impossible and after a few years she had to stop working altogether.

At first, Adele had no idea what was happening to her, and nor did any of the doctors she consulted. But the symptoms she had were quite different from anything she had felt before she started the drug, so it soon dawned on her that she was experiencing paroxetine withdrawal. With this realisation, Adele started to read everything she could find on antidepressant withdrawal and she searched for evidence that other people were reporting the same problems.

In 2005 she joined paxilprogress.org, one of half a dozen peer-support websites for antidepressant withdrawal then in operation, which already had around 20,000 members. In 2011, she used her tech skills to set up her own website, now one of the most long-lasting online communities for people undergoing psychiatric drug withdrawal: Surviving Antidepressants.

As well as connecting her to the thousands of people in the same situation, survivingantidepressants.com enabled Adele to put her accumulating knowledge about withdrawal to good use (and she is one of the most knowledgeable people I know on this subject). The website contains information about how to withdraw from antidepressants and other psychiatric drugs slowly, to reduce the risk of severe and protracted withdrawal, and hosts forums that enable people to exchange advice and tips. Survivingantidepressants.com has had 20,000 members since it was launched, and Adele estimates she has personally helped thousands of people who have contacted her via the site for advice and support.

Her symptoms lasted eleven years and cost Adele her career and much else. She was 54 when she came off paroxetine. 'When I recovered,' she wrote, 'I was a white-haired retiree.'[15]

When I first heard of people reporting antidepressant withdrawal symptoms persisting for years after stopping the drug, I was surprised and probably a bit incredulous. Withdrawal symptoms were traditionally thought to subside rapidly as the drug is washed out of the body. Alcohol withdrawal is over in a few days, for example, or at least it appears to be. Antidepressants are eliminated more slowly, but still most of them will have dissipated almost entirely within a week, on average, although Prozac lingers for a few weeks.[16]

But then I remembered there were papers published in the late 1980s describing protracted withdrawal states following the cessation of benzodiazepines. These papers were written by an old teacher of mine from Newcastle University, pharmacologist Heather Ashton.

Ashton started the first NHS clinic dedicated to helping people come off benzodiazepines in the 1980s, and she is well known among people who have become dependent on benzodiazepines and other psychiatric drugs because she was one of the first people to take the issue of withdrawal seriously. She worked out careful tapering regimens to help people get off their medication smoothly and published them in what became known as the *Ashton Manual*, which is still a valuable resource for those seeking help with getting off these drugs.[17]

Ashton noticed early on that benzodiazepine withdrawal symptoms could last for months and sometimes longer after the drugs were stopped. Along with anxiety and depression, which Ashton felt were part of the withdrawal state, persistent symptoms typically included tinnitus (buzzing in the ears), muscle jerks, restless legs, pain, numbness and pins and needles. The nature of the symptoms suggests benzodiazepines 'reset' the sensory and motor nervous system, rendering people hypersensitive and hyper-responsive following withdrawal. Ashton concluded that not only could benzodiazepines produce 'slowly reversible functional changes in the central nervous system', the generally accepted mechanism of drug withdrawal, but they could 'occasionally cause structural neuronal damage' – brain damage, in other words.[18]

Other drugs may also give rise to protracted symptoms following withdrawal. Although the most dramatic manifestations of alcohol or heroin withdrawal are over relatively quickly, more subtle symptoms, such as problems with mood, sleep and concentration, can persist for months and possibly years.[19] The trouble is we rarely look for them, so there is little data.

Our survey suggested around 10 per cent of people had symptoms that lasted for longer than a year, but it is difficult to be sure exactly how many people are affected. Tens of thousands of sufferers have come together on internet sites like Adele's, however. Most had been taking antidepressants for years when they tried to stop; many were advised that coming off antidepressants was not difficult and they could stop in two to four weeks, as suggested by official guidelines. Yet, when they tried this, like

Adele, they were catapulted into a state of physical and mental upheaval, with terrible consequences in some cases.

In 2021, I conducted another survey (together with Mark Horowitz and John Read), this time of the experiences of members of these online support groups. Over 1,000 people took part. Most of them had gravitated to these groups because they had found their doctor's advice unhelpful.[20]

When they were asked about the consequences of protracted withdrawal, a quarter said they had suffered a relationship breakdown, a fifth had had to give up work, and a third had cut down their hours or duties. Some people described how they had been 'bedridden' or 'unable to cope with normal daily responsibilities' for weeks or months during or following withdrawal, and the process of coming off an antidepressant had 'ruined' or 'permanently changed' their lives. They had missed out on time with their children, had had to give up promising careers and shut down businesses, and many had lost confidence and self-esteem. Some ended up socially isolated and 'reclusive'; many described feeling suicidal.[21]

In 2015, major national newspapers in the UK started to print stories about how difficult antidepressant withdrawal could be. One of the first was that of Luke Montagu, son of the Earl of Sandwich, a member of the British House of Lords. Luke had suffered catastrophic withdrawal symptoms after undergoing a rapid and unorthodox detoxification from a benzodiazepine and subsequently stopping an antidepressant. Luke had never had significant emotional problems and had been prescribed psychiatric drugs when he developed neurological symptoms following surgery on his sinuses.

Luke knew the editor of *The Times* newspaper, who was interested in Luke's experiences and published some articles on benzodiazepine withdrawal. Later, the *Daily Mail* ran a series of features on the topic of withdrawal from prescribed medicines in general, including antidepressants. Luke also raised the issue among Members of Parliament and helped set up the All Party Parliamentary Group on Prescribed Drug Dependence. In 2018, this group instigated a major review on the subject undertaken by Public Health England.[22]

Media coverage of antidepressant withdrawal increased from this point. Well-known figures, such as British journalist Sarah Vine, described her experiences in the *Daily Mail*, and the *New York Times* series ran in 2018.[23]

In 2019, after a debate on Twitter (now X) between the then President of the Royal College of Psychiatrists, Wendy Burn, and several campaigners, the college commissioned Mark Horowitz to rewrite the antidepressant withdrawal section of its website. The new guidance acknowledged that withdrawal could be severe and prolonged for some people and advised that antidepressants should be stopped gradually, especially when people had used them for a long time.[24]

The professional reaction

Still there was pushback from some members of the profession. Using tactics that would become all too familiar to me, two young academic psychiatrists – Joseph Hayes, from my department at University College London, and Sameer Jauhar of King's College London – attacked Davies and Read's review. They alleged it was full of 'errors' and 'mistakes' and did 'not accurately portray the data'.[25] These sound like damning criticisms, and scientists don't generally use this sort of language unless they are certain a paper has fundamental flaws. However, as Davies and Read showed in their reply, many of the accusations were mistaken; others were trivial.[26]

Hayes and Jauhar accused Davies and Read of missing out five relevant studies, for example. Davies and Read explained that these studies, which were conducted by the drug companies

Lundbeck and Forest pharmaceuticals (makers of the SSRIs citalopram and escitalopram) were not included because none of the reports contained any data on withdrawal effects. Hayes and Jauhar also suggested that Davies and Read had omitted certain studies from their estimate of the severity of withdrawal. Yet again, Davies and Read explained they had not omitted anything; the studies they were accused of missing out didn't present any data on severity.

Hayes and Jauhar criticised Davies and Read for lumping all the studies together, but then performed their own combined analysis, adding in data from the Lundbeck–Forest trials that was available in a subsequent analysis produced by the company. Adding in these trials, which involved people who had only taken antidepressants for a few weeks or months (therefore underestimating the likelihood of withdrawal in longer-term users), still produced an overall rate of withdrawal symptoms of 44 per cent. This is not a million miles away from the 56 per cent found by Davies and Read, who pointed out that given the extent of use of antidepressants, 44 per cent still represents 3.2 million adults in England alone. The point is, however you cut the cake, a lot of people experience antidepressant withdrawal symptoms.

Hayes and Jauhar were not alone in their opposition to the review. At the same time as their blog was published, a senior UK psychiatrist close to Hayes and Jauhar wrote to *Addictive Behaviours* (the journal the review was published in) demanding the review be retracted. At one point, the journal was told if this didn't happen, a large proportion of the editorial board would resign. The journal didn't cave into the pressure and advised the complainant to submit their criticisms in an academic response, which would be considered for publication in the usual manner of scientific debate. The psychiatrist never did this.[27]

It seems the review's critics were not just trying to fine tune our knowledge on withdrawal, they were attempting to adjust the scientific record. It's not immediately obvious why psychiatrists should take such exception to a paper setting out the research on antidepressant withdrawal, especially when the Royal College of Psychiatrists was in the process of acknowledging the problem. The fact that James Davies and John Read are vocal critics of psychiatric drugs most likely had something to do with it. Had the review been written by members of the British Association of Psychopharmacology, it's unlikely it would have drawn the same fire. No one was denying the existence of antidepressant withdrawal; rather, the review's critics were quibbling about methodological minutiae and exact numbers in what looked like an attempt to undermine the credibility of a widely publicised paper. Ironically, the debate they provoked only drew further attention to the extent of the problem of antidepressant withdrawal.

In 2024, the proponents of antidepressants had a further opportunity to talk down the extent and significance of withdrawal effects. The occasion was the publication of another systematic review of antidepressant withdrawal studies, led by two German psychiatrists from the University of Cologne. As Mark Horowitz and I pointed out in *The Conversation*, the review was based on a set of poor-quality studies, most of which were sponsored by drug companies, involved people who had only used antidepressants for a few weeks or months, and made no attempt to assess withdrawal symptoms in a reliable or systematic way. Despite these drawbacks, it still found that about one in six people had pharmacological withdrawal symptoms when stopping an antidepressant, after accounting for the fact that some people experience symptoms after coming off a placebo. Only 3 per cent were reported to have severe symptoms, but the assessment of severity was even more haphazard than the assessment of withdrawal per se.[28]

The review was immediately hailed as showing that the risks of withdrawal had been exaggerated. Sameer Jauhar believed he was vindicated and told the Science Media Centre, which helped publicise the review, it is 'gratifying to know rates of withdrawal are nowhere near as high as reported'. Other expert commentators lined up to applaud the review for providing reassurance that there was nothing to worry about with antidepressants. UK psychiatrist Paul Keedwell comforted people by claiming 'that withdrawal symptoms are not dangerous, and the risk of experiencing them at some future date should not be a reason for refusing antidepressant treatment'.[29] Another declared the 'myth that antidepressants are addictive has been debunked – they are a vital tool in psychiatry' and suggested people 'should be reassured by the very low incidence of severe discontinuation symptoms'.[30]

In contrast, people who had struggled to get off antidepressants expressed their concern on social media about the way the review was being interpreted.[31] The closer I looked at the review, the worse I realised it was. Very few of the studies included in the review had even bothered to ask people about withdrawal symptoms specifically. Yet, it was proclaimed to demonstrate that withdrawal is nothing to worry about.

One user of X compared this whitewashing exercise to Pfizer's attempt to suppress information about withdrawal, revealed in an old memo obtained by the BBC for its 2023 *Panorama* programme. Pfizer's memo read, 'We should not volunteer to describe the withdrawal symptoms [of its drug sertraline] but have an agreed list prepared in case they [the regulators] insist'.[32]

Admitting its most widely used and emblematic remedy causes significant dependence and withdrawal problems has been challenging for the psychiatric profession to accept. Many of those suffering from protracted withdrawal have been told they are having a relapse of their psychological problem. Others are diagnosed as having 'psychosomatic' complaints, adding insult to injury.[33] Before his untimely death following his own experience of withdrawal, Ed White[34] described the profession as being in a state of 'vehement denial', and reacting in a way that exhibited 'professional arrogance, protectionism, denial and minimisation'.[35]

It is worrying that it was only when the son of a member of the House of Lords (Luke Montagu) experienced antidepressant withdrawal that the issue got into the newspapers and onto the Parliamentary agenda, eventually forcing the medical profession to acknowledge the problem. Pharmaceutical companies have no interest in uncovering quite how difficult it is to stop taking their products. Psychiatric researchers and research funders also prefer to concentrate on the positive developments in medical treatment and not its downsides. So, it is left to 'consumers' to highlight the damaging effects of drugs like antidepressants, and they have to contend with professional scepticism and denial.

The fact that antidepressants can produce long-lasting and debilitating withdrawal symptoms and can suppress people's sexual and emotional sensitivity long after they have been stopped suggests they are profoundly disrupting the way the brain functions. We may not know exactly what this disruption consists of, but, as Heather Ashton observed, the prolonged nature of the symptoms raises the possibility that the drugs can cause lasting or even permanent damage to the brain tissues themselves.[36]

Weighing up the effects of antidepressants

So, how can we weigh up the various effects of antidepressants? The emotional numbing described in the last chapter may, in theory, be helpful for people who are in acute distress or experiencing emotional pain or anxiety. It may reduce the intensity of such feelings. It might provide someone with a buffer against the things that are getting them down or causing them concern. If it does this effectively, it might enable that individual to engage with therapy or make changes to improve their situation that they couldn't otherwise manage. It might also reduce people's sensitivity to situations they don't need to be so sensitive to. These may be the effects that Peter Kramer observed in his patients and that are described by some participants in the Oxford research.

The randomised trials suggest that, ultimately, it is the amplified placebo effects that distinguish an antidepressant from a placebo, however, not these effects. So, I think we should be cautious about assuming that emotional numbing can be useful. There is also the problem that numbing our emotions might obscure the source of the problem: it might enable us to go on functioning in a situation that makes us – and *should* make us – unhappy, like the frustrated and no doubt sometimes abused 1960s housewives who got through the day on 'Mothers' Little Helper' (Valium).

Everyone agrees that antidepressants have unpleasant and sometimes debilitating side-effects, like all other drugs, but these are not always explained to patients. However, many doctors are not aware of the serious legacy effects of antidepressants – the persistent sexual dysfunction and severe and prolonged withdrawal – and, therefore, these are rarely discussed. But no one should be prescribed antidepressants now without being warned about these potential consequences. If people choose to take antidepressants knowing the risks, they are making an informed choice, but we must avoid more people becoming unsuspecting victims.

For anyone taking antidepressants, hearing about these effects must be frightening. Although people describe persistent sexual dysfunction after short-term use of antidepressants, it is likely that long-term use carries the most significant risks of both persistent sexual dysfunction and protracted and severe withdrawal. Therefore, my advice to anyone who feels they must try an antidepressant is to take it for the shortest possible time. Once the worst is over, consider coming off it – with professional support, of course.

For people who are already taking antidepressants, especially those who have been taking them for more than a year or so, undertaking withdrawal in a slow and measured fashion is important to minimise the severity of withdrawal symptoms and the likelihood of suffering prolonged symptoms. One of the lessons from the thousands of people who have been suffering on the sidelines in online communities is that the medical profession needs to be better trained to help people come off medication like antidepressants.

Fortunately, Mark Horowitz and David Taylor, Professor of Psychopharmacology at King's College London and author of the gold standard *Maudsley Prescribing Guidelines*, have published the *Maudsley Deprescribing Guidelines*. These aim to help doctors guide people in coming off a range of psychiatric medications, including antidepressants, in as safe and as harmless a way as possible.[37]

Professionals also need guidance on how to support people who are currently suffering from drug-induced complications. As illustrated by the personal stories I have set out here, antidepressants have deprived some people of years of a healthy and fulfilling life – it is the least we can do.

Part 4

Reactions

13

Moving the Goalposts

Having presented the evidence on antidepressants, I want to come back to the various responses to our paper on the serotonin theory of depression. I wrote this book partly because I was so shocked by the way my profession, the profession of psychiatry, reacted. Before I describe the nature of that reaction, let me just pause to set out what a reasonable response might have looked like, one that 'follows the science'.

The profession might have used the publication of the paper as an opportunity to reflect on why it had not acknowledged the lack of evidence sooner. It might have worried that it had misled people into believing the biological basis of depression was established when it is not, or that it had not stopped other parties, such as the pharmaceutical industry, from misleading people. It might have expressed concern that many people had made decisions about whether to take antidepressants on the basis of misinformation.

Psychiatrists might have questioned what the lack of evidence for a neurochemical cause of depression means for our understanding of depression. They might have wondered what antidepressants are doing to the brain if they are not correcting an underlying chemical imbalance, and how this might affect the millions of people using these drugs. They might have called for research to establish this. They might have reconsidered the evidence that claims to support the idea that 'antidepressants work' and paid more attention to the harmful effects people have been reporting in recent years. At the very least, there might have been an open-minded debate about these issues.

Sadly, none of this happened, at least not at the top levels of the profession. I was invited to speak at a few meetings by some broader-minded colleagues, but there was no professional reckoning. While the public reacted with dismay to finding out they had been misled for more than three decades, the profession tried to neutralise the findings and divert people's attention from their implications for our understanding of antidepressants.

I will describe the profession's tactics and motivations in Chapter 15, including how they culminated in an orchestrated campaign to discredit the paper, led by a group of aggrieved psychiatrists from the UK. But, here, I want to focus on the arguments put forward to counteract the paper's impact, and to describe research that was proposed to salvage the serotonin theory, along with alternative theories about the biological basis of depression.

The publication of our paper threw members of the psychiatric establishment into panic. They knew it would open up a public debate about antidepressants and they didn't want that to happen. The UK's Science Media Centre coordinated the initial response. The centre's mission is to improve the public understanding of science – a laudable aim – but it receives funding from numerous pharmaceutical companies, as well as from the industry's trade association, the Association of the British Pharmaceutical Industry.[1] Its spokespeople on mental health regularly include vociferous advocates of drug treatments and other biological interventions.

Ironically, the Science Media Centre had originally been approached by the press office at my university to collaborate on publicising the paper, as they do for other important papers. To our surprise, at first, the centre offered to help, but then it changed its mind and withdrew its offer. Instead, the centre released a press briefing featuring seven 'experts', all psychiatrists, criticising and dismissing the paper. A spokesperson for the Royal College of Psychiatrists was also quoted, reassuring people about the use of antidepressants.[2]

The experts said no one believed the serotonin theory of depression anyway, but at the same time, serotonin *is* involved. They said the studies we looked at were inadequate because they only measured serotonin indirectly, or because they were too diverse. Some said there was new evidence to support the role of serotonin, and others that the serotonin theory has been supplanted by more up-to-date ideas about the biology of depression. And finally, everyone said again and again and again that it didn't matter what we had found because antidepressants 'work'.

The responses were reminiscent of Freud's story of the borrowed kettle. Freud relates how a man is accused by his neighbour of returning a kettle in a damaged condition. The man offers three conflicting excuses: that the kettle wasn't really damaged, that it was already damaged when he borrowed it, and that he never borrowed it in the first place![3]

The reactions to our paper reveal a profession trying to uphold the idea, with whatever contradictory arguments come to hand, that depression has biological roots. This reflects the real objective of being able to justify the use of antidepressants according to the disease-centred model: being able to say that antidepressants act on the biological mechanisms that supposedly produce depression. This is the sacred cow that must be kept alive at all costs. People mustn't get a hint of the evidence we have just uncovered – the evidence that suggests antidepressants are doing nothing of the sort, and are most likely ineffective and harmful.

'We knew it anyway'

The first argument made by those who wanted to challenge the paper was that it wasn't important. People already knew the serotonin theory of depression was not supported by evidence, they claimed. David Curtis from Dundee told the Science Media Centre, 'It is certainly not news that depression is not caused by "low serotonin levels". The notion of depression being due to a "chemical imbalance" is outmoded.'[4] It may not have been news to David Curtis, but it was news to other people, including, presumably, the American Psychiatric Association, which was, at the time (and still is, as of February 2024), telling people that 'differences' in brain chemicals may be involved in depression.[5]

Two weeks after publication of the paper, Ronald Pies and another US psychiatrist, George Dawson, wrote an article in *Psychiatric Times* entitled 'The Serotonin Fixation: Much Ado About Nothing New'. In 2011, in the same publication, Pies had had to admit 'there certainly are psychiatrists, and other physicians, who have used the term "chemical imbalance" when explaining psychiatric illness to a patient, or when prescribing a medication for depression or anxiety'.[6] Yet, in 2022, Dawson and Pies claimed the serotonin theory of depression had 'never' been 'espoused by academic psychiatrists; psychopharmacologists; standard psychiatric textbooks; or professional psychiatric organizations, at least in the US'. They added that four other reviews had already concluded that 'the total evidence was inconclusive or inconsistent'. They likened assessing the evidence for the serotonin theory of depression to exploring the theory that depression is caused by excessive 'black bile' or 'an imbalance in the 4 bodily humors'.[7] In other words, even though Pies had already been called out for making this argument, he continued to suggest it was ridiculous to take the serotonin theory seriously.

David Hellerstein, Professor of Clinical Psychiatry at Columbia University Medical Center and director of Columbia's Depression Evaluation Service, claimed our review 'was largely met with yawns from the psychiatric community' and invoked the same black bile analogy, with the sarcastic comment, 'Wow, next she'll [meaning me] tackle the discrediting of the black bile theory of depression'.[8]

The hypocrisy of these comments is astounding. It is well known that the psychiatric profession has promoted the serotonin theory of depression. Pies defended a version of it himself, and academic literature and public information has been presenting the theory for decades as a credible, if not certain, explanation of depression.[9] As we have seen, numerous organisations have until recently suggested depression is caused by a chemical imbalance, and many, including the American Psychiatric Association, continue to do so (see Appendix 1).[10]

It may have been the case that, if pressed, some psychiatrists would have admitted the serotonin theory of depression is not supported, but no one from the psychiatric establishment had disseminated this fact. As Canada's *National Post* put it, 'Doctors have stopped believing that "chemical imbalance" causes depression. They didn't tell us.'[11] The vast majority of the public had continued to believe the serotonin theory was proven, as surveys have shown.[12] And although there had been previous reviews of the area, no one had surveyed the evidence systematically and comprehensively in the way we did, which enabled us to say, with certainty, that the theory has no clothes.

'Serotonin is involved'

At the same time as saying that disproving the serotonin theory of depression was nothing new, the critics of our paper maintained that serotonin *is* involved in depression, but it's 'complicated'.[13] Pies and Dawson suggested 'more recent integrated theories incorporating 5-HT [serotonin] systems with other depression hypotheses are under active development' and some research on serotonin and its metabolites did support the role of serotonin in depression.[14] Of course, some studies have yielded positive results, but we showed that when you look at the data overall, these are cancelled out by negative ones. Research on serotonin and its metabolites, in particular, gave no indication that serotonin is involved in depression.

Phil Cowen of the University of Oxford also wanted to stress that there were some positive findings, even though he agreed with our conclusions that the serotonin theory of depression is not supported. 'I studied the role of serotonin in people with depression for three decades and I'm broadly in agreement with the authors' conclusions about our current efforts,' he said. Cowen concluded by suggesting that 'it would be surprising if a such a widely distributed brain neuromodulatory system was completely uninvolved in the complex experiences that make up clinical depression'.[15] This is likely to be true, of course, because there is serotonin in the brain and we need a brain to feel anything, including depression. But it is not an informative or testable proposal. It's the equivalent of saying that blood is involved in depression because it is 'widely distributed' all over the brain.

So, at the same time as claiming the serotonin theory of depression was never credible, Pies, Cowen and others suggested that serotonin does, in fact, play a role in depression. They were careful to avoid specifying quite what that role consists of, however. They also failed to add that there is little evidence to support their assertions. David Curtis, on the other hand, boldly alleged, 'It is very clear that people suffering from depressive illness do have some abnormality of brain function', but then admitted, 'We do not yet know what this is'.[16]

A version of the 'it's more complicated' line of argument is the suggestion that serotonin is involved in *some* people with depression or in some *types* of depression. A response to our paper by two Hungarian psychiatrists and a British psychiatrist claimed, for example, 'The decreased activity of serotonin, which undoubtedly plays an essential role in the pathogenesis of depression, is characteristic of only a subgroup of depressed subjects.'[17]

It is possible serotonin is involved in producing depression in people with certain subtypes of depression – anything is possible – but there is simply no evidence to support this idea. In fact, there is no agreement about whether there *are* any distinctive subtypes of depression. As we saw earlier, since the publication of the third edition of the *Diagnostic and Statistical Manual of Mental Disorders* (*DSM*) in 1980, depression has officially been regarded as a single disorder that can present with varying degrees of severity, and not as a set of different conditions. Research has followed suit; hence, few studies distinguish different types of depression.

Suggestions that serotonin is involved in a more complicated causal scenario were also put forward in scientific letters sent to the *Molecular Psychiatry* journal in response to our paper. Like Cowen's proposal, they were vague and overinclusive – impossible to test and impossible to disprove. They were not scientific theories, in fact, they were conjectures. The authors of one of the letters, for example, suggested that depression is the result of a complex 'dysbalanced dynamic system involving genetic, epigenetic, environmental and stress vulnerabilities initiating a cascade of neurobiological alterations in and beyond the serotonergic functioning'. They went on to propose that these alterations involve neurotransmission, neurogenesis (the formation of new brain cells), 'neural circuitries' (a vague term meaning the connectivity of different parts of the brain), hormonal systems, inflammation and blood vessels, and were mediated by serotonin along with noradrenalin, dopamine, glutamate GABA and numerous other chemicals.[18] In other words, they suggested everything in the brain is involved in producing depression, which is like saying we need a brain to feel depressed. We surely do, but this does not explain the causes of depression and nothing they proposed represents a testable claim.

Other research on serotonin and depression

The authors of another letter claimed that 'leads from emerging new research point towards serotonin as playing an essential role within complex brain systems that are affected in major depression and implicated in response to antidepressant treatment'.[19] They proceeded to set out an array of studies from a variety of different research areas that might, if you employ a lot of imagination and overlook glaring inconsistencies, indicate that serotonin is involved in depression.

One example of this 'emerging' research consists of a bizarre series of experiments conducted by some of the authors of the letter. These experiments are said to test whether antidepressants modulate normal 'emotional processing' – meaning our ability to recognise and interpret emotions in other people. They consist of giving healthy volunteers a dose of an antidepressant or a placebo and asking them to identify, as rapidly as possible, various facial expressions presented to them using photographs of unknown people. In some experiments, they are also asked to classify personality characteristics as either positive or negative, again under pressure of time. The theory is that antidepressants increase people's receptivity to positive emotional states and personality characteristics and reduce their sensitivity to negative ones – the opposite of what is presumed to happen in depression. Since antidepressants are thought to increase serotonin activity, it is inferred that any observed effects are mediated by serotonin.

In one of the first of these experiments, published in 2004, people given antidepressants were less likely to identify expressions of fear correctly than those who were given a placebo, so this was in line with predictions, although results for other emotions, including happiness and sadness, showed no effects or were inconsistent. Several studies have produced opposing results, however. Two found that people given antidepressants were *more* likely to identity fearful expressions than people given a placebo, and another that they were better at recognising expressions of disgust. A couple of studies found people on antidepressants were slightly superior in identifying happy faces, but in every study there was no effect for the majority of emotional expressions that were tested. Moreover, the few contradictory effects that were detected are likely to be 'false positives' (random positive results) due to the large number of tests that must have been conducted involving various combinations of emotional expressions, reaction times and correct and incorrect responses.[20]

Yet, these studies are frequently represented as showing that antidepressants work by rectifying underlying abnormalities in 'the way we see the world around us', as one psychiatrist put it, stopping us from 'seeing it in such a negative light'.[21] They are far from convincing, even if you accept the questionable premise that identifying facial expressions from photographs of random people provides a valid measure of our emotional reactions. Consequently, this research does not establish that serotonin is involved either.

A new study

A few months after our review was published, a new study hit the headlines, which was proclaimed to have found 'the first direct evidence of a link between low serotonin and depression'.[22] Needless to say, people had not been informed that previous research was merely 'indirect' when they were told they had a chemical imbalance, but, in reality, the new evidence was far from direct – and far from compelling.

The study involved giving people with depression and healthy volunteers a dose of amphetamine, which stimulates the release of serotonin (along with other substances). The idea was to measure whether amphetamine stimulates more serotonin release in healthy volunteers than in people with depression. This was measured by giving people an injection of a radioactive tracer substance that attaches to one of the serotonin receptors in the brain and which can be detected using a Positron Emission Tomography (PET) scan. Changes in the concentration of the tracer were assumed to reflect the amount of serotonin being released because serotonin can displace the tracer from the receptor (and the tracer is only detected when attached to the receptor).

In fact, the authors admitted they were not measuring serotonin directly, describing how they '*conceptualise*' the change in radio-tracer as an 'index' of brain serotonin.[23] Their justification for this assumption was a study involving four pigs, which showed some correlation between a similar technique and serotonin concentrations in the pigs' brains, measured by sampling brain fluid (not something you can do in humans). However, the correlation was far from perfect, and the study was much too small to confirm that the two measures are actually related.[24]

In any case, the new study only involved seventeen people with depression altogether, a third of whom had used antidepressants and five of whom also had Parkinson's disease. Parkinson's disease destroys the brain's capacity to produce dopamine most markedly, but it also affects other brain chemical systems, including serotonin.[25]

Even so, the results were not convincing. Only after excluding one participant, whose results were extreme, and using an unconventional 'one-sided' statistical test was it possible to demonstrate a difference between people with depression and people without.[26] Moreover, the difference still depended on three outlying values, and if these were removed the difference disappeared.[27] In a published response to the paper, psychologists Michael Hengartner (who was part of our serotonin review team) and Martin Ploederl analysed the data in another way and used the recommended 'two-sided' statistical test. They found no difference.[28]

Alternative theories about the biological origins of depression

Following the publication of our paper, along with trying to shore up the serotonin theory, various other options were hauled out to take its place. There are scores to choose from. A psychiatrist on X (then Twitter) listed fifty-nine different theories about the biological origins of depression – and there are more.[29] Many were popular for a while and then quietly forgotten, either because the evidence was contradictory or because the researchers got bored and moved onto other ideas.

Brain cells and brain cell connections

A currently fashionable theory, quoted in several responses to our paper,[30] is that depression involves an impairment of 'neurogenesis' (the generation of new nerve cells) or 'neuroplasticity', a term that encompasses neurogenesis but can also refer to the growth of nerve cell projections or spines. This theory also holds that antidepressants, along with ketamine and psychedelics, work by stimulating the production of new nerve cells or nerve cell projections and connections.

The Johns Hopkins University website page on esketamine, for example, claims, 'Research suggests that untreated depression causes long-term brain damage'. You'd think you'd need pretty strong evidence to make such a frightening pronouncement, but you need to know that the Johns Hopkins Drug Discovery Unit and some individual Johns Hopkins academics receive funding from Janssen, makers of esketamine.[31] The website goes on to tell people, 'Esketamine may counteract the harmful effects of depression'.[32]

So, is there any basis to such worrying claims? The neurogenesis theory of depression is vaguer than the serotonin theory and, therefore, it is not even clear what evidence would be required to prove it. It originates from a study published in the 1990s showing the formation of new nerve cells in part of the brain called the hippocampus in five people who had died of cancer.[33] Prior to this, it was generally believed no new brain cells were made in the mature human brain. A few years later, an animal experiment suggested that injecting antidepressants into the brain, as well as administering electric shocks, increased signs of neurogenesis in parts of the hippocampus.[34]

There is no direct evidence of an impairment of neurogenesis in depression, however, and the effects of antidepressants are not certain either. Support for the theory is sometimes said to come from research on the size of the hippocampus, which is frequently claimed to be smaller in people with depression, but this has not been confirmed. Studies have produced variable results, and bigger and better studies show no difference in the size of the hippocampus between people with depression and healthy volunteers.[35] Moreover, evidence suggests that stress, child abuse, poor physical health and antidepressants (notwithstanding the animal research on neurogenesis) can all reduce the volume of the hippocampus, which likely accounts for the effects found in many studies.[36] In fact, large, well-conducted studies indicate that differences between the brains of depressed patients and healthy individuals are 'remarkably small' and that 'similarity' predominates.[37]

The evidence that antidepressants stimulate neurogenesis is also inconsistent and ambiguous. A review of animal research found widely different results across studies as well as evidence of publication bias (selective publication of positive findings). When this bias was accounted for, antidepressants appeared to have no effect on neurogenesis.[38] Trials of antidepressants for the treatment of neurodegenerative conditions, such as multiple sclerosis and Alzheimer's disease, have failed.[39] Moreover, if antidepressants do stimulate neurogenesis, this might indicate they are harming the brain, not restoring it. Brain injuries, such as stroke, provoke various aspects of neurogenesis in a compensatory process,[40] and evidence that electric shocks to the brain (as are administered during ECT) are associated with signs of neurogenesis also suggests it may be a reaction to injury or disruption.[41]

In other words, there is no direct evidence that depression involves an abnormality in the generation of new nerve cells or nerve cell connections. The size of the hippocampus, where the nerve cell regeneration is thought to occur, is not reliably related to depression. Evidence that antidepressants provoke neurogenesis is inconsistent; if they do, this may be a cause for concern, not a beneficial effect. Finally, the whole premise of this area of research is still debated, and some studies have found no evidence that neurogenesis occurs in adult humans after all.[42]

The Inflammatory Theory of Depression

Another frequently cited candidate for the biological basis of depression is an abnormality in the inflammatory response.[43] Inflammation is a natural process by which the body heals itself from infections and injuries. Inflammatory mechanisms can become overactive, however, and turn against normal parts of the body. This is what happens in auto-immune diseases, like rheumatoid arthritis, in which a chronic inflammatory process in the joints causes pain, swelling and damage.

Some studies show differences in levels of inflammatory chemicals between people with depression and healthy volunteers, but, like the hippocampus, the inflammatory system is affected by almost everything, including obesity, exercise, sleep deprivation and social class, not to mention antidepressants.[44] All these are linked with depression and may account for the results of such studies.

As it happens, Mark Horowitz studied the relationship between inflammation and antidepressants for his PhD at the prestigious Institute of Psychiatry, Psychology and Neuroscience in London. He used nerve cells treated with inflammatory chemicals to mimic the state of the nervous system under stress, and he added antidepressants to the cells to see whether they neutralised the effects of the inflammatory substances. Mostly, the drugs had no effect, and when they did show effects, these were contradictory, with some antidepressants leading to increased levels of inflammation.[45] Mark later described the research as a 'giant disaster'. The experience convinced him that looking for depression in the brain is looking in the wrong place.

Quite apart from the outcome of these experiments, it is interesting to note the sort of research on which claims about the biological origins of depression are based. If you think studying people's reactions to contrived photographs of emotional expressions is a questionable way of understanding human emotion, then studying the behaviour of cells in a Petri dish is surely beyond ridiculous. Yet, when Mark started to question whether you could tell anything about 'the mind' from these methods, he was told he was being a nihilist. He obtained his PhD and was awarded a prize for his research from the British Association of Psychopharmacology. In the process, he contributed to the vast amount of biological research that finds nothing, but by its existence seems to suggest the field is advancing.

OTHER BIOLOGICAL THEORIES OF DEPRESSION

Abnormalities in other brain chemical systems, such as the glutamate system, have also been suggested to be the origin of depression, particularly by people involved in marketing or advocating for the use of ketamine and esketamine. For instance, John Miller, who sits on Janssen's advisory board and gives presentations about esketamine, wrote an article entitled 'Depression's Journey From Monoamines to Glutamate', in which he proposed various deficits in the glutamate system in depression that these drugs might be targeting.[46] Johns Hopkins University also suggests that esketamine produces its effects through its actions on glutamate.[47]

Research on glutamate is sparser and more confusing than research on serotonin, however, and is also influenced by the effects of antidepressants. A recent meta-analysis found that depressed people taking antidepressants had lower levels of glutamate than volunteers, but those who were not taking antidepressants did not.[48] Moreover, ketamine and esketamine (whose antidepressant effects are doubtful, in any case) exert effects on many other brain chemical systems, not just glutamate.[49]

None of the evidence for these alternatives to the serotonin theory holds up under scrutiny; nor does it come close to demonstrating a causal connection. But theories are not advanced on the basis of scientific merit. The ones that persist, at least, are those that align with marketing imperatives and the latest fashions in medical panaceas.

Many theories about the biological origins of depression and actions of antidepressants have come and gone. What the responses to the serotonin paper illustrate so neatly is the longstanding tactic of moving the goal posts. This has been going on for seventy years now, since the field of modern biological psychiatry first started to take off in the 1950s. Thousands of studies have been conducted on every imaginable aspect of brain function in depression. The volume of research creates an illusion of progress and provides the basis of so many theories, it is impossible for anyone to thoroughly evaluate every one of them. As soon as one theory is discredited, the advocates of the biological paradigm turn to another, putting forward a new set of ropey, inconclusive and ambiguous studies as putative evidence. Challenging the biological model of depression feels like a game of whack-a-mole: as soon as you put one theory to bed, another one sprouts up.

Conclusions

It remains the case that the serotonin theory of depression is one of the most well-tested theories of recent times. Moreover, it forms the principal justification for the use of antidepressants. Whether the serotonin theory of depression holds up under scrutiny or not is important, and the research we examined was, and remains, the main body of research designed to test the theory. Evidence for the most popular contenders to the serotonin theory is sparse and unconvincing, and many other so-called theories are too vague even to be testable.

Attempts to obscure this situation may not be an active conspiracy, plotted by people sitting in dark, smoke-filled rooms, but there is a confluence of interests and power that make it almost impossible to defeat the consensus position on the biology of depression, however weak its evidence base might be. Researchers, funding bodies, journal editors and media commentators are all invested in the belief that depression is a biological condition, and they control access to resources and infrastructure for research, to academic publication and to publicity.

The psychiatric establishment and its allies appeared to be deeply frustrated that our paper called this position into question. They attempted to neutralise the threat by deluging the academic literature and the public with a host of other unconvincing studies and alternative theories, dressed up with complex language and technical details. It looked as if there was life left in the biological approach to depression, yet what was proposed was wishful thinking dressed up in scientific terminology.

As we said in our response to the first set of letters sent to *Molecular Psychiatry* about the serotonin paper:

> There are always further studies that can be presented to support the serotonin theory, and research on other possible biological mechanisms, which may or may not involve serotonin [...] The onus is on others to present a convincing case based on other types of research or alternative hypotheses, not on us to disprove every speculation.[50]

Yet, the speculations go on and they continue to be confidently presented as if they are scientific facts backed by strong and undisputed evidence. People are still being given the impression that the biological cause of depression has been identified, when this is patently untrue.

14

Battening Down the Hatches: Public Reactions

I had never even thought about trying to publicise our paper. I had done the research so there was something in the scientific record, but I expected it to go unnoticed. It was Mark's suggestion to ask the UCL media office to help with publicity, but even then I didn't expect it to get much attention. The public reaction was extraordinary and a huge surprise to me. The way it played out also provided glimpses of some of the interests that operate behind the scenes to shape the way science is packaged for public consumption.

The weeks following the paper's publication were hectic and surreal. My clapped-out mobile phone could barely keep up with the requests I received for appearances and interviews. For a few weeks I was doing a dozen interviews a week, often late into the evening or in my lunch break. Mark was doing them too.

At first it was exciting – tearing round to television studios, having makeovers, doing interviews on my phone in the street. It was also heartening. At last, the world was getting a chance to hear what I had to say, and millions of people had been disabused of the false story they had been fed. But then the hatches started to come down and I realised I was witnessing a scientific cover-up taking place in real time.

Antidepressants are too big to fail. There are pharmaceutical company interests and professional reputations at stake; but, as well as those, many people in the media, as in other areas of life, are taking antidepressants themselves. For all these people, our paper raised uncomfortable questions: 'Don't we *know* that depression is a brain problem?' and 'Have I been really ingesting potentially harmful chemicals for no good reason?'

One of the people I spoke to in the weeks following the publication was Caroline (not her real name) from the USA. Caroline is a journalist and initially she told me she wanted to write about the paper. However, when I met her, she simply seemed to want to tell me her story and how angry she was that she had been lied to – as she saw it. She had gone to the doctor during a stressful time in her life and she had been informed, she remembered, that she had a chemical imbalance in her brain and she should start taking an antidepressant. She had taken antidepressants religiously ever since and encouraged members of her family to take them too.

Now that Caroline had read about our research, she wondered what the drug was doing to her brain. She decided to come off it as soon as she could. She was shocked to discover that she had been taking a potentially harmful chemical on the basis of an unproven theory that had been misrepresented to her as a fact. In retrospect, she felt she had been misled into seeing the normal ups and downs of life as a medical condition. She had wasted years of her life thinking her low mood was an inevitable consequence of her biology, when she could have been doing other things to sort out her problems.[1]

In a similar vein, a British man emailed me to say he was disappointed with the medical profession. He now felt he had been 'wrongly' prescribed an antidepressant, and the serious side-effect he had suffered could be considered a 'crime in itself'. 'I'm very pleased that this new information has been made public,' he continued, 'and would like to thank you for speaking up about this problem.'[2]

Other people were angry with me, though. Had I not considered how publishing our research would upset millions of people, one emailer asked me, adding a sarcastic 'congrats'? Another felt our findings could be 'extremely dangerous' and one suggested we were causing people distress for no reason because, echoing the 'experts' we met in the last chapter, scientists already know the serotonin theory is an oversimplification and the important thing was that antidepressants 'do work'.[3]

Some people felt the research undermined their choice to take medication, and this filled them with fear and anxiety. Some searched for another biological theory that could fill the gap, some looked for reasons why the research could be ignored. Speaking to *Vice* magazine, Jake Jackson, a philosopher from Temple University, Philadelphia, described how the chemical imbalance theory had offered people a 'raft to cling to while drifting around' in the uncertainties that constitute the nature of mental health problems and appropriate ways to respond to them. In this context, 'People gravitate to whatever half-truths or inconclusive theories appear sensible to them,' he said.[4] Removing the raft left people feeling adrift, no longer sure of what they were experiencing or even who they were.

But there was something more at work. Antidepressants and the idea that depression is a medical problem have become part of the narrative of the current political and cultural establishment – part of a world view that is presented as an indisputable consensus backed by science. In this scenario, it is essential that the public continue to believe the supposed experts who tell them what the science shows. The narrative must be shored up, and how this is done and what is sacrificed in the process is not important.

The first wave: surprise and curiosity

On the day of publication, our serotonin paper was covered in all the major national newspapers in the UK, on national television and radio.[5] I was invited to discuss it in person on *GB News*[6] that morning, where the presenters were keen to debate the use of antidepressants and be open to the idea that they were overprescribed, and that perhaps we misunderstood the nature of depression.

I have had little media training, but by fortunate coincidence I had attended a session led by the organisation Safely Held Spaces the week before.[7] I was incredibly grateful for this, as I soon found myself in the midst of a media furore.

The day after the paper's publication, I was invited to appear on the UK's popular morning television show *This Morning*. I was nervous because I was coupled with resident GP Dr Ellie Cannon, whom we met earlier. Dr Ellie (as she is referred to) uses antidepressants herself and had confidently told viewers just a few weeks earlier that depression is due to a chemical imbalance. So, I knew she wasn't likely to welcome our research or to like my view of antidepressants. The two presenters were open and curious, however. They expressed their astonishment at finding out that depression is not caused by low serotonin and, like everyone else, they wanted to know what this meant about antidepressants.

I explained the findings of our paper, the lack of evidence for the benefits of antidepressants and the fact they change our normal brain chemistry and can make us emotionally numb. We all agreed that people shouldn't stop their antidepressant abruptly and should consult their doctor if they were thinking about doing this.

Dr Ellie expressed her view that antidepressants 'work' and that it doesn't matter that we don't understand how. This was not unexpected, but I was glad of my brief media training when she accused me of having 'cherry picked' the studies for our review. Using the assertive but gentle interruption technique I had been taught, I challenged the point and explained that our research was a *systematic* review, meaning we had ensured we had not done this. The presenters listened attentively to both our perspectives and, overall, it felt like a good discussion that gave viewers a chance to understand the issues involved.

I was exhilarated. I had had a chance to pass on information that many viewers would not have heard before. At last, it seemed, people would be able to hear a balanced view about the science on antidepressants. I should have known it wouldn't last.

In the same week, Mark appeared on Sky News in Australia, I appeared with the genial psychiatrist Andrew McIntosh on BBC Scotland, and we were both interviewed by numerous, lower-profile media outlets. The article we wrote about the research for the online site The Conversation was read by more than 1.3 million people in the first month after it was published, and our review itself was fast becoming one of the most widely read scientific papers of modern times.[8]

At this point, it felt as if people were re-evaluating what they had been led to believe about the nature of depression and antidepressants. But signs that the mainstream media were nervous about the story soon started to emerge. I was invited to discuss the study on the BBC's *Today* programme and then suddenly uninvited. The research was mentioned briefly on the programme, but other than this, the main arm of the BBC didn't cover the story at all at this point. The discussion on *This Morning* never appeared on YouTube as an official clip, as is standard and as I was assured it would.[9] Then we heard that the *New York Times*, which had commissioned an article for which Mark and I had both been interviewed, had decided to drop the story. The reporter was disappointed and apologetic; the editor who had commissioned it wouldn't answer my emails.

As coverage progressed, a political rift started to open up between the hesitancy and sometimes hostility of centre and centre-left publications and the enthusiasm of some sections of the right-wing media. This was a strange experience for me, having always regarded myself as on the left of the political spectrum. The *Daily Mail*, for example,[10] covered the serotonin story sympathetically in four separate articles across its print and online versions[11] and I was invited back to the right-leaning *GB News* several times over the summer. I was reassured the channel was reasonably balanced when I bumped into the left-wing former mayor of London, Ken Livingstone, who was being interviewed on the same programme. I turned down the opportunity to be interviewed by *Epoch Times*, however, which has been accused of taking extreme right-wing positions and supporting conspiracy theories.[12]

One of the few major media outlets that covered the research early on in the USA was *Fox News*. A few days after publication, Tucker Carlson discussed it in his popular primetime show in an episode entitled 'Drugs are not the answer to every human problem'. While acknowledging that some medical drugs are undoubtedly useful, Carlson used our research as a pivot to consider the malign influence of the pharmaceutical industry and the overuse of drugs for all sorts of human problems they cannot solve. 'First we were told that SSRIs would save lives,' Carlson said. 'Now we learn they don't actually work as intended. In fact, the whole idea behind the drug was completely wrong.' Carlson aligned the misrepresentation and mis-selling of antidepressants with the prescription opioid crisis, and he also discussed what he perceived as the inappropriate and dangerous programmes to give children the Covid vaccines.

Throughout the programme Carlson questioned why important scientific findings were being ignored. 'How can that happen in a country based on science?' he asked. Towards the end of the programme, he interviewed British author Johann Hari about the social and environmental causes of depression. Carlson wound up, concluding, 'People are more than just a collection of chemicals that could be manipulated to produce a desired result. They're human beings. They have souls. If they're sad or sick or alienated from other people, it's just possible that Pfizer is not the solution.'[13]

Carlson has promoted agendas I do not agree with, including opposition to gun controls. However, in my view, he described our research accurately, he drew reasonable conclusions about the nature of depression and the overselling of antidepressants, and he asked important questions about the role of the pharmaceutical industry in promoting drug treatment for social and personal problems.

The BBC finally published a full-length feature on the research two weeks after it came out. The article, published on the BBC website, entitled, 'Did we all believe the myth about depression?', warned readers in its opening lines that our research 'has provoked a wave of misleading claims about antidepressant drugs', but reassured them it didn't 'show the drugs aren't effective'.[14] The same day, BBC Radio 1's *Newsbeat* website put up an article featuring several young people who felt antidepressants had been useful for them and complained that coverage of the research had been 'fearmongering'. An array of young psychiatrists were quoted, criticising anyone who had used the serotonin paper to question the usefulness of antidepressants.[15]

The US national radio programme *On Point*, which devoted a programme to the research and its implications in August 2022, was also keen to ensure people did not question the usefulness of antidepressants.[16] The programme was a curious blend: it managed to be critical of pharmaceutical marketing practices and of the collusion between the industry and the medical profession, yet it still strongly endorsed the drugs. In the opening line, the presenter, Meghna Chakrabarti, reassured the audience that 'antidepressants have been a godsend for millions of people who suffer from depression, so todays show is not about whether antidepressants work because they do, for some people'. The mantra that 'antidepressants work' was repeated about every ten minutes throughout the hour-long programme, just in case anyone in the audience thought to question the fact; at one point, the presenter and her studio guest, the psychiatrist Daniel Carlat, both acknowledged that they took, or had taken, antidepressants themselves. Carlat was gracious about our paper and admitted that 'biochemically we do not know what the cause of depression is', but also argued that it doesn't matter how they work. His patients didn't care about this, he said, and if they did, he would tell them that some other brain chemical might be involved.

The beginning of the programme featured a clip of me explain ing the findings of our research, and when I did the recording I tried to persuade the producer to ask more probing questions about antidepressants. If the programme was going to be critical of the way the industry and the medical profession had misled the public about the scientific research, which it was, how could it also conclude this didn't matter, I suggested? Might it not be pertinent to ask *why* millions of people had been deceived?

Looking back, the programme's makers knew their audience was not ready for a more radical message. Several listeners got in touch to say the programme would 'freak people out who are suffering and getting care from these mediations' and it should have stressed how 'antidepressants work and save many lives'. It's difficult to believe the programme could have advocated for antidepressants any more strongly than it did (as the presenter rather indignantly pointed out). But at least it alerted listeners that you cannot trust drug advertising and, less obviously, that your doctors' advice may also be unreliable.

I also realised the public was not ready to hear that antidepressants don't work when I went on *Weekend Prime*, a primetime news programme on the US channel Newsnation.[17] Because of the time difference, I had to get up in the middle of the night and when the presenter asked me, 'But you're not suggesting antidepressants don't work are you?', with a look of utter disbelief on her face, I realised I couldn't just say, 'Yes I am'. So, I blearily stammered something about how we don't know what they do exactly, but they are only marginally different from a placebo in randomised trials. The presenter's reaction brought home how the idea that depression is a brain problem that requires drugs to set it right has become a fundamental part of our collective belief system.

The second wave: on the attack

Those involved in *On Point* and Newsnation came across as genuinely interested in the serotonin research and in trying to explore what it meant, notwithstanding their reluctance to contemplate the horrifying possibility that antidepressants might not be useful. Then the reaction started to set in.

On 30 July 2022, *Rolling Stone*, the famous music and culture magazine, published an article entitled 'Who Is the Psychiatrist Behind the Antidepressant Study Taking Over Right-Wing Media?'[18] In a subsequent response to the article in the online, left-leaning publication *CounterPunch*, psychologist and writer Bruce Levine described it as a 'hatchet job', which he explained was 'not necessarily libel or false but is a maliciously destructive critique that routinely includes extraneous and irrelevant points aimed at unfairly casting its victim in a bad light'.[19]

The piece about me was one of a number published by *Rolling Stone* in recent years criticising people who have raised concerns about antidepressants[20] and it used a mixture of techniques to shed doubt on the reliability of my work, presumably to reassure readers there was no need to question the use of antidepressants. It wrongly accused me of making inaccurate claims and promoting 'fringe' views; it quoted my work out of context; and it irrelevantly brought up the Scientologists (the cultish group who oppose the use of psychiatric drugs – with whom I have never had any dealings), a standard trope employed by those who want to shut down critique of psychiatry. In the end, however, the article acknowledged that what our serotonin paper showed was correct. It admitted that 'even critics of the paper believe that the meat of the conclusions it draws – i.e., that the serotonin hypothesis is potentially inaccurate – is reasonable'.

I wrote a detailed response to the article on my blog, but here is a sample of the tactics used.[21] As I was reading the article for the first time, for example, I was surprised to learn that I had supposedly 'inaccurately linked' Transcranial Magnetic Stimulation (TMS) to a risk of cognitive impairment (TMS is a procedure that involves applying magnetic currents to the brain). I was surprised because I have never written about this procedure. Then I realised the article was referring to one of my tweets, in which I cited an online article describing side-effects of TMS reported by hundreds of members of a Facebook group, including problems with concentration, thinking and memory.

In another part of the *Rolling Stone* piece, I was said to have 'inaccurately connected' severe Covid-19 to the use of antidepressants and antipsychotics. This statement linked to a tweet in which I shared the results of a scientific paper reporting research conducted on behalf of the Public Health Scotland COVID-19 Health Protection Study Group.[22] It showed that people taking common antidepressants were almost three times more likely to develop severe Covid symptoms, after adjusting for other known risk factors. There is other research on Covid and antidepressants that is not all negative, but that does not make my tweet 'inaccurate'.

In recent years, *Rolling Stone* has become a 'liberal cheerleader', as the *Guardian* once dubbed it – pro-Democrat, pro-gun controls and anti-Trump.[23] The thrust of the article was that I was aligned with 'far-right commentators' and helping them to further their nefarious agendas, particularly resisting gun controls. In particular, I was accused of having 'promoted' the idea of a link between SSRIs and aggression, which *Rolling Stone* claimed was a 'fringe view'.

It is true that Tucker Carlson and other right-wing spokespeople have drawn attention to a number of mass shootings in which the killer was taking an antidepressant and discussed the possibility that the drugs may have contributed to the causation of these horrific events. I agree that they have stressed the connection with antidepressants over and above more important issues, such as gun availability and the alienation produced by adverse socioeconomic conditions. Yet, it is surely not outrageous, as the article implied, to consider that the drugs may occasionally play a role in such events. Moreover, I have never 'promoted' the idea that SSRIs cause aggression, and this is not a 'fringe view', in any case. The only time I have addressed this issue in print is when I commented on the results of the Danish meta-analysis I described in Chapter 12 (which revealed an association between antidepressants and aggressive behaviour in young people) in an editorial I was invited to write for the *British Medical Journal* – hardly a fringe publication. I concluded the editorial cautiously, by suggesting that with 'evidence that they [antidepressants] can produce such serious adverse reactions as suicidal and aggressive tendencies, regulators and the public need access to more comprehensive and reliable data'.[24]

There is a legitimate scientific debate to be had about whether antidepressant use is relevant in the case of any particular mass shooting or killing, but none of the right-wing commentators mentioned by *Rolling Stone* had used our serotonin research in that debate. So, I was bemused when the *Rolling Stone* journalist, who emailed me some questions before the piece was published, asked me what I thought about the fact that my research could potentially be used to argue against gun controls. I said I would be upset, because I, like almost everyone in the UK, support gun controls, but I did not believe this was a good reason to withhold important scientific findings.

The attack felt personal at the time, but it wasn't really. It was just that I had briefly become too prominent to ignore. I called my response to the article, 'First they ignore you. Then they ridicule you. And then they attack you.'[25] I was a punchbag because I had been making an evidence-based case against the widespread use of antidepressants for many years, and when people got to hear it, many found it compelling. The *Rolling Stone* article was the equivalent of putting cotton wool in your ears to block out a noise. And the noise was the question that some people don't want to have to ask: 'Have we got it all wrong about antidepressants?'

Constructing consensus

Along with several other publications, *Rolling Stone* painted a picture of a cosy consensus on mental health issues that it was unreasonable to challenge. It suggested that criticising the pharmaceutical industry or the motives of the medical profession were tantamount to 'light conspiratorial thinking', as if debate about the nature and validity of scientific findings, part and parcel of the normal practice of science, is the equivalent of doubting that men walked on the moon. Yet, leading doctors, including psychiatrists, have condemned the activities of the pharmaceutical industry.[26] Some have also criticised their own profession, such as Canadian psychiatrist Joel Paris, ex-editor-in-chief of the *Canadian Journal of Psychiatry*. Paris told Canada's *National Post* that the 'toxic relationship between industry and academia' had prevented the truth from coming out.[27] *Rolling Stone* would no doubt brand him a conspiracy theorist.

In *Vice* magazine, US psychiatrist Awais Aftab was quoted as saying, 'A different team of researchers could've taken the same findings and discussed them differently, and the reception would've been very different'.[28] It is true, many psychiatrists would have interpreted our research differently (many did, as we have seen), but that's because they have an agenda to defend the use of antidepressants and the biological approach to depression, not because they have superior access to the truth.

Everyone has views or 'biases' about the research they do; the idea that scientists work in a subjective vacuum is a myth. The problem is the message people have been given up to now has only been one side of the story, told by one camp with one set of biases. There is another way of interpreting the evidence – the one I have set out here – and people need access to this view if they are going to make up their own minds.

The Left–Right divide

The politics of mental health has gone through a curious metamorphosis in recent decades. People on the Left used to be the most vocal critics of Big Pharma. They were not afraid to challenge the big corporations and the professional and political establishment. Now that job has fallen to Carlson. The Left used to be concerned that the medicalisation of mental health problems obscured the social and political causes of discontent such as poverty, inequality, injustice, racism and child abuse.[29] Now, much of it is pushing medical diagnoses and antidepressants.

Some sections of the Left were more positive about our research, however. There were those for whom, like Carlson, it confirmed suspicions that there is more to human feelings than chemicals and brain events. In an article in the left-leaning online magazine *The Slate*, for example, the philosopher Sahanika Ratnayake described how the issues of *whether* antidepressants work and *how* they work are inextricably linked for most people, and it is 'disingenuous to pretend otherwise'. She described how a female friend, who had been taking antidepressants, had been 'devastated' by news of the research. It had undermined the friend's view of herself as someone with a malfunctioning brain. Ratnayake, on the other hand, who described how she had also suffered from depression, had related her moods to problems in her life, rather than her brain chemistry. Her friend's reaction led Ratnayake to reflect on how the chemical-imbalance narrative, as embodied in antidepressants, 'has altered how people understand themselves and their lives', leaving some feeling helpless and at the mercy of their brains.[30]

Motivations

After the first wave of interest and questioning, positive takes on our serotonin paper became exceptions to the general trend. Each time a new article came out, we were braced for another attack. Maybe this is not surprising given just how many people take antidepressants at the moment, including those working in the media. I am sure the individuals who covered the serotonin research in the media were acting with good intentions and wanted the best for people suffering from depression. Hearing such opposed opinions must have been confusing for anyone who had had no previous inkling that there was a debate about the nature of depression and antidepressants.

As both Jake Jackson and Sahanika Ratnayake pointed out, the idea that depression is a brain condition, embodied in and symbolised by antidepressant tablets, has become a crucial part of some people's identity.[31] Our paper threatened to take that away, pulling the rug from under people's feet and leaving some feeling anxious and confused. When people asked themselves whether they had been misled, some, like Caroline and others, were angry they had been deceived, but some wanted the question to go away.

I was asked once or twice if I thought we should not have published or publicised our research because of the distress it might have caused people. But this question assumes that the current situation, in which millions of people are taking antidepressants all over the world, is harmless. I don't believe it is, for all the reasons I have outlined – including the physical and psychological harm antidepressants can inflict.

There are more systemic reasons for the negative media coverage, however. In the USA in 2018, the pharmaceutical industry was the fourth-largest spender on television adverts and, in 2022, the industry spent a total of $8.1 billion on advertising.[32] Media companies are increasingly dependent on this revenue.[33] Along with advertising, social media is increasingly filled with promotional content from 'patient influencers', who are paid by pharmaceutical companies to promote their products but who do not always disclose their funding.[34] Money, often lurking behind the scenes, shapes what we hear and read about medicines.

Professional pride and status are also at stake. The psychiatric profession has invested its reputation in antidepressants and could not let a challenge like our serotonin paper ride. From the start it was defensive, particularly about antidepressants, but the strength of feeling was only revealed later in the day.

15

The Profession Strikes Back

People often ask me how I have survived within the academic establishment of psychiatry, given my views, and the answer is I have largely been ignored. The serotonin paper changed that: I couldn't be ignored any longer.

But it's also the case that psychiatry used to be more tolerant of dissension and controversy. Although not exactly embraced by the profession, famous critics of the medical approach to mental distress, such as Thomas Szasz and R.D. Laing, were still taken seriously when I was a medical student and junior psychiatrist in the 1980s and 1990s. Psychoanalysis, which provided a completely different explanation of the nature of mental disturbance from biological psychiatry, was also influential, and there was a tradition of scepticism about new treatments (including antidepressants).[1]

The appetite for debate remains among many practising psychiatrists. When I have managed to get through the selection process to run a symposium at the principal psychiatric conferences in the UK and USA, my sessions have been jam-packed with psychiatrists eager to ask questions and join in discussion. But some of the leaders of the profession do not want such issues discussed in public, especially anything that questions the biological view of depression or the supremacy of antidepressants. They were horrified at the public debate ignited by our paper.

Initially, I was requested to reassure people about the benefits of antidepressants, and when I explained that I couldn't because I didn't believe it was true, I was asked not to talk about antidepressants or preferably not to talk to the press at all. Instead of highlighting important work by a member of its staff, my university department published a feature on previous studies that supposedly supported the use of antidepressants.[2]

Such mild attempts to silence me were only the beginning though. A more belligerent confrontation was to come.

Poland

Before I come to that, let me tell you how the psychiatric profession in Poland treated the author and journalist Beata Pawlikowska. Beata is an elegant and articulate woman, who is a fluent English speaker and has published popular books on travel, cookery, how to learn English and self-help. She reached out to me in the early part of 2023, and we met online. She was flanked by the beautiful artefacts she has collected on her various travels.

In 2016, Beata published a memoir called *Heal from Depression. The Mind, Body and Soul Solution: A Personal Journey* (in its English version) about her own struggles with mental health problems.[3] She wrote the book, she said, so that 'other people should know this is possible – to change your life, to become healthy and happy, no matter what happened to you in the past'. This was the first time she realised how contentious the area of mental health can be.

The book became a bestseller, but it was attacked by sections of the press and by some Polish psychiatrists, who insisted depression is a brain chemical problem that could only be cured with drug treatment.[4] It seemed that 'the very idea that you can change the way you think and behave, improve your life, and become healthy and happy, was quite offensive,' Beata reflected.[5]

The criticism she received inspired Beata to look into the state of scientific knowledge about depression. This led her to my work and other research that cast doubt on the conventional psychiatric view of depression and antidepressants. Beata realised the Polish doctors who had criticised her were wrong. Naïvely, she thought they might simply have been unaware of this work, so she thought she would perform a public service by presenting it in Polish. In January 2023, she released a video entitled 'Depression: Latest scientific research'.[6]

'I'm used to getting criticized for telling the truth,' Beata recalled in a blog she wrote after the event, 'but nothing could have prepared me for the vehement attacks that followed my video. It made me the No. 1 public enemy in Poland.'

The video described our research on serotonin, the disease- and drug-centred models of drug action and evidence about the effectiveness of antidepressants. Everything she said was scrupulously evidenced with reference to scientific papers. She made it clear she was not a doctor or scientist and explained that her aim was to present information so people could make up their own minds about their medical treatment, and not to 'replace individual medical advice provided by a doctor'. She finished the video with a warning to people not to stop antidepressants abruptly, to follow their doctors' instructions and 'if necessary, work with your doctor to gradually stop taking them'.[7]

The day after the video was posted, a psychiatrist and President of the Polish Medical Media Association, Maja Herman, started a campaign to take legal action against Beata for publishing 'untrue information that poses a threat to the health and life of hundreds of thousands of people suffering from depression'. Herman set up a funding page, which carried the following astonishing message:

> I'm a doctor, psychiatrist, CEO, and I'm honestly sick of celebrities talking about health. Especially about mental health. On January 16, 2023, on the YT channel, Ms. Beata P., a journalist fluent in English, published a video in which she gives false information that poses a threat to the health and life of hundreds of thousands of people suffering from depression. I've had enough. I need your help to raise funds and show all her possible successors that this type of content is over. It is time to start punishing.[8]

In a subsequent interview, Herman explained, 'All we want to do is get this lady banned from talking about mental health', and she repeated the threatening language, 'Time to start punishing ... Enough fighting with just the written word, it's time for judgement'.[9]

The media and the general public weighed in too. They accused Beata of being responsible for the possible deaths of people who might stop their medication, they wished her dead and hurled insults at her on Facebook, Instagram and YouTube. For several weeks, she was afraid to go out of her house in case she was attacked. This was when she got in touch with me. When we met, she was visibly shaken and upset.

Beata knew the legal action had no chance of success because she had not presented any false information, nor made illegitimate claims about her qualifications or experience. Nevertheless, she felt intimidated and alone with everyone baying for her blood, so she briefly took the video down and issued an apology for causing offence. She was not going to be cowed into silence, however, and gradually she found allies.

A lawyer offered to defend her for free if the lawsuit ever took place and one of the journalists' associations in Poland confirmed her right to write and speak about mental health in a public statement. At the suggestion of her lawyer, Beata filed a suit against the psychiatrist for 'infringement of personal rights', demanding an apology and acknowledgement of her right to publish her video.

But after a few days, Beata had second thoughts. She worried about inflicting the same ordeal on the psychiatrist that she had been put under herself. 'I thought she must be feeling terrible,' Beata told me, 'knowing that she made a huge mistake and now being threatened with a lawsuit like I was before.' So, Beata made a personal approach to Dr Herman, and asked if they could discuss the situation woman to woman.

She told me the meeting was amicable and they both agreed not to proceed with the lawsuits. They each published a statement, Beata admitting to some minor inaccuracies, such as showing a picture of barbiturates when talking about benzodiazepines (yes, they were that trivial!) and Herman explaining that it was not the content of Beata's video that she objected to but the way it was presented. This is difficult to understand, but allowed Herman to save face and Beata was able to put the video back up and get on with her life. Beata remained effectively cancelled in the eyes of the Polish public, however, and, of course, nothing could undo the months of stress she had endured.[10]

Beata's kindness and willingness to forgive makes the behaviour of the Polish psychiatric establishment look particularly ugly. It was determined that people should not hear an alternative to the mainstream story about antidepressants and it was prepared to intimidate those who dared to dissent, regardless of the case for scientific debate or the personal welfare of those it confronted.

The case of esketamine

When our serotonin paper was published in July 2022, I was braced for a challenge by the British psychiatrists who had condemned the review of antidepressant withdrawal. They had criticised my work in the past too. In 2021, Mark Horowitz and I published a paper on esketamine in the *British Journal of Psychiatry*. Esketamine had just been licenced for the treatment of 'treatment-resistant depression' (depression that hasn't got better with the usual treatments) and was being positioned as a new pharmaceutical blockbuster by its makers, the drug company Janssen.[11] We pointed out there was little evidence that esketamine had worthwhile benefits and that it had a worrying lack of data on its long-term effects.[12]

We had expected to get responses to this paper because it started out as an online exchange about an editorial published in the *British Medical Journal*, which had welcomed esketamine as 'probably the first truly new and effective psychiatric therapeutic agent of the 21st century'.[13] The lead author of the editorial was Sameer Jauhar, one of the two psychiatrists who had challenged the antidepressant withdrawal review. As expected, Jauhar and some colleagues submitted an online response to our esketamine article and another response was received from a group of psychiatrists with extensive ties to drug companies, including Janssen.

Both responses made several debatable points, such as disputing the relevance of withdrawal effects and other side-effects we had highlighted (such as bladder problems and suicidal behaviour – all of which have been clearly documented).[14] We prepared to address all these points in the usual 'author's reply'. So far, it seemed like an ordinary, if heated, exchange of views in the scientific press. But then we were informed that the *British Journal of Psychiatry* had received demands that the paper be retracted.

A call for retraction of a paper is a serious matter, and only usually done where there is evidence or strong suspicion of fraud. Having a paper retracted is a significant embarrassment to the authors and, as the scientific publisher Elsevier point out, can 'affect future employment, funding and, of course, the reputation of the researcher'.[15]

We never knew who made this demand, but, in the process that followed, we were required to defend ourselves against the accusations made in these two online responses. Eventually, the *British Journal of Psychiatry* decided there were no grounds for retraction and the responses were published in the journal itself, alongside our detailed reply.[16] However, the episode illustrates again the appetite to dictate what is published and to delete articles that are perceived as a threat to the biological or pharmaceutical approach to depression.

The leaky umbrella

So having been through this gruelling process in 2021, I expected a similar response to the serotonin paper. Yet, despite the media furore, following the initial reaction from the Science Media Centre, there was an unsettling silence from those I expected to be our most vocal critics. However, I was right to suspect they would not take this blow to the reputation of biological psychiatry lying down. It turned out they were biding their time.

At some point, a group of thirty-six biological psychiatrists, mainly from the UK, submitted a letter to the editor of *Molecular Psychiatry*, the journal that had published our paper. The lead author was Sameer Jauhar, and the group included many leading lights of British biological psychiatry. As with the attack on the antidepressants withdrawal paper, the letter disputed minor points of methodology and, while not contradicting our conclusion that the serotonin theory was unproven, claimed there was some evidence for the role of serotonin in depression. The journal received several other letters and, after sending them out for peer review, we were requested to write an 'author's reply'. This was also subject to peer review, and by the time this lengthy process was concluded, the first batch of letters, including our reply, was set to be published in June 2023.

As I discovered later, the day the letters were published, King's College London, Jauhar's employer, issued a press release about his and his colleagues' letter, which, it turned out, had been published as a stand-alone 'comment', rather than a letter. This meant it wasn't obvious that we had replied to it. I emailed King's to request they add a link to our reply to the press release, in the interests of providing the media and the public with balanced information, but no one responded.

The *Daily Mail* picked up the story with an article that carried the headline 'Demands for flawed study that cast doubt on the effectiveness of antidepressants to be axed'. The piece quoted the psychiatrist David Nutt, who said of our serotonin paper that he was particularly concerned it 'has been frequently cited and people believe it is true'.[17] Nutt previously promoted the chemical imbalance theory of depression on behalf of the pharmaceutical industry, as we saw earlier.[18]

The medical press, reluctant to cover the original research, seemed delighted to be able to report that the review had been questioned. The *British Medical Journal* covered the piece in a page-long article in its 'News' section (our original review had only been given a small paragraph) without contacting me for comment or citing our reply.[19] Our point of view was only added after I complained.

The general press were less interested and the *Daily Mail* was the only major British newspaper or media outlet to cover it, which was ironic, given the paper's extensive and enthusiastic coverage of our original article.

Around the same time, the Mental Elf blogsite, which specialises in providing detailed analyses of important papers in mental health research, released a piece on our serotonin paper, eleven months after it had been published. The piece was written by Sameer Jauhar, along with another young psychiatrist, and it made essentially the same points as the 'comment'.[20]

On X, Jauhar released dozens of posts spread over a few days, in which he detailed the criticisms contained in the 'comment'. He included a hashtag[21] he created called 'leaky umbrella'. Co-authors reposted his posts, seemingly keen to ignite an exchange. I was reluctant to get drawn in but, at one point, I reflected on the reasons for the sudden rush of attention to our research by posting, 'The public have been misled by Pharma and sections of the medical profession into believing depression has an established biological cause. Our serotonin paper exposed this but Jauhar and co want the situation to continue.'[22] One of the 'comment' authors demanded that I 'respond' to the 'concerns and criticisms' and insisted I 'play the ball, please', despite the fact I had already highlighted our published response in several posts.[23] An observer of this exchange commented, 'Is it really a "scientific debate" if one side spends 50 years promulgating an unproven hypothesis on behalf of drug companies, despite no evidence? Continuing to play the ball at this point seems like a waste of time. It's the man that is the problem.'[24]

Several people advised me that not replying to the accusations in detail gave the impression we had something to hide, even though our response was freely available. So, I spent a sunny weekend squirrelled away composing a series of posts and released them the following Monday. My hands were shaking as I typed them out and pressed the 'post' button. It was gratifying to see some of the replies. Peter Sterling posted, 'Moncrieff et al. defend their case that depression is not caused by deficit of serotonin and that SSRIs cannot fix what is evidently not broken. Calm and clear as a bell. Thank you!'[25]

No doubt the authors of the 'comment' felt they were acting in the interests of science, but as one member of X pointed out, why was anyone 'so agitated about an unproven hypothesis remaining unproven?'[26]

Let me show you what Jauhar and his colleagues' criticisms amounted to, and you can decide for yourselves whether our 'conclusion was overstated', as they suggested, even though everyone had agreed with it a few months earlier and the 'comment' does not actually refute it.[27] You can also read our published response on the Nature website, which contains more details.[28]

The criticisms

The authors of the 'comment' made several inaccurate accusations, including that we had omitted data, which was actually included in our tables, and we had missed out studies when, in fact, the studies they mentioned were irrelevant or ineligible. They made unsubstantiated allegations that we had not followed standard methods for umbrella reviews. Yet, as we explained in our reply, we had followed the guidelines for umbrella reviews assiduously. We had pre-published our protocol, used systematic methods to identify and select studies and evaluated the quality of studies and the certainty of the evidence as recommended. Our team member, Ruth Cooper, is an expert in systematic reviews and worked in a well-respected team specialising in this methodology, so I am confident we used the best and most up-to-date methods available for this sort of review.

One of their main criticisms of our methods was the way we assessed the certainty of our findings. We had added a 'certainty' measure after publishing our protocol to be consistent with emerging standards in systematic reviews; yet, rating the certainty of findings is an inherently subjective process and there is no standard method of assessment for the sort of research we looked at. For this reason, we adapted the most commonly used system, known as GRADE, which was devised for use with randomised controlled trials,[29] to suit the sort of studies we looked at. We followed the example of other umbrella reviews that had done this or devised similar systems of their own. The certainty ratings had little impact on our conclusions, as it turned out, except to highlight that the only decisive area of research was the genetic research, which was resoundingly negative.

The 'comment' authors also took issue with our interpretation of some of the research we looked at, although without challenging our findings per se. In relation to the tryptophan depletion research, for example, they didn't dispute that lowering brain serotonin via the tryptophan depletion technique has no effect on mood in people who do not have depression to begin with. Everyone agrees about this. Yet, they felt we hadn't given enough weight to the studies of tryptophan depletion in people with a history of depression, and wrongly accused us of omitting data on some of these studies. We had included all this data, in fact, but we had pointed out how it was highly inconsistent, derived from small numbers of people, and not supported by the two studies in our sample of more recent research that involved people with a history of depression. They also acknowledged the results were imprecise. The most important aspect of this research, however, remains that tryptophan depletion does not produce depression in healthy volunteers, because if lowered serotonin is the underlying cause of depression then this procedure should be able to induce it in anyone.

On the subject of serotonin receptors, Jauhar and colleagues argued we had 'misinterpreted' the data and ignored the complexity of the area. Like Freud's man with the kettle, on the one hand, they argued the studies we examined had used inadequate methods and a better study found higher levels of the inhibitory receptor (the 5HT1a receptor), consistent with lower levels of serotonin. On the other, they claimed the receptor is not inhibitory after all (or that not all variants of it are inhibitory), so that lower levels of the receptor, as suggested in some studies we looked at, would imply lower serotonin. It is true there are different forms of this receptor, which may have different effects on serotonin, although these have not been clearly defined. However, a considerable amount of evidence suggests the overall effect of this particular receptor is to inhibit or oppose the effects of serotonin. For example, when animals are given a drug that stimulates this receptor, they become *more* sexually active – the opposite effect to serotonin.[30]

Overall, research on serotonin receptors, like the 'comment' authors' summary of it, is inconsistent and confusing. What it definitely does not provide is persuasive evidence that serotonin is reduced in people with depression.

Another criticism was that we should have included studies of the concentration of the 'parent' molecule of serotonin, tryptophan. We had focused our review on serotonin and not tryptophan for good reason, however. Tryptophan's relationship to brain serotonin levels is unclear. Only 1 per cent of dietary tryptophan contributes to serotonin in the brain and tryptophan plays numerous biological roles that are independent of serotonin or only distantly related to it. It is also highly sensitive to the sort of diet we have, which may well vary between people with depression and people without. The authors cited two meta-analyses of studies of tryptophan that reported reduced levels in people with depression, but there was evidence of publication bias (negative studies not being published) in both,[31] and they were small and exclusively involved studies of people who were taking or had taken antidepressants. In any case, it is unclear whether this data has any relevance to serotonin.[32]

The conclusion of the 'comment' was that 'a more accurate, constructive conclusion would be that acute tryptophan depletion and decreased plasma tryptophan in depression indicate a role for 5-HT [serotonin] in those vulnerable to or suffering from depression, and that molecular imaging suggests the system is perturbed'.[33] Rather than admitting that the research was highly inconsistent, Jauhar and colleagues tried every which way they could to imbue it with significance. But there being 'a role for' serotonin or the system being 'perturbed' are untestable and, therefore, scientifically meaningless claims.

When Michael Hengartner, a member of my team of authors, told Jauhar on X, 'Your whole campaign against us is ridiculous and you haven't been able to make a strong and convincing argument', Jauhar protested, 'No campaign, sorry'.[34] Yet, he had issued a press release about the 'comment', coordinated publication with a piece on the Mental Elf blog, accompanied it by prolific coverage on X, created a hashtag to ensure all the activity would be linked – and the 'comment's' authors congratulated each other on X for the publicity their piece had received.[35] That seems like a campaign to me.

Of course, there is nothing wrong with seeking a scientific debate or wanting to publicise your work, but the fact that a group of psychiatrists felt so strongly about a paper that a few months before had been dismissed as saying nothing new, including by some of them, is remarkable. The authors' sentiments were shared by other biological psychiatrists. I was reliably informed by an attendee that cheers went up at the British Association of Psychopharmacology Conference in 2023 when the 'comment' was mentioned. It seems that challenging our paper had become a cause célèbre in some professional circles.

Motivations

This extraordinary reaction reflects the importance of maintaining the illusion that the biological basis of depression has been established for some sections of the profession. The concern about our paper was that it might raise questions in people's minds about whether depression is a biological condition and whether taking antidepressants is such a sensible idea. These questions had to be shut down. So, as we saw earlier, as soon as we showed the serotonin theory had no clothes, its defenders wheeled out numerous other half-baked theories to replace it. Then they attacked us and tried desperately to revive the moribund serotonin theory from the dead. The bottom line was always that 'antidepressants work' and not to question how.

A large proportion of the profession do not want to contemplate that there might be other explanations for what drugs, like antidepressants, are actually doing – that they might be dampening emotions or producing amplified placebo effects – and they do not want the public to do so either. The view that depression is a predictable reaction to life events and that drugs act as chemical pacifiers, which was so successfully suppressed by pharmaceutical industry marketing, must be kept at bay.

Antidepressants and Professional Identity

Psychiatry came of age in the asylums – the huge Victorian institutions that loomed over the landscape and housed a motley crowd of the distracted, distressed and neurologically diseased. The medical superintendent of the asylum was the prototype psychiatrist. The Royal College of Psychiatrists started life in 1841 as the Association of Medical Officers of Asylums and Hospitals for the Insane and the *British Journal of Psychiatry* was originally the *Asylum Journal*.

By the middle of the twentieth century, the asylums had started to be perceived as a drag on the profession. They were overcrowded, full of people with chronic conditions and, despite efforts at reform, they were still perceived as places of incarceration and control. Psychiatrists felt stigmatised by their association with asylums, just like their patients.[36]

When the new drugs that came to be known as antipsychotics and antidepressants were introduced in the 1950s, there was enormous enthusiasm that the prognosis of mental illness would be transformed and psychiatry would at last become a proper branch of medicine.[37] The profession saw itself moving away from the asylum into outpatient practice, giving people pills to make them better – something psychiatrists had not been able claim to do before.

The asylums were closed, eventually, but people with severe mental disorders were not cured, they were moved to different sorts of institutions: privately run residential homes and secure facilities, homeless hostels and sometimes prison.[38] They did become less visible, however, as a result of their dispersal, and psychiatrists did become increasingly concerned with people who had less-severe problems. The prescription of drugs and the idea that these drugs were working by targeting an underlying disease process (the disease-centred model) was crucial for justifying this expansion into the realm of 'everyday nerves', as David Healy dubbed it.[39]

The pharmaceutical industry had long recognised that medicating misery is a lucrative market. As we learned, barbiturates and benzodiazepines were prescribed in vast quantities in the middle of the twentieth century; but most prescriptions were issued by GPs, and psychiatrists were never too enthusiastic about drugs that clearly acted, and were marketed, as tranquillisers. The introduction of the SSRIs and other new drugs in the late 1980s brought the profession and the industry closer together, however. Psychiatrists became an important target audience for the industry and they became accustomed to drug company inducements.

When I started working in psychiatry in the early 1990s, drug company paraphernalia was everywhere. Doctors wrote with drug company pens on drug company sticky notes, drug company calendars hung on the walls and every hospital kitchen was stocked with drug-company-embossed mugs. At least once a week, a lavish lunch would be provided, courtesy of one company or another, followed by a promotional talk, dressed up as education, provided by the drug company representative or a senior psychiatrist in the company's pay. Senior doctors were regularly taken out to dinner in fancy restaurants. Conferences took place at expensive hotels in attractive locations and 'key opinion leaders' among the profession were flown out and paid generously for giving presentations about a company's product.

The money helped psychiatrists to feel important. It massaged the profession's vulnerable ego. This was brought home to me at the Royal College of Psychiatrists' Annual Conference in the summer of 2008. The president of the college at the time was Sheila Hollins, a psychiatrist whose career had been in the field of learning disability. Hollins is a quietly principled person, who has supported efforts to reduce unnecessary prescribing of antidepressants and establish services for people harmed by prescribed drugs.[40] She was not willing for the college to accept pharmaceutical company sponsorship under her watch. So, instead of being held at an expensive hotel or conference centre subsidised by advertising revenue, the annual college conference in 2008 was held at the Imperial College campus in west London. Lectures and presentations took place in scruffy lecture theatres and classrooms, and attendees had to sit on uncomfortable benches and endure student toilets. I realised that psychiatrists had been lured into a false sense of their importance by the ubiquity of drug company money. This was what the conference fee bought in reality – without subsidy.

You can have a perfectly good conference in scruffy surroundings, but the inconsistent results of small studies of brain processes might not be as persuasive as when they are delivered on the main stage at a flashy, brand-new conference centre with high-tech equipment and multiple screens. Psychiatry is only able to act like a big player because of pharmaceutical cash.

Drugs such as antidepressants brought the psychiatric profession the kudos it craved. They enabled it to construct a narrative that psychiatrists are real medical doctors, using sophisticated medical treatments, just like physicians and surgeons. Psychiatrists fought hard to achieve this, as they see it. For years, they had endured the ridicule of colleagues and the stigma of the public. Glossing over the leg-up they had from the pharmaceutical industry, they finally saw themselves as enjoying the status they needed and deserved. Of course, the profession did not want its new self-image to be punctured.

The pharmaceutical industry is not such a big player in psychiatry any more and, to be fair, psychiatry was never its sole target (although it was an important one for many years).[41] Most antidepressants are now off patent and therefore no longer big money spinners. Yet, the industry has helped establish drugs as the standard treatment for most situations, and it has woven a web around medicine and psychiatry that continues to resonate.

A 2021 investigation by journalist and mental health campaigner Robert Whitaker showed how the financial ties between psychiatrists and the pharmaceutical industry remain significant. By examining the United States Open Payment System, Whitaker revealed how:

> Money flows to the consultants and advisors who help the companies design their trials and author articles on the results; it flows to those who publish reviews and further analyses of the new drug once the trial results are published; and it flows to those who serve on speaker bureaus.

Individual psychiatrists benefit to the tune of hundreds of thousands of dollars. Their value lies in how they lend credibility to pharmaceutical-friendly research and help give it traction.[42]

The industry also influences medicines regulators, which now receive a significant part of their funding from the companies whose products they are meant to scrutinise. The UK regulator, the MHRA, derives 86 per cent of its budget from industry payments.[43] The industry also funds patient groups and 'grassroots' campaigns that lobby for the licensing and adoption of particular drugs.[44]

This is not meant to impugn anyone's motives. The industry does develop useful products, and working with it to bring genuine therapeutic innovations to the public is not inherently wrong. But pharmaceutical companies are ultimately interested in profit, and we know that money talks. It influences what people say and write as academics, and what they do as doctors or regulators – even when they think it doesn't.[45] It is unlikely that a product as ineffective as antidepressants would ever have captured a mass market without significant industry backing.

Several people on X highlighted the long list of 'conflicts of interest' (payments or connections with pharmaceutical or other commercial companies) listed by the authors of the 'comment'. One suggested it was longer than the 'comment' itself and, because I thought this couldn't be true, I cut and pasted the article into a Word document using a uniform font. It turns out the claim was not far off. The text of the 'comment' is about two and half pages long and the 'declaration of interests' just over two. It records payments to many of the authors from most of the major drug companies in the world.

* * *

If I was a psychiatrist who thought that antidepressants work swimmingly and there is no problem with a fifth of the population taking them, I would most likely never have done the serotonin research in the first place. As we have seen, many leading psychiatrists were perfectly happy for people to go on believing in the myth of the chemical imbalance. No doubt, they genuinely believe antidepressants are useful and that depression has a biological cause, even if they would admit, if pressed (as they surely must), that we don't know what that is. But they rarely do admit this, in public anyway. I can only assume this is because they think it doesn't matter, as eventually the biological basis of depression *will* be identified – and it will just happen to be rectified by antidepressants.

But to maintain these beliefs, they must resolutely set themselves against a multitude of scientific data. They must ignore the lack of consistent evidence of *any* biological mechanism in depression and they must turn a blind eye to the poor results of antidepressants trials. They must ignore the fact that antidepressants, like other psychiatric drugs, are psychoactive substances that disrupt normal brain functioning and modify people's normal thoughts and feelings. And they must overlook the unnecessary harm people suffer as a consequence of taking such substances on a daily basis for weeks, months and often years on end.

Understandably, doctors like to offer people hope, especially people who are miserable or distraught. Telling someone there is no miracle cure is not easy, but giving people potentially harmful substances in order just to do *something* is not doing them any favours. Not only does it expose people to the unpleasant and sometimes dangerous and incapacitating effects that arise when the body has to deal with an alien substance, it lets society off the hook. Instead of encouraging us to work together to create a more compassionate and supportive culture and environment, it enables us to carry on as we are, leaving those who struggle with their mental health to the mercy of the latest medical fad. And there are some worrying ones in the pipeline.

Part 5

The Future

16

Hope or Hype? Psychedelics and Other New Drugs for Depression

Although conventional antidepressants remain by far and away the most commonly prescribed drugs for emotional distress, they are fast being eclipsed in terms of interest and media coverage by a range of new drugs, including the psychedelics and psychedelic-like substances such as ecstasy (MDMA) and ketamine.[1] Ecstasy is the preeminent party drug and ketamine, which makes people high and puts them into a sort of trance, is also widely used on the recreational drug scene.

The hype around these drugs is reminiscent of the early days of Prozac. They are presented as swift-acting, highly effective drugs with few or no side effects – 'antibiotics for the mind,' an Australian professor called them.[2] Yale University psychiatrists describe esketamine (an inhaled form of ketamine) as a 'game-changer' and a 'unique' antidepressant, and ketamine clinics promote ketamine as a 'groundbreaking solution' for people with depression.[3] The University of Cambridge's psychedelic medicines group suggests psychedelics provide a rapid and lasting cure with no downside. On its website, it asks: 'If someone told you we have a remedy with nearly no relapse, no long-term side effects, and life-altering potential, wouldn't you be curious?'[4]

Psychedelic drugs are certainly interesting chemicals. The dream-like state produced by classical psychedelics such as LSD and psilocybin (the active ingredient in magic mushrooms) has no parallel in our ordinary waking lives and, consequently, they have been a subject of fascination since they were discovered. Yet are they really a useful treatment for emotional problems? Are they safe, and what does it mean for them to be a medical treatment as opposed to a drug one might take for fun or inspiration?

The combination of a potentially exciting and pleasurable drug-induced experience and the authority conferred by a medical setting and stamp of approval is an enticing prospect, especially for someone who is intensely unhappy and has tried lots of different antidepressants without experiencing improvement. This is the opportunity that has been spotted by investment capital, which is funding most of the burgeoning ketamine and psychedelic treatment services.[5] It seems a toxic mixture of desperation and profiteering.

The power and wealth of these organisations are propelling the field of 'psychedelic medicine' forward before there is convincing evidence that it does, in fact, help people, let alone proper studies of safety and side effects – just as happened with antidepressants in the early days. There is by now an extensive industry of private ketamine clinics across the USA; ketamine can be provided without special regulations because it has a medical licence as an anaesthetic, and esketamine, which is essentially an inhaled preparation of ketamine, has been licensed in the US and Europe. In the UK, a national ketamine service has been operating for over a decade, run by the National Health Service Trust in Oxford, although it requires people to fund the treatment themselves.[6] Several other clinics, run by private companies and other health service trusts, have opened recently.

Two states in the US have legalised the use of classical psychedelics, such as psilocybin (the active ingredient in magic mushrooms), in therapeutic settings. Clinics in Oregon now offer 'professionally guided mushroom experiences' in private sessions or a group retreat. Potential customers are encouraged to come and experience a 'safe journey inspired by psychedelic therapy clinical trials'.[7] In Australia, a group called 'Mind Medicine Australia' successfully lobbied the Australian drug regulator to legalise the use of psychedelics for medical treatment and is now offering this treatment throughout the country to people with 'treatment resistant depression' or post-traumatic stress disorder. The organisation sees itself as leading the world and 'pioneering a new paradigm' in the treatment of mental health.[8]

It is a familiar playbook: talk up the benefits, get the treatment established – however feeble the evidence is – and hope that it takes a couple of decades for complications to become apparent and the penny to drop that it doesn't do any good.

It is, nevertheless, astounding, particularly after the opioid crisis, that the scientific community is spearheading the promotion of substances that are widely used for recreational purposes with little acknowledgement of their risks and side effects. And despite the fact that the psychedelic experience is the unique selling point of these substances, it is increasingly glossed over or ignored altogether in the scientific literature. The paradigm of a one-off transformative experience is gradually morphing into one of long-term treatment targeted at underlying brain deficiencies, just like regular antidepressants.

The irony of this situation is brought home by doing a quick internet search for 'ketamine services', which, along with clinics offering ketamine treatment, brings up 'rehab' clinics providing help for people who have become dependent on ketamine. Presumably most of these customers become dependent through use of illicit ketamine, although it is not necessarily easy to distinguish recreational use from therapeutic use, and one can easily merge into the other.

As the drug-centred model of drug action reminds us, these substances exert their mind-altering effects by disrupting normal brain activity. The experience they induce is distinctive and for some pleasurable, unlike those of standard antidepressants, yet, as they come to be positioned as medical treatments, their mind-altering effects start to be forgotten along with their dangers – just as happened with antidepressants back in the 1960s.

Psychedelic-Assisted Psychotherapy

After years of being regarded as an eccentric pastime for hippies, taking psychedelics started to be rehabilitated in the context of what is called 'psychedelic-assisted psychotherapy': the practice of administering a psychedelic substance alongside psychotherapy sessions. Although this is still emphasised by some services, there is an increasing tendency to drop or minimise the therapy and simply offer the drug.

Psychedelic-assisted psychotherapy has been trialled for a variety of problems, including depression, post-traumatic stress disorder (PTSD), alcohol and drug problems, and anxiety about death in the terminally ill. The idea behind it is that the psychedelic experience – the 'trip' or 'high' – can provide people with new understandings of past experiences and feelings, which enable them to develop their 'inner healing intelligence', and overcome emotional difficulties. In theory, psychotherapy should be offered before, during and after the 'trip' to help prepare people properly, to support them through the drug experience and then to help them 'process' and 'integrate' their drug-induced insights.[9]

There is a logic to the idea of drug-assisted psychotherapy. It acknowledges the mind-altering effects the drugs have, for a start. Indeed, the psychedelic 'trip' has long been advocated as a means of expanding one's consciousness – of seeing the world in a different way – and inspiring creativity. MDMA, or ecstasy, which produces intense feelings of warmth and connectedness, has been proposed as an aid for 'couples therapy',[10] and in his book, *Manufacturing Depression*, author and psychotherapist Gary Greenberg describes how this worked for him. Greenberg recounts a time when he and his girlfriend took a tablet of ecstasy while attending a concert. Although they took it simply to enjoy the music and the occasion, under the influence of the drug Greenberg realised, for the first time, the depth of his feelings for his girlfriend. The revelation led him to overcome his chronic ambivalence and hesitancy, and he subsequently asked her to marry him. In a sweet, fairy-tale ending, they settled down and had a family.[11]

Personal development through drugs does not have to be limited to psychedelics or related substances, however. One patient told me that the effects of alcohol had shown him how to overcome his shyness and social inhibitions, and this helped him to socialise without it. Another described how her experience of taking a stimulant-like drug for Parkinson's disease taught her to loosen up and do things for herself, instead of focusing solely on her family's needs. She, too, was able to maintain this new attitude after she had to stop the drug for medical reasons.

Yet what Greenberg and my patients are describing is best understood as a process of personal development aided by the feelings induced by drugs, rather than a medical process (whether Greenberg might have come to the same realisation through other means is a moot point). It is akin to the personal insight others may gain from travelling, dancing, being in nature, sports and many other things.

Although some people enjoy the 'high' induced by psychedelics and ketamine, not everyone does, and occasionally these drugs give rise to experiences that are frightening, even terrifying

– colloquially known as the 'bad trip'. They also produce a 'come down' when the acute effects wear off, much like an alcoholic hangover, which can make people depressed and emotional.[12]

Moreover, it seems improbable that a few drug-induced experiences will resolve the underlying personal and social problems that make most people feel depressed, distressed or anxious in the first place. And if the aim is to learn more about oneself, there are probably safer and more enduring ways of doing this.

The Evidence

Much of the coverage of psychedelics suggests they have already been shown to be effective. Organisers of the 2026 Festival of Genomics in Boston, for example, told potential attendees 'the evidence is clear' psilocybin shows 'significant effectiveness in treating depression' as well as anxiety and 'addictive symptoms'.[13]

The Mind Medicine Australia website features emotive videos in which individuals tell of family members whom they think may have been prevented from committing suicide if only they had had access to psychedelic therapy. Dr Brian Walker, who lost his son to suicide in 2023, says, 'This was preventable. The medication that is currently being offered does not work. Psychedelic assisted therapy does.' And he adds, 'People are suffering, people are dying needlessly.'[14]

These claims are simply not supported by the current evidence. In the first place, studies with psychedelics are riddled with problems, including short-term follow-up, selective reporting of positive results, statistical manipulations and inconsistent reporting of side effects.[15] Although, with the exception of esketamine, they are not being marketed by traditional pharmaceutical companies, most of the research is being conducted or funded by companies aiming to commercialise psychedelic treatment. One of these is Compass Pathways, a UK-based biotech company producing a synthetic version of psilocybin.[16] Many researchers in the field have extensive financial ties with these companies.

Perhaps the most critical issue with the research is that it is impossible to do a clinical trial of psychedelics that is properly double-blind. The effects of psychedelics are so dramatic and distinctive that participants quickly recognise whether they have received the real drug or the placebo in a placebo-controlled trial. In a recent trial of psilocybin in people with alcohol problems, for example, 94–95 per cent of people correctly guessed whether they had received the psilocybin or the placebo.[17] Participants can also distinguish the effects of a psychedelic from the effects of other drugs. In a trial comparing ketamine with the opioid drug (remifentanil), 88 per cent of participants and 89 per cent of the researchers correctly identified which drug was which.[18]

Psychedelic trials often attract people who have used the drugs before and want to try them again.[19] They enter the trial hoping to be allotted the psychedelic substance, and will be happy if they think they are and disappointed if they suspect they are getting the placebo. This will boost the apparent effect of the drug and depress the effect of the placebo.

Yet, even despite these biases, the evidence doesn't look convincing. Several trials of psilocybin in people with depression have failed to show that it is better than a placebo or different from regular antidepressants, which, as we have seen, are minimally helpful at best.[20] The largest study so far was conducted by Compass Pathways and found that people experienced a greater elevation in mood after a single administration of high-dose psilocybin compared to a tiny, placebo dose, but this was a temporary effect and had worn off by the end of the twelve-week follow-up period. A medium dose had no effect. There were also indications that people who were given high or medium doses were more likely to develop suicidal thoughts and to harm themselves compared to people who only had the tiny dose.[21]

A German study published in 2026, which found no difference between psilocybin and a placebo on the main outcome ('response' to treatment), also suggested that psilocybin might make people suicidal. Moreover, one of the participants developed a severe and persistent reaction to psilocybin consisting of anxiety, panic attacks and visual disturbances – a recognised complication of psychedelics.[22]

Numerous studies of ketamine have been conducted, mostly involving giving people one or two doses intravenously (it has minimal effect when taken orally) and following them up for a few days or weeks. Most studies involved minimal, if any, psychotherapy. The majority show that ketamine has an immediate effect on mood, which is predictable in view of its euphoriant effects. However, illustrating how easily the mind-altering properties of these drugs can be overlooked, researchers have instead concluded that ketamine has a remarkably 'rapid' antidepressant action and argued this might give it specific anti-suicidal properties.[23] Studies exploring this possibility show that ketamine and, to a lesser extent, esketamine can temporarily reduce the strength of people's suicidal ideas, but this effect is not sustained and they do not reduce actual suicides or suicide attempts.[24]

In some cases, the positive effects of ketamine persist for a few weeks, but the likelihood that this is an amplified placebo effect is demonstrated by studies in which people have been given ketamine while they are having a general anaesthetic. For example, one study was conducted in people who had depression and were scheduled to have surgery. When they had their operation, they were given ketamine along with a regular anaesthetic.[25] In this scenario, people are less likely to detect whether they have had ketamine or not, because they are anaesthetised for the period during which ketamine would exert its psychoactive effects, although there may be some lingering effects when they wake up. In any case, the study found no difference in mood ratings between people who were given a ketamine injection during their anaesthetic and people who were given a placebo injection.

On the other hand, as in antidepressant studies, people who guessed they had been given ketamine improved more than people who guessed they had been given the placebo, confirming that people's expectations significantly influence their mood ratings.[26]

Esketamine is intended to be used repeatedly, but even so the main clinical trials only lasted four weeks and showed it to be barely distinguishable from a placebo. In fact, five of the first six completed trials of treatment initiation were negative and in the one positive study the difference between the drug and the placebo was small. Indeed, the evidence was so weak, the US regulator, the Food and Drug Administration (FDA), had to make various concessions to Janssen in order for it to pass the licensing process, as revealed in the FDA report.[27]

Long-Term Use

The relevance of trials that investigate a single treatment or a short course of treatment, are not double blind, include participants with high expectations and show, at best, a temporary elevation in mood (likely due to the direct euphoriant effects of the drugs or an amplified placebo effect) is questionable. In practice, we know that people will end up taking these drugs on a long-term basis and, as so often happens, we have very little data to tell us whether this is safe or not.

The ketamine industry in the US has already cultivated a base of returning customers. People rarely have just one or two treatments but return repeatedly, with some clinics offering high-dose, intravenous treatment twice a day.[28] Even if people are not physically dependent, they can become psychologically dependent. When Hannah's local ketamine clinic shut down, she told *The Guardian*: 'It's devastating ... it feels like my life is on hold.'[29] Other people go back for more because they are chasing the miraculous transformation they were promised that never materialised.[30]

At the same time, the therapy element of these treatments is being pared down or removed. Financial imperatives are driving these trends in what is becoming an increasingly competitive business environment. Psychotherapy is labour intensive and costly, and many ketamine clinics in the US no longer offer it.[31] Some UK services do, some don't. In the Oxford clinic therapy is 'optional'.[32] The tendency of ketamine treatment has been towards the provision of the drug for the longest possible time in the cheapest possible way, and this will inevitably be the pattern for other psychedelics when they are marketed as medical interventions.

There is also evidence that psychedelic businesses are capitalising on the increasingly blurred line between recreational and medical use. Some of the burgeoning online ketamine services are simply acting as 'glorified drug dealers', one ketamine therapist told *The Guardian*, sending drugs out by post for people to take on their own.[33]

The fashion for microdosing LSD or other psychedelics represents another trend towards long-term use. Microdosing involves people using small doses of the drug on a daily or frequent basis, and people report that they do it to enhance their mental performance, creativity, reduce anxiety and improve their mood.[34] However, microdoses of psychedelics have not been shown to improve cognitive performance or creativity in 'proper studies'. Moreover, effects appear to fade with repeated use, suggesting the body adapts and therefore that withdrawal effects of some sort would be expected.[35]

The tragic death of *Friends* star Matthew Perry, who died in his jacuzzi after being injected with ketamine by his assistant, highlights the addictive properties of the drug and the thin line between therapeutic use and misuse. Perry was having ketamine treatment for depression once every one or two weeks, but was also using vast quantities on top of this that he obtained from corrupt local doctors and drug dealers.[36] What started as a treatment seemed to have become a compulsion.

Neurospeak

Although the ideas behind psychedelic-assisted psychotherapy are still prevalent, as treatment morphs into routine, long-term use with minimal therapy, the way psychedelics are explained as working is also changing. They are increasingly discussed in terms of what they do to the brain, such as enhancing brain 'connectivity', 'neuroplasticity' or repairing the 'neurotoxic effects of depression'.[37]

Yet, these apparently scientific explanations often simply reframe a psychological explanation in speculative neurological terms. Researchers often talk about psychedelics having a 'snow-globe' effect, for example, which refers to them shaking up thinking processes and re-setting rigid thought patterns, comparable to the way cognitive behavioural therapy (CBT) aims to stop people focusing on negative thoughts. These ideas are increasingly translated into 'neurospeak' – so the drugs are said to '"shake up" the brain's communication networks', disrupt existing nervous pathways and stimulate new connections between different parts of the brain.[38]

This sounds much like the old habit of kicking the television set to see if it brings it back to life (don't try this with a flat screen TV!). You use a chemical to stir up the brain and hope some good may come of it, but you have no idea what you're doing and the consequences could be dire.

One effect of explanations in terms of brain activity is that they enable the mind-altering effects of taking psychedelics to be played down; the drugs can then be presented as working in a disease-centred manner, by targeting an underlying brain abnormality. This helps position the drugs as bona fide medical treatments, counteracting doubts that might arise due to their established recreational status.

Serotonin is implicated in this account, too. Psychedelics, such as psilocybin and LSD, influence the serotonin system, although whether this is related to their most distinctive effects is not known since they modify numerous other brain chemical systems too. Nevertheless, a video by Compass Pathways explains that psilocybin activates the serotonin 2a receptor, which 'may make the brain operate with more flexibility'. In this way, 'connections underlying unhealthy brain states, such as depression, can re-set in a healthier way'.[39] In other words, although the nature of the 'unhealthy brain state' is not spelled out, the claim is that it can be rectified by psychedelics' action on the serotonin 2a receptor. In an interview published in *Nature*, David Nutt put it slightly differently, claiming that psychedelics 'turn off parts of the brain that relate to depression' and 'reset the brain's thinking processes' via their actions on brain serotonin receptors.[40]

None of these theories have been proven so far and even calling them theories seems generous. They are far too nebulous to translate into experiments that could prove them one way or another. Yet, the disease-centred view is useful because it enables psychedelics to be positioned not as one-off stimulus to personal development – a model that is unlikely to generate large profits – but as treatments that need to be taken regularly on a long-term basis. It also helps divert attention from the side effects and dangers associated with their use.

Most people have forgotten the 'bad trip' in the current hype, but a recent recipient of ketamine described the experience as 'terrifying'.[41] More worrying still is the fact that these effects may persist. Science journalist John Horgan, for example, describes months of depression and flashbacks following a 'bad trip'.[42]

Recent research found that 3.5 per cent of people who had used psychedelics recreationally had experienced adverse effects that lasted more than a month, and over 1 per cent had had them for more than a year.[43] The most common symptoms included anxiety, social disconnection and perceptual disturbances.

Ketamine and esketamine are known or suspected to be associated with a long list of physical and psychological complications, including heart instability, bladder damage, liver toxicity, accidents, cognitive impairment, dependence, depression and suicide, but these have received little attention.[44] The consequences of long-term, regular use of other psychedelics simply hasn't been studied.

Other New Antidepressants

Alongside psychedelics, there is a worrying trend to develop other recreational substances and related molecules as antidepressants. One, Auvelity, licensed in 2022, consists of a combination of the antidepressant and smoking-cessation drug bupropion, with a cough medicine ingredient, dextromethorphan, known as DXM. DXM has ketamine-like effects and is a popular drug of abuse among young people in the US and Europe (taking it is referred to as 'Robo-tripping', after the brand-name preparation, Robitussin). It is known to produce a withdrawal syndrome when used on a regular basis.[45] The dose of DXM in Auvelity is small, which may have encouraged regulators to wave it through, but bupropion increases the concentration of DXM in the body, so the combination is not as innocuous as it might first appear.[46]

A version of the chemical imbalance story has been recruited to market Auvelity. The Auvelity website proclaims, 'experts believe that depression involves certain brain chemicals', and then, 'While the exact way that Auvelity works to treat depression is unclear, it acts on multiple receptors in the brain, which affect certain brain chemicals'. The website doesn't mention risks of misuse or dependence, and the prescribing information sheet explicitly states that Auvelity 'has not been systematically studied in animals or humans for its potential for abuse, tolerance, or physical dependence', a stunning admission.[47]

Another newly licensed antidepressant, zuranolone (Zurzuvae), has been introduced for the treatment of post-natal depression and is being tested for general depression. Although it was developed to mimic the effects of a pregnancy hormone, its main action is similar to benzodiazepines. In line with this, it is claimed to work by rebalancing levels of the brain chemical GABA, the main target of the benzodiazepines. Researchers with links to zuranolone's manufacturer, Sage Therapeutics, have postulated that GABA may be 'low or reduced' in people with depression.[48] Although concerns about dependence and misuse were initially downplayed,[49] they are now well-acknowledged hazards.[50]

Scepticism

Despite the predominantly enthusiastic coverage of psychedelics in the scientific literature and the media, it is not all plain sailing. Although esketamine and zuranolone were licensed in the UK, they were not approved for use in the National Health Service. Mark and I submitted evidence to the National Institute for Health and Care Excellence (NICE) panel that rejected the use of esketamine and attended the appeal hearing requested by Janssen, the manufacturer. It was impressive to see public officials stand up to the pressure of Janssen's no doubt highly paid lawyers. But the NICE staff had done their homework and would not let themselves be swayed. They decided the long-term benefits of esketamine were uncertain and did not justify the costs of the treatment.[51] Zuranolone was also provisionally rejected by NICE in 2025, but a draft consultation is still pending.[52]

In 2024 the FDA refused to grant a licence for MDMA (ecstasy) to be used as a treatment for post-traumatic stress disorder and in 2026 it refused Compass Pathway's application for an expedited review process for its psilocybin analogue.[53] It issued guidance to help companies hoping to develop psychedelic treatment to do more rigorous studies, highlighting some of the flaws of recent research, including the ineffectiveness of blinding, short-term follow-ups and the lack of data on important side effects, including dependence.[54] Whether it will maintain an independent and appropriately inquisitory perspective, or whether it will fold under pressure as appears to have been the case with esketamine, remains to be seen.

The scientific literature, although remaining predominantly enthusiastic about ketamine and psychedelics, is also starting to discuss the inadequacies of the evidence and sound notes of caution.[55] An editorial in the *Journal of Clinical Epidemiology* in 2026, for example, expresses concern that the coverage has run away from the facts and cautions people to be suspicious of 'interventions that are launched with the most fanfare and media hype'.[56]

Conclusion

Signs of scepticism are welcome, especially as the psychedelic-assisted psychotherapy paradigm is being replaced by an ostensible neuroscientific model that reverts to the idea that the drugs are rectifying an underlying brain defect, encouraging the development of a mass market of long-term users. Other compounds, derived from or related to established recreational substances, are presented as targeting chemical imbalances and positioned for regular, long-term use, just like conventional antidepressants.

There is something fascinating about psychedelics drugs: they take people out of the humdrum everyday world into one of vivid colours, sounds and sensations – an experience that some find profound and inspiring, others just enjoy and some find unsettling and sometimes frightening. The debate about whether these drugs should be legalised is different from the question of whether they are useful medical treatments, however.

The trouble is that when they are designated as medicines, we forget they are drugs. Nowadays, you can read hundreds of scientific papers on ketamine and barely be aware that it produces dramatic alterations in people's mental and physical state. If psychedelic drugs become established as routine treatments, no doubt their subjective effects will also be relegated to the footnotes of scientific papers. And when we forget the mind-altering effects of these drugs, we forget their potential dangers, too.

Most likely there are customers and potential customers of ketamine and psychedelic services who want to take the drugs for fun but are inhibited from sourcing them from drug dealers. The companies that offer mushroom 'retreats' undoubtedly recognise this. But there are also many unhappy people who are looking for something to numb or distract them from their feelings, or waiting for the promised solution that antidepressants didn't deliver.

Just like antidepressants, the psychedelic business and other new or repurposed compounds thrive on the vulnerability of people who have been led to believe that somewhere there is a magic bullet that will resolve their difficulties. And just like antidepressants, we are ignorant of the range of physical and psychological consequences of taking these drugs on a long-term basis. Once again, the medical-scientific community is keen to make these drugs available before there is adequate data on the harm this might do. Another unofficial experiment is being launched on an unsuspecting public.

17

Forging a New Self: An Alternative Approach to Recovery

Amidst the jungle of research and media headlines about biological mechanisms and new pharmacological approaches, it is easy to lose sight of the fact that we do not need to think of depression and emotional problems as medical conditions that need medical solutions. The quest to find the brain pathway that causes depression and the drug that can fix it may promise a quick fix, but it doesn't deliver one. Consequently, it ultimately prolongs people's suffering.

Instead of viewing depression, anxiety and other unpleasant emotional states as a nuisance or a threat – as things that need to be eradicated like an infectious disease or inflamed appendix – there is another narrative that goes back to the ordinary sense of depression and emotional problems I described earlier. This is the idea that they are an understandable reaction to life events and circumstances and can therefore be understood as signals that something needs changing.

In this framework, what people need is not 'treatment', in the medicalised sense of the term, but support to enable them to get through difficult times and tap into their own resources. This approach may not be as sexy as giving people brand-new drugs and other neuroscientific paraphernalia, but it doesn't give people side effects or leave them with persistent sexual dysfunction.

People react differently to this message. Some, like Krishnan Murphy, who interviewed me for the Channel 4 podcast *Ways to Change the World*, suggest it is depressing to think there isn't – and isn't going to be – a pill that effectively eliminates depression. Others see it as a hopeful message that suggests people can recover from depression and emotional problems through their own efforts, and, in the process, create better lives for themselves and others.

In Chapter 3, I presented the view that depression is a sort of emotional state, and that these states are, by their nature, reactions to our circumstances, coloured by our previous experiences. In other words, our emotions are an integral part of who we are – of our character. Pharmaceutical advertising and health awareness campaigns have tried to persuade us of exactly the opposite. The slogan of one – 'Depression is a flaw in chemistry not character' – has spawned an industry of merchandise, including sweatshirts, car stickers and gifts.[1]

Thinking of depression as part of who we are doesn't have to mean it is a 'flaw', however. Many things in the world *should* make us depressed, and many people have good reasons to be depressed. Adverse social and economic conditions and life experiences have a profound impact on people's chances of becoming depressed, as we have seen.

Moreover, if some people are less well buttressed against the stresses and strains of modern life than others, this is a cause for sympathy, not blame. Challenging the biological model of depression doesn't negate the importance of empathising with, and being compassionate towards, those who are unhappy. In fact, thinking of depression as a meaningful emotional reaction better equips us to imagine each other's pain and to appreciate where it comes from. And because our emotions are so often a spur to action, it highlights how people can change and develop, which is why the idea that depression is not a disease is an inherently optimistic message.

Campaigns such as 'chemistry not character' are premised on the widely held assumption that viewing depression as a brain condition reduces stigma. However, there is a considerable volume of research showing that regarding mental health problems as brain diseases leads to *more*, not less, stigma. Numerous attitude surveys show that when people are presented with biological explanations for mental illness, as compared to psychological or social explanations, they are more likely to think of the sufferer as being dangerous, as having no chance of recovery and they are less likely to want to get acquainted with them. Biological explanations do not result in people blaming the individual any less, either.[2]

Depression and Change

A few years ago, I supervised Maev Conneely, a promising student who studied what people with depression wrote on internet blogs. Most of the bloggers embraced the chemical imbalance theory of depression – one described how she did not have enough 'happy chemicals' in her brain. However, when these bloggers discussed their recovery, they revealed a different understanding of depression.

Bloggers discussed how depression had acted as an opportunity to identify what was wrong with their lives – what they lacked and what they wanted. For several, this involved re-evaluating the role of their job or career and of conventional standards of success. They recognised that working for long hours to earn more money and obtain promotion and higher status had not brought fulfilment. They started to ask themselves what it meant to lead a 'good life'. For some, this involved appreciating little things and being more present in the moment; for others it involved the rediscovery of religious faith. It was an active process that could only be instigated by the individual sufferer – they had to take hold of 'the steering wheel', as one put it. Another described it as forging a 'new self'.

These bloggers described recovering from depression as a journey that involved changing their circumstances but also changing fundamental aspects of themselves – what they valued and how they lived. It was a positive process that led them to become 'better versions of themselves' – it was a process of growth.[3]

Recovery from Depression

This is how Joe Tudor sees his recovery from depression, too. Joe is a man in his early thirties, who kindly agreed to let me tell his story. Joe grew up in the north of England and, when he was 23, he moved to London and took a job in a recruitment agency. He worked hard and was good at his job, got on well with his workmates, played football several times a week and went out drinking with his friends. He was a 'completely normal bloke', he told me.

Occasionally he had problems sleeping, however, and after an amicable but sudden break-up with his girlfriend, this got worse. He was so deprived of sleep on some days that he started to make mistakes at work, and on one occasion he gave a job candidate the wrong time for an interview. The client was mildly annoyed with him, but he was devastated he'd messed up. He went home and cried. He started to feel he was worthless, and despite the support of his football team, he felt lonely too. He was finding it increasingly difficult to cope at work and at home, so eventually he did what he thought he ought to do and went to see his GP.

Joe said his doctor was sympathetic, but the meeting was brief. She asked him the nine questions of the Patient Health Questionnaire, a questionnaire that is commonly used to screen for depression in General Practice (the development of which was funded, incidentally, by Pfizer, makers of the SSRI sertraline).[4] Then she told him calmly and authoritatively, 'Joe, you have severe clinical depression.' He was taken aback. He knew he was distressed, but didn't think he had a severe medical condition. On the other hand, he felt vulnerable and he needed help. He asked why he had it and she told him not to worry: 'You have a chemical imbalance.' He left with a prescription for sertraline.

Joe wasn't sure whether to take the antidepressant. He tried to contact various mental health organisations to ask their advice, but no one got back to him. He turned to his friends, and several told him they were taking antidepressants too and it was nothing to worry about. Joe should take them, they suggested. So he did.

For a few weeks, he felt better, but soon the negative feelings crept back. He went back to his doctor and she increased his dose. It didn't help, so it was increased again. He was on the waiting list for therapy, but he couldn't see how this would help if he had a chemical imbalance. Yet, he wanted to connect with people who would understand his situation. He wanted somewhere to go where he could get advice and discuss his worries, but he couldn't find anywhere.

He felt worse than before. Now he thought he had a severe medical condition and that the recommended treatment wasn't working. He thought he would never get better, that he would have to quit his job and move back to his mum's. The antidepressant affected his coordination, so he was struggling to play football, but he didn't care any more. When he mentioned the possibility of giving up football, his lifelong passion, to his mum, she was alarmed. Maybe he needed to do something different, she suggested. Maybe he should think about quitting his antidepressant.

So Joe went back to his doctor to ask about coming off the medication. By coincidence, at the same time, the practice therapist had a cancellation and Joe took the appointment. Joe says the therapist provided him with support while he was reducing his medication and helped him to reflect on the causes of his problems. This enabled Joe to realise the job he was doing was not helping. He had enjoyed it and it paid well, but he wanted to do something more meaningful.

So Joe gave it up and went travelling. It's a cliché, but the experience opened his eyes to other cultures and other philosophies. He volunteered in a Sikh temple and spent time in a Buddhist monastery. He learnt the importance of simple communal activities, like taking a meal together, and he was exposed to a different view of suffering – one that suggests it can be a stimulus to personal growth.

One morning, watching the sun rise over Mount Everest, he realised how far he had come. And he knew that, if it hadn't been for his depression, he wouldn't have been there, witnessing the beauty of that sunrise. Depression had taught him what he didn't want in life and helped set him on the route to finding what he did.

When Joe eventually returned to the UK, he had the idea of setting up an organisation that would combine the different things he had found helpful under one umbrella. For a year, he worked out of his mum's house and then he obtained funding for a pilot project. He returned to London and set up the Reconnect Club.

The Reconnect Club describes itself as an 'inclusive community that helps people find hope through the tough times'.[5] With help from Gillian Bowden, a clinical psychologist and the lead author on the British Psychological Society's *Understanding Depression* report,[6] Joe started by running a six-week pilot programme co-designed by the club members. The intention was for people to discuss issues, such as 'what is depression', in a safe and supportive environment so each individual could develop their own understanding of their particular difficulties. It was also intended as a way of linking people up, so they could provide mutual support and validation, and of introducing people to a range of activities and resources so each person could decide what was helpful for them.

The NHS's 'social prescribing' initiative also aims to connect 'people to activities, groups, and services in their community to meet the practical, social and emotional needs that affect their health and wellbeing'.[7] Social prescribing is done in different ways in different places, but a common model involves a member of staff employed by a GP surgery who directs people to appropriate community facilities. It lacks the element of personal and mutual support, but people can be directed to other places that provide this.[8]

The problem is that community facilities are patchy, and as Joe had experienced himself, places that fulfil people's needs to meet other people in a mutually supportive setting are not easy to find. Yet, when we spoke, Joe was keen to stress that the Reconnect Club wasn't intended as an end in itself. He didn't want it to become a crutch for people. He wanted people to use it to develop confidence, friendships and routines that would help them move on with their lives. He didn't want others to feel broken and hopeless like he had when he thought he had an imbalanced brain. And, most of all, he wanted people to realise that their experiences of depression could enable them to grow.

Helping People with Depression

Understanding depression as an emotional reaction that is entwined, as all emotions are, with our individual history and character means there is no universal substitute for antidepressants. Recovering from depression is a personal process that is different for each individual, depending on the circumstances that led them to feel depressed in the first place. Supporting people on this journey, whether as a professional, friend or relative, is about helping people to identify the causes of their discontent, worry or despair and how to address these. When circumstances cannot easily be resolved, it may involve making people feel accepted and supported as they wrestle with their emotions.

'Treating' depression must, therefore, be first and foremost about helping people to address the problems in their lives. Some people need relationship counselling, some social activities to combat loneliness, some debt advice, some help to find work, some guidance from a trade union for work-based problems or bullying. Some people might benefit from formal psychotherapy with a professional who can help them come to terms with previous traumatic or stressful experiences. And some people need the space and support to work out what they want from life. Therapy can help with this process in some cases, as it did for Joe, but some people find other ways of figuring it out. For each individual, the methods and answers will be different.

There are some general steps people can take to improve their mood, too, though. The 2022 NICE depression guideline lists nine interventions for 'less severe' depression and eight for 'more severe' depression that do not involve drug treatment and have been demonstrated to be effective in randomised controlled trials. These include various forms of psychotherapy, including cognitive behavioural therapy (CBT) and problem-solving therapy, as well as things people can do on their own, such as exercise and meditation or mindfulness.[9] Different forms of exercise have been shown to be beneficial, including running, walking and dancing, and short-term effects are generally larger than those obtained with antidepressants.[10] Things that haven't been tested in randomised trials but are likely to be useful, or at least cause no harm, include eating a healthy diet, being active and having a regular daily routine.

I asked Joe what had helped him. He listed – in no particular order – his therapist, playing football, his teammates and other friends, his family, keeping busy, leaving his job, travelling, experiencing other cultures and being among people with different values, doing things he'd never done before (like meditating), running, reading Johann Hari's book *Lost Connections*,[11] managing his sleep problems and ultimately doing something to help other people and finding a new purpose in life.

Joe's Reconnect Community is aiming to help people find their own unique solutions, along with probably the most powerful ingredient of all: human kindness and understanding.

What If This Doesn't Work?

As I write this, I can hear protests from people who say they have tried all these things, but they still feel depressed. What do I have to offer them? Many people feel some sort of intervention *must* be on offer. 'Without a firm explanation, or an alternative [to anti-depressant medication ...], I consider the publication of your findings to be potentially extremely dangerous,' an email correspondent told me angrily.

I admit I don't have another blanket solution up my sleeve, but that doesn't mean that taking antidepressants or any other questionably effective and potentially harmful medication is necessary or advisable. In the words of the Hippocratic oath, 'First do no harm'.

This is the case even for people with severe depression, including people with 'melancholic' or psychotic states that require hospitalisation. Antidepressants rarely help in this situation. As I explained earlier, occasionally, electroconvulsive therapy (ECT) can temporarily override people's underlying gloom, but it has no lasting benefits. There simply is no magic bullet. What is needed in this situation is care – looking after people, helping them to eat and drink, keeping them safe, providing company and reassurance, and supporting them to gradually engage with the world again. The vast majority of people with depression will recover of their own accord in the end. It may take months, sometimes longer, but there is no evidence that antidepressants, ECT or any other medical intervention shortens the ultimate duration of the problem.

Cathy, who we met in Chapter 3, shows how people can put their experience of depression to good use, even when it has been prolonged and severe. Cathy now devotes some of her time to supporting health professionals from medical departments and accident & emergency services to interact more positively and sensitively with people with mental health problems – people who are often regarded as a nuisance by busy staff dealing with other medical emergencies. She encourages staff to take a collaborative approach – to work with the individual to look beyond the immediate crisis, to consider what the root causes might be and to identify the right kind of help.

A New Service

For decades now, people have been advised to go and see their doctor if they feel depressed or anxious and led to expect the doctor will have a treatment that will make them feel better. It is difficult for the doctor not to try to fulfil this expectation.

Although 'talking therapy' is freely available through the National Health Service in the UK, people have to wait a few weeks for it to start. Initially, at least, it is administered online or over the telephone and increasingly, due to the huge demand, it is delivered in a group setting. Social prescribers can direct people to other services that might be helpful, such as exercise classes and social groups, but this might not feel like enough for someone who is acutely distressed.

So doctors prescribe antidepressants because that is what they can do. This is why we have come to the state of affairs in which almost a fifth of the adult population of England and a quarter of women take antidepressants.[12] If we want to change this, we need a completely new sort of service based on a new outlook – one that is not centred around doctors and health professionals, and not modelled on treating physical illness or disease.

Such a service would most logically be located within social services. This would emphasise how our mental health reflects our social situation, and how what most often needs addressing is not the individual's brain or mental attitude, but their circumstances. The service could include or be linked with financial, employment and housing advice, and relationship counselling, and it could host or introduce people to clubs like Joe's. Psychotherapy could be provided to people who would benefit from it. Locating the service outside the health service – a service that, despite its name, is designed to deal with disease – could help foster people's inherent strengths and gradually repair the damage done by decades of convincing people they have a broken brain.

The Politics of Distress

Understanding emotional problems, like depression, as understandable reactions to life events and adversity highlights the political nature of mental health. Indeed, several writers have suggested the current epidemic of mental illness is related to the modern era of souped-up capitalism that many refer to as neoliberal capitalism, and what therapist and writer Oliver James calls 'selfish capitalism'. They highlight how, in contrast to the more redistributive capitalism of the mid-twentieth century, neoliberal capitalism is highly competitive, has led to soaring rates of inequality, is based on insecurity of employment and income, has eroded traditional sources of support, including trade unions, and damaged community cohesion.[13]

At the same time as creating the conditions for rampant distress, neoliberal society encourages us to see our reactions as problems of our biology – whether that's our brain chemistry, our genetics or our neural make-up. This conveniently diverts attention from how features of the current system might be to blame. It prevents us from understanding our emotions as 'commentaries on social life', as James Davies put it.[14] Antidepressants are the perfect intervention from this perspective. As well as purporting to resolve a social or personal problem in a medical manner, they dampen our sensitivity and therefore potentially numb us to the suffering, injustice and exploitation around us, as well as to our own problems.

But whether it is neoliberal capitalism, or some other economic system, the relocation of social, political and personal problems into the medical domain is profoundly conservative (with a small 'c'). It buffers whatever political philosophy and economic regime currently exists – whether that be of the Left or Right – against legitimate criticism.

Moreover, medicalisation, or what sociologist Nikolas Rose called the 'psychiatric re-shaping of discontent',[15] is not, in the end, a compassionate approach for the individual. Rather than supporting people with mental health problems, it isolates them. It turns people into 'patients', who need to be cured of their internal, biological or cognitive defects. Far from exculpating them of blame, it focuses on their individual deficiencies, which is most likely why it's been found that medical explanations increase rather than reduce stigma.

The medical approach doesn't help people find solutions to their problems either; it substitutes a careful understanding of each individual's predicament with a diagnostic label. And rather than providing the social support and community that most people need, it discourages people from understanding the social implications of their feelings and hinders them from reaching out to others to find collective solutions. It undermines the redemptive power of taking action and the power, friendship and creativity that is fostered when people tackle the social causes of discontent together.

Conclusions: Nurturing Recovery

We should welcome the fact that depression, anxiety and other forms of distress are not, as far as we know, caused by brain abnormalities – that they are not diseases. Although this means there will not be a simple biological remedy, it also means we can learn to manage these states ourselves and, in some instances, we can gain and learn from them.

Our emotions provide us with clues about our lives. They signal to us that something is amiss, when the circumstances we find ourselves in, or something we are doing, isn't good for us or doesn't align with our aims and values. Emotions can be overwhelming and difficult to interpret, but if we can work out what they are telling us, they can be a spur to change our lives for the better.

Depression can be profound and debilitating, and nothing I have said is meant to trivialise it. It is also a vicious circle –the lower you feel, the less you want to do anything, the more you withdraw from life, the lower you get. Recovery sometimes needs to start with small steps to break this cycle: taking regular exercise, having a routine and taking opportunities to see other people. Sometimes you have to do this before you have the capacity to work out what has gone wrong in your life and what you can do about it.

Recovering from depression is not like flicking a switch. It is a process, it takes time and it needs nurturing.

Friends and family can help with this process, but it can be hard. It may be necessary to take over the depressed person's responsibilities, as well as looking after them, which is often draining. It is also difficult to know whether to 'push' the person who is depressed to do more, get out more or go back to work, for example, or whether to let them be. In my experience, gently encouraging them to re-engage with the world and become more active is the best attitude. Sometimes this could start with simple things like encouraging them to do household chores, go for a walk or watching television together.

Professionals can also support this process, as well as help people to address their underlying problems. If this were done in a non-medical setting it would dissolve the current temptation to give people pseudo-medical labels like 'clinical depression', tell them they have an abnormal brain and give them an ineffective pill with side effects.

At the social and political level, reducing depression, anxiety and other emotional problems will not be achieved by expanding mental health services or increasing awareness of mental health problems. Instead, it requires society to tackle the sources of people's unhappiness. It needs political measures to combat poverty, inequality, job unavailability and insecurity, and the strengthening of families, communities and social activities that bring people together where they can help each other.

18

Informed Consent

So, what have we learnt? From the beginning, the chemical imbalance theory of depression was more wishful thinking than science. Modern evidence has not supplied confirmation, but the medical establishment has been reluctant to let the theory go. This is because it serves the purpose of representing depression as a medical condition and portraying the drugs that are used to treat it as targeted treatments. The dubious effects of antidepressants can then be claimed to be worthwhile; indeed, to be necessary and life-saving.

By exposing that the serotonin theory of depression is unproven – that it is speculation rather than fact – the publication of our paper brought the edifice that supported antidepressant use crashing down. It turns out antidepressants do not do what they were designed to do – that is, reverse the underlying cause of depression, at least there is no evidence this is the case.

What's more, despite the robotic claims to the contrary, the results of clinical trials and other studies suggest that antidepressants do not work: they do not make people better. They have placebo effects and they numb people's emotions, but there are no grounds for believing that they help people in any meaningful way.

The pharmaceutical research community has been beguiled by the idea that antidepressants are magic bullets and has forgotten that they are foreign chemical substances that change our usual biological state and mental activity with potentially damaging effects. This means that research on the human costs of taking antidepressants has been woefully inadequate. Serious consequences, including prolonged withdrawal symptoms and persistent sexual dysfunction, are only now coming to light, and only through the bravery and persistence of people whose lives have been turned upside down by these drugs. Although most of the medical profession continues as if these problems don't exist, they are the predictable, unpredictable consequences of using chemicals that interfere with the normal functioning of a delicately balanced organ like the brain.

What followed the publication of our serotonin paper was a concerted and, at times, coordinated effort by sections of the psychiatric profession and the media to keep evidence about the nature of depression and antidepressants away from the public and suppress debate about all the issues this book has raised. It was a graphic example of how powerful interests shape what passes as scientific knowledge.[1] This situation is a scandal and it needs to be challenged because it prevents people from exercising one of their most basic rights: informed consent.

* * *

As I sat in the Royal College of Psychiatrists HQ on that cold February day in 2022, working my way through ten boxes of papers relating to the Defeat Depression Campaign, it dawned on me what a seismic change there has been in our views about emotions and our mental life more generally. While we used to think of our moods as reflecting our lives and depression as being the understandable consequence of hardship, loss, failure, isolation, stress, boredom and lack of purpose, we have come to see it as a neurochemical state – as a feature of the brain, not of the person.

The shift occurred, in part, as a result of massive propaganda orchestrated by the pharmaceutical industry, with the collusion of the medical profession. Psychiatrists and other doctors not only failed to stop the industry from spreading the myth about the chemical imbalance theory, frequently they joined in, because, despite knowing the theory was unproven, they desperately wanted to believe it themselves.

Mark and I came of age on different sides of this transformation. When I looked through the results of the surveys commissioned by the Defeat Depression Campaign, I realised my adolescent self had not been alone. Before the advent of the SSRIs and the deluge of marketing that accompanied them, the majority of the British population resisted the medicalisation of their feelings and were wary of the way that drugs that were presented as treatments for emotional problems might cloud one's mind and subtly change one's personality.

But generations who have grown up since the 1990s have been drip-fed the idea that unwanted thoughts and feelings are medical conditions, resulting from faulty brain mechanisms and requiring medical treatment – usually in the form of a drug. Crucially, people have been persuaded that this view has been proven.

The subsequent erosion of people's natural caution and suspicion has led to the epidemic of medication use we have today, with millions of people taking antidepressants and other drugs prescribed for common mental health problems. Many remain on the drugs for years on end, despite the fact there is almost no formal research on the consequences of taking these drugs for such a duration.

Thankfully, most people survive their encounters with antidepressants relatively unscathed, especially if they don't take them for too long. Many are grateful for having taken antidepressants. For some, the emotion-blunting effects of the drug may genuinely have been useful, but we know the main reason people feel better when they take antidepressants is down to the placebo effect – that is, through the hope they provide. In the short term, this hope improves people's mood, but in the long run, we don't know how it plays out. On the contrary, it may lead to disillusion and dejection, as people realise the promised solution doesn't work after all, and it may prolong and worsen depression by discouraging people from taking a more active role in their recovery.

It is difficult to know how many people have been harmed by antidepressants exactly, but there are at least tens of thousands of people, like Mark, Audrey, Roy and Adele, who have suffered years of disabling symptoms, and many more, like Tom, who have endured shorter-term discomfort. They are all victims of a mass programme of misinformation. They were sold an idea of themselves as biologically flawed, alongside a simple but scientific-sounding remedy. They were not told the pills on offer were barely better than a placebo for reducing symptoms or that the long-term effects were essentially unknown and untested. They were encouraged to take and keep taking their medication and they were not warned how difficult it would be to get off it, or of the risk of enduring complications.

This situation continues. Despite the media coverage of our review, people are still being told that depression is due to a chemical imbalance,[2] or to some other speculative biological mechanism, and that this mechanism can be corrected or ameliorated by antidepressants. Adverse effects are still presented as if they are a trivial inconvenience. Not surprisingly, prescriptions continue to rise.

The history of the serotonin theory shows how the supposedly scientific story we have been fed for the last few decades is a fanciful concoction of an insecure profession, disseminated by the marketing departments of powerful pharmaceutical companies. Working in the midst of academic psychiatry, I have long known that much of what is written in textbooks, what fills the pages of academic journals and what is taught to students and trainee doctors about the nature of depression and antidepressants is a misleading and partial picture. But I knew there were other people, some in influential positions, who, like me, believed the scientific evidence tells a different story. Naively, as I now see it, I had faith the truth would eventually come to light.

It was shocking to witness the process of constructing and defending the current narrative in action as I did after the publication of the serotonin paper. The lengths to which sections of the psychiatric profession went to prevent the public from hearing another view about depression and antidepressants were astounding. They tried to curtail public discussion of the paper (because it's not important). They hounded an innocent Polish journalist, they tried to discredit our research with spurious and irrelevant criticisms (despite never seriously disputing our conclusions), they blinded their audience with a torrent of vague and often impenetrable speculations dressed up as science, and they repeatedly and authoritatively declared that antidepressants 'work' and 'save lives', never acknowledging the meagre evidence such proclamations are based on.

While I don't doubt such people believed they were acting in the public's best interests, they were reluctant to let the public decide what these are for themselves. Sections of the psychiatric profession are deeply committed to the idea that depression is a biological condition: they have built their temple on this foundation and will defend it tooth and claw.

The mainstream view of mental health problems as medical conditions requiring medical treatments is rooted in long-standing commercial and professional interests – it is not impartial, as its proponents would have you believe. It has been maintained by an informal alliance of institutions and people with power: drug companies, doctors, research institutions and media outlets.

The immediate publicity surrounding our paper allowed a different view to slip out for a fleeting moment, but this only showed how effectively the message had been controlled in the first place. The lid was quickly shut back down.

It seems that medical history endlessly repeats itself. Barbiturates, benzodiazepines and opioids have all been liberally distributed to unsuspecting and vulnerable patients at different points until their dangers were finally acknowledged. Now it transpires that antidepressants, the most popular mental health treatment of modern times, have caused untold misery to tens of thousands of people for little, if any, gain. Besides, just like their predecessors, many people can't stop them.

The result is that people need to inform themselves about what the evidence indicates. To facilitate this, I have presented a different but scientifically supported way of explaining antidepressant effects, which highlights how they alter normal conscious awareness and mental experience. This view reflects our instinctive understanding of how drugs that disrupt our brain chemistry are likely to impact on our feelings – the understanding that was drummed out of us by marketing campaigns. This information, along with data on withdrawal effects, sexual dysfunction and other health consequences, is essential to enable each individual to evaluate the pros and cons of taking an antidepressant in their own unique situation.

Knowledge can be painful, however, especially when it makes us re-evaluate the beliefs we have adopted about ourselves and the choices we have made. Moreover, learning about the previously little-known risks of antidepressants will be frightening for those who are taking them. But knowledge is also power, as the saying goes. It opens up choices we would not have had without it.

As long as people are unhappy, anxious and insecure, there will be other people trying to make money out of their misery. A flood of new technologies and substances are on offer or in the pipeline – psychedelic-assisted psychotherapy, ketamine and opioids among them – each accompanied by the same hype with which Prozac was launched decades ago. Like antidepressants, they show modest, if any, benefits and no one has invested in researching the consequences of taking these substances for year on year, as many will inevitably do. You can bet the companies that offer these 'breakthrough' treatments will be happy to keep their customers coming back for more. And as the range of ways of meddling with the brain expands, the casualties will only accumulate.

When you are offered a solution to a complex problem in life that sounds too good to be true, it probably is.

Despite what your doctor may tell you, despite what the experts say, despite the endless media headlines, there is no credible evidence that depression is caused by a biological abnormality, whether it is to do with brain chemicals like serotonin, nerve cell growth or neural connections, the inflammatory system or anything else. Therefore, there is no justification for the idea that antidepressants, or anything else, target an underlying brain dysfunction, rather than dumbing people down in more or less subtle ways in the manner of other mind-altering drugs. In the vast majority of situations, antidepressants are the wrong solution to the wrong problem. Not only are they unlikely to help, but they may well make the situation worse. The fact that they are recommended and endorsed by respected and trained professionals does not change this.

Sometimes people want to be dumbed down – sometimes what they are going through is just too intense to bear – and that is fine. But I want to ensure that if people do decide to take an antidepressant, or another drug on offer for mental health problems, they do so on the basis of all the evidence and information currently available and not on a selected batch filtered by people who are defending particular interests. I want people to be able to make truly informed decisions about what they take into their bodies. We must demand nothing less.

Epilogue

The widely propagated idea that depression is a chemical imbalance with a chemical solution has created a huge problem for our society and for the generations to come. It has shaped the life stories of millions of individuals, left many with significant drug-induced complications and created a culture in which people have come to explain the difficulties of life in terms of the brain. In this sense, depression has acted as the template for the creeping medicalisation of a widening array of life problems. This process is increasingly taking place using diagnoses such as bipolar disorder, adult ADHD and neurodiversity,[1] as well as depression and anxiety.[2] And, as we have seen with depression, when something is presented as a medical condition, it is possible to persuade people it has a neurological basis, regardless of the science.

Nothing in this book is meant to suggest that depression, anxiety and other psychological problems are not real or that people don't need help and support with them at times. But the process of medicalisation only makes things worse. It gives people false hope and leads to the over-prescription of potentially harmful drugs that, at best, offer ways to stifle uncomfortable feelings. We have to find better ways to help people.

There is no simple or universal alternative, but understanding depression as a meaningful human reaction points to more fruitful and enduring solutions. There is much about modern life to make us worried and depressed: although Western countries are richer than ever before, many people struggle to make ends meet and others struggle to find meaning in what they do. The ubiquity of the media and the internet means we are constantly comparing ourselves to those who seem to be richer, happier and more successful. We worry that we don't measure up to some impossible ideal, and then blame ourselves when we don't. Stress and disappointment are inevitable.

Yet, our moods and emotions are reflections of our nature as complex, biological organisms that have the ability to make choices. Within the varying constraints of our lives, we are free to shape who we become. This freedom is both a burden, when we realise the responsibility is on us, and an opportunity. For, unlike with a brain disorder, we can change at least some of our circumstances and we can change ourselves. We may be able to do this on our own, we may need help from family, friends or professionals, and sometimes we may need to take collective action to change society.

This is why, ultimately, mental health problems like depression and anxiety are social and political problems. If we wish to tackle them, we need as a society to prioritise addressing the circumstances that give rise to them. We need to provide people with financial security, stable employment and housing and to create a healthy and sustainable environment. We need to foster communities and opportunities for collective activity that can provide fellowship and a sense of purpose. Everyone deserves the chance to flourish.

Forging a life in today's world is not easy. Most of us will experience anxiety, uncertainty and disappointments; for some, these will be difficult to overcome. Emotional crises are the understandable result. The meaning of these is not in our brain chemistry, it is in the world. And that is where the solutions lie too.

Appendix 1

Public Information Suggesting Depression is Linked to a 'Chemical Imbalance'

Source	Quote
Drug Company Information	
Lexapro website, Forest Laboratories, 2009[1]	Whatever the circumstances, depression is caused by an imbalance of certain chemicals in the brain. Normally, these 'chemical messengers' help nerve cells communicate with one another by sending and receiving messages. They may also influence a person's mood. In the case of depression, the available supply of the chemical messengers is low, so nerve cells can't communicate effectively. This often results in symptoms of depression.

Paxil CR website, GlaxoSmithKline, 2009[2]	Scientific evidence suggests that depression and certain anxiety disorders may be caused by a chemical imbalance in the brain. Paxil CR helps balance your brain's chemistry.
Prozac website, Eli Lilly, 2007[3]	A growing amount of evidence supports the view that people with depression have an imbalance of the brain's neurotransmitters [...] many scientists believe that an imbalance in serotonin may be an important factor in the development and severity of depression.
Effexor website, Wyeth, 2006[4]	[Effexor] works by affecting the levels of two chemicals in the brain – serotonin and norepinephrine. Correcting the imbalance of these two chemicals may relieve symptoms of depression.
Zoloft television advertisement, Pfizer, 2005[5]	While the cause is unknown, depression may be related to an imbalance of natural chemicals between nerve cells in the brain. Prescription Zoloft works to correct this imbalance. You just shouldn't have to feel this way anymore.
Celexa website, Forest Pharmaceuticals, 2005[6]	Celexa helps to restore the brain's chemical balance by increasing the supply of a chemical messenger in the brain called serotonin. Although the brain chemistry of depression is not fully understood, there does exist a growing body of evidence to support the view that people with depression have an imbalance of the brain's neurotransmitters.

Health Company Information	
Package leaflet for escitalopram by Accord Healthcare, Ireland, 2020[7]	Escitalopram is an antidepressant which belongs to the 'SSRI' group (selective serotonin reuptake inhibitors). These medicines act on the serotonin-system in the brain by increasing the serotonin level. Disturbances in the serotonin-system are considered an important factor in the development of depression and related diseases.
Very Well Mind website, 2023[8]	The body needs serotonin, but too much or too little can lead to health issues. For example, too little serotonin can cause depression. Medications can help treat low serotonin. These include SSRIs, which help the body make better use of serotonin.
Cleveland Clinic, USA, 2024[9]	Serotonin in your brain regulates your mood. It's often called your body's natural 'feel good' chemical. When serotonin is at normal levels, you feel more focused, emotionally stable, happier and calmer. Low levels of serotonin are associated with depression. Many medications used to treat anxiety, depression and other mood disorders often target ways to increase the level of serotonin in your brain.

National Health Service, UK, 2024[10]	It's thought they [antidepressants] work by increasing levels of chemicals in the brain called neurotransmitters. Certain neurotransmitters, such as serotonin and noradrenaline, are linked to mood and emotion. It's thought that SSRIs work by increasing serotonin levels in the brain. Serotonin is a neurotransmitter (a messenger chemical that carries signals between nerve cells in the brain). It's thought to have a good influence on mood, emotion and sleep ... It would be too simplistic to say that depression and related mental health conditions are caused by low serotonin levels, but a rise in serotonin levels can improve symptoms and make people more responsive to other types of treatment, such as CBT.
Medical Organisations	
American Psychiatric Association, USA	
'Let's Talk Facts About Depression', 2005[11]	Antidepressants may be prescribed to correct imbalances in the levels of chemicals in the brain.
'What is Depression?', 2024[12]	Differences in certain chemicals in the brain may contribute to symptoms of depression.

Royal College of Psychiatrists, UK	
'Depression', 2006[13]	Two neurotransmitters (serotonin and noradrenalin) are particularly affected [in depression] [...] antidepressants increase the concentration of these chemicals at nerve endings, and so seem to boost the function of those parts of the brain that use serotonin and noradrenalin.
'Antidepressants', 2014[14]	How do antidepressants work? We don't know for certain, but we think that antidepressants work by increasing the activity of certain chemicals in our brains called neurotransmitters. They pass signals from one brain cell to another. The chemicals most involved in depression are thought to be serotonin and noradrenalin.
The Royal Australian & New Zealand College of Psychiatrists, 2022[15]	Medications work by rebalancing the chemicals in the brain. Different types of medication act on different chemical pathways.
Center for Disease Control and Prevention, USA, 2023[16]	What causes mental illness? There is no single cause for mental illness. A number of factors can contribute to risk for mental illness, such as [...] Biological factors or chemical imbalances in the brain.

Appendix 2

What to do if you are taking antidepressants: advice and resources

IT IS REALLY IMPORTANT THAT YOU DO NOT STOP YOUR ANTIDEPRESSANTS SUDDENLY OR TOO FAST.

Many people taking antidepressants today have been told by their doctor they have a chemical imbalance and their antidepressant will help put that right. If this is you, you might want to reconsider whether you need or want to continue taking your antidepressant, in the light of the information in this book and elsewhere.

If you are reassessing the use of antidepressants, and before making any change yourself, I would encourage you to take time to reflect on how exactly antidepressants might be affecting you. What side-effects are you experiencing? Make a list of what you think are the positive and negative effects of being on them. It will be helpful to discuss this information with your family and friends and with your doctor or prescriber.

We know that many people suffer from withdrawal symptoms when they try to stop their antidepressant, and these can be severe and prolonged for some people, especially those who have used antidepressants for a long time. If you are considering stopping your antidepressants, you should do this gradually with the support of a doctor or knowledgeable health professional.

There is useful guidance on how to manage this process on the Royal College of Psychiatrists website (www.rcpsych.ac.uk/mental-health/treatments-and-wellbeing/stopping-antidepressants) and in the new *Maudsley Deprescribing Guidelines* (available at www.wiley.com/en-gb/The+Maudsley+Deprescribing+Guidelines%3A+Antidepressants%2C+Benzodiazepines%2C+Gabapentinoids+and+Z-drugs-p-9781119823025).[1]

Other resources that might be helpful include the British Psychological Society's report 'Understanding Depression', which can be found at www.bps.org.uk/guideline/understanding-depression, and the All Party Parliamentary Group on Prescribed Drug Dependence's 'Guidance for Psychological Therapists', available at https://prescribeddrug.info/guidance-for-psychological-therapists.

Glossary

Conditions

Attention Deficit Hyperactivity Disorder (ADHD): A condition characterised by lack of attention and hyperactivity, originally characterised in children, now increasingly diagnosed in adults.

Bipolar disorder: A condition in which someone suffers from recurrent episodes of mania and depression (the most severe form of bipolar disorder was previously known as manic depression).

Mania: An episode of extreme overarousal, with reduced sleep, excitement and overactivity lasting weeks or sometimes months.

Manic depression: A condition in which someone suffers from recurrent episodes of mania and depression (now usually referred to as bipolar disorder).

Melancholia: A severe form of depression, sometimes accompanied by delusions.

Obsessive-compulsive disorder (OCD): A disorder characterised by obsessions and compulsions.

Parkinson's disease: A neurological disease consisting of loss of nerve cells in certain parts of the brain.

Post-traumatic stress disorder (PTSD): A disorder characterised by anxiety and other symptoms following a traumatic event.

Psychosis: An episode of mental disturbance, during which people lose contact with reality and develop delusions and hallucinations.

Schizophrenia: The concept is much debated. It generally refers to the situation in which people have episodes of psychosis recurrently or have chronic symptoms of psychosis, sometimes accompanied by 'negative' symptoms, such as social withdrawal and loss of motivation.

Social anxiety disorder: A disorder characterised by anxiety in social situations (previously known as social phobia).

Tardive dyskinesia: A neurological condition caused by antipsychotic drugs.

Drugs and treatment procedures

Amitriptyline: An early drug of the tricyclic antidepressant family.

Amphetamine: An early stimulant drug prescribed for depression, ADHD and as an appetite suppressant; also used as a recreational drug.

Antipsychotics: Drugs used for the treatment of psychosis and schizophrenia, among other things (also referred to as 'major tranquillisers').

Auvelity (dextromethorphan and bupropion): A drug licensed as an antidepressant in 2022.

Barbiturates: Sedative drugs prescribed for anxiety, among other things.

Benzodiazepines: Sedative drugs prescribed for anxiety, among other things.

Bupropion (brand name Wellbutrin): A drug used as an antidepressant and for smoking cessation.

Buspirone: An anti-anxiety drug.

Chlorpromazine: An early antipsychotic drug (or 'major tranquilliser').

Citalopram: An SSRI.

Dextromethorphan (DXM): A drug with ketamine-like effects.

Drinamyl: A combination of a barbiturate and amphetamine.

Duloxetine (brand name Cymbalta): An SNRI.

Ecstasy: A recreational drug that induces feelings of warmth and happiness.

Efexor (venlafaxine): An SNRI.

Electroconvulsive therapy (ECT): Application of electrical currents to the brain to stimulate an epileptic fit.

Ephedrine: An early stimulant drug used particularly to relieve nasal congestion.

Escitalopram: An SSRI.

Esketamine: A close relative of ketamine, delivered by a nasal spray.

Fenfluramine: An appetite suppressant drug thought to have actions on serotonin.

Fentanyl: An opioid.

Fluoxetine (brand name Prozac): An SSRI.

Imipramine: The first drug of the tricyclic antidepressant family.

Iproniazid: A drug considered to be an antidepressant; an inhibitor of monoamine oxidase.

Ketamine: A drug that is used as an anaesthetic. It has 'dissociative' effects (feeling disconnected from your body or the world) and is also used as a recreational drug.

Librium: The first benzodiazepine drug.

Methylphenidate (brand name Ritalin): A stimulant used for the treatment of ADHD.

Monoamine oxidase inhibitors: An early class of drugs considered to be antidepressants, including iproniazid.

Opiates: Drugs derived from opium, such as morphine and heroin.

Opioids: Synthetic drugs that mimic the actions of opiates.

OxyContin (oxycodone): An opioid.

Paroxetine (brand names Paxil or Seroxat): An SSRI.

Prozac (fluoxetine): An SSRI.

Psilocybin: A hallucinogenic drug (the active substance in 'magic mushrooms').

Reboxetine: An antidepressant with mildly stimulant properties.

Reserpine: A tranquillising agent used in the 1950s and 1960s as an antipsychotic and for high blood pressure.

Selective Serotonin Reuptake Inhibitor (SSRI): A class of drugs considered to be antidepressants; inhibitors of serotonin reuptake.

Serotonin and Noradrenaline Reuptake Inhibitor (SNRI): A class of drugs considered to be antidepressants; inhibitors of noradrenaline and serotonin reuptake.

Sertraline (brand names Zoloft and Lustral): An SSRI.

St John's Wort (hypericum): A biologically active plant extract used as an antidepressant.

Stimulants: Drugs that increase wakefulness and energy (such as amphetamine).

Tianeptine: A drug used as an antidepressant that enhances serotonin reuptake.

Transcranial magnetic stimulation (TMS): Application of magnetic currents to the brain.

Tricyclic antidepressants: An early class of drugs considered to be antidepressants.

Valium (also known as diazepam): An early benzodiazepine drug.

Venlafaxine (brand name Efexor): An SNRI.

Zelmid (zimelidine): An early SSRI.

Zoloft (sertraline): An SSRI.

Zuranolone (brand name Zurzuvae): A benzodiazepine-like drug licensed for post-natal depression.

Biochemicals and processes

Adrenaline: A body chemical involved in the arousal and stress response (not found in the brain).

Cerebrospinal fluid (CSF): The fluid that surrounds the brain and nerves in the spine.

Deoxyribonucleic acid (DNA): The constituent of genes.

Dopamine: A body chemical that is present in the brain and acts as a neurotransmitter chemical.

Forced swim test: An animal model of depression.

Gamma-aminobutyric acid (GABA): A body chemical that is present in the brain and acts as a neurotransmitter chemical.

Glutamate: A body chemical that is present in the brain and acts as a neurotransmitter chemical.

Noradrenaline: A body chemical, related to adrenaline, that is present in the brain and acts as a neurotransmitter chemical.

Monoamine oxidase: A chemical (enzyme) that breaks down monoamines.

Monoamines: The name given to adrenaline, noradrenaline and serotonin.

Neurogenesis: The growth of new nerve cells.

Neuroplasticity: Encompasses neurogenesis but can also refer to the growth of nerve cell projections or spines.

Neurotransmission: The process by which an electrical impulse is transmitted from one nerve cell to another in the brain and the rest of the nervous system.

Neurotransmitter: A chemical that transmits electrical impulses from one nerve cell to another across the synapse.

Positron Emission Tomography (PET): A scan procedure that traces the metabolic activity of parts of the body.

Reuptake: The process by which neurotransmitter chemicals are transferred out of the synapse into the body of the nerve cell.

Serotonin (also known as 5-HT, 5-hydroxytrypamine): A body chemical that is present in the brain and acts as a neurotransmitter chemical.

Serotonin transporter protein (SERT): The chemical that transports serotonin out of the synapse.

Synapse: The gap between nerve cells across which electrical impulses are transmitted from one nerve to another.

Tryptophan: The chemical precursor (building block) of serotonin.

Tryptophan depletion: An experimental process designed to lower tryptophan levels and thereby lower brain serotonin levels.

5-hydroxyindoleacetic acid (5HIAA): A breakdown product of serotonin.

Other terms

American Psychiatric Association: The USA's professional body for psychiatrists.

ANTLER study (ANTidepressants to prevent reLapse in dEpRession): A UK-based, government-funded clinical trial of antidepressant discontinuation and placebo substitution versus antidepressant continuation.

British Association of Psychopharmacology: A UK-based 'learned society'.

British Psychological Society (BPS): The UK's professional body for psychologists.

Clinical Global Impressions Scale (CGI): A scale to measure the overall state of someone's condition.

Cognitive Behaviour Therapy (CBT): A form of psychotherapy, usually short term, focused on changing thought patterns.

***Diagnostic and Statistical Manual of Mental Disorders* (*DSM*):** Manual produced by the American Psychiatric Association.

European Medicines Agency (EMA): The European medicines regulator.

Food and Drug Administration (FDA): The US medicines regulator.

Grading of Recommendations, Assessment, Development, and Evaluations (GRADE): A system for assessing the certainty of medical evidence.

Hamilton Depression Rating Scale (HRDS): A depression symptom rating scale.

***International Classification of Diseases* (*ICD*):** Manual produced by the World Health Organization.

Medicines and Healthcare Products Regulatory Agency (MHRA): The UK medicines regulator.

Meta-analysis: A statistical combination of the results of several individual trials.

Montgomery–Åsberg Depression Rating Scale (MADRS): A depression symptom rating scale.

National Health Service (NHS): The UK's publicly funded health service.

National Institute for Health and Care Excellence (NICE) – formerly the National Institute for Clinical Excellence: UK Government organisation that makes decisions about what treatments will be available within the NHS and produces treatment guidelines.

Patient Health Questionnaire (PHQ): A questionnaire commonly used to screen for depression in General Practice.

Post-SSRI Sexual Dysfunction (PSSD): Sexual dysfunction that persists after an SSRI or other antidepressant is stopped.

Public Health England: A UK Government agency that existed from 2012 to 2021.

Quality of life: A concept that is measured in some clinical trials using various scales.

Randomised controlled trial (RCT): A clinical trial in which people are allocated to different treatments randomly.

Royal College of Psychiatrists: The UK's professional body for psychiatrists.

STAR-D Study (Sequenced Treatment Alternatives to Relieve Depression): US Government-funded study of gold-standard medical treatment of depression (including the use of antidepressants).

Statistically significant: When the results of a statistical test strongly suggest the result is not due to chance (usually defined as a 95 per cent probability it is not due to chance).

Treatment for Adolescents with Depression Study (TADS): US Government-funded trial of fluoxetine and psychotherapy for depression.

Umbrella review: A review of previous reviews or meta-analyses of studies in a defined area.

Acknowledgements

First of all, I would like to offer my gratitude to all the people who shared their stories with me. Mark, Joe, Cathy, Tom, Adele and Beata, thank you – without your courage and generosity this would not be the book that it is. Thanks especially to Mark, for not only sharing his story, but for reading parts of the book, coordinating the publicity of the serotonin paper, providing encouragement and support through what was at times a gruelling process, and for reminding me of how important our work is.

Thank you to the other people who read all or part of the book and offered useful advice and editing tips: Richard Millwood, Ursula Moncrieff, Ann Moncrieff and Peter Hacker. Peter Hacker has been generous with his time and wisdom – it has been an honour to know him. Thank you to Richard Millwood for productive conversations about the approach of the book, general support and producing the neurotransmission figure.

It has been a privilege to work with my agent, Andrew Lownie, whose enthusiasm and persistence has been a great help. Claire Hartley, my editor at FLINT and The History Press, also read the book and has skilfully steered it and me through the publication process, offering commitment, positive feedback and general support. Thank you to the rest of the team at FLINT and The History Press.

The original serotonin study that sparked this book was conducted with Ruth Cooper, Michael Hengartner, Tom Stockmann and Simone Amendole, as well as Mark Horowitz. Thank you all for your hard work on the project and your collegiality.

I have had productive exchanges and collaborations with many people over the years, who have all contributed to my research and ideas, including Pat Bracken, Richard Byng, David Cohen, James Davies, Duncan Double, Adele Framer, Peter Gøtzsche, Anne Guy, David Healy, Paul Higgs, Peter Kinderman, Lucy Johnstone, Jon Jureidini, Irving Kirsch, Glyn Lewis, Hugh Middleton, Luke Montagu, Martin Plöderl, Sally Porter, John Read, Graham Scambler, Sandy Steingard, Sami Timimi, Robert Whitaker and others.

I am also grateful to all the people who have drawn attention to previously unrecognised or underrated adverse effects and challenged misleading mental health information – the public and the scientific community are indebted to you.

Finally, I would like to thank my family for their continual interest in and support for what I am doing, including my late father, Martin, my mother, Ann, and the rest. All of you are a constant source of encouragement and inspiration.

Notes

Preface

1 A systematic review is a comprehensive synthesis of the research in a particular area, conducted according to a pre-specified protocol using transparent methods. Our review is: Moncrieff, J.; Cooper, R.E.; Stockmann, T.; Amendola, S.; Hengartner, M.P.; & Horowitz, M.A. (2022). 'The Serotonin Theory of Depression: A Systematic Umbrella Review of the Evidence', *Molecular Psychiatry*: doi:10.1038/s41380-022-01661-0. Available at: www.nature.com/articles/s41380-022-01661-0.

Chapter 1

1 Some recent examples include: https://mentalhealth-uk.org/help-and-information/conditions/depression/diagnosis/; https://adhduk.co.uk/diagnosis-pathways/; www.theguardian.com/society/2020/sep/30/my-treatment-for-add-changed-my-life-so-why-cant-i-stop-worrying-about-it; www.verywellmind.com/the-chemistry-of-depression-1065137; www.theguardian.com/society/2022/oct/22/it-is-a-flaw-in-our-cells-that-becomes-a-flaw-in-love-doctor-siddhartha-mukherjee-on-the-search-for-a-cure-for-depression (accessed 25 February 2023).

2 'Girl in Red – Serotonin' (2021), www.youtube.com/watch?v=Gh8Gl2GwB6s (accessed 6 February 2024).
3 Kalin, N.H. (2020). 'The Critical Relationship Between Anxiety and Depression', *American Journal of Psychiatry*, **177**(5): 365–67.
4 See Horwitz, A.V. (2010). 'How an Age of Anxiety Became an Age of Depression', *Milbank Quarterly*, **88**(1): 112–38; and Healy, D. (2004). 'Shaping the Intimate: Influences on the Experience of Everyday Nerves', *Social Studies in Science*, **34**(2): 219–45.
5 Caspi, A.; Houts, R.M.; Ambler, A.; Danese, A.; Elliott, M.L.; Hariri, A. et al. (2020). 'Longitudinal Assessment of Mental Health Disorders and Comorbidities Across 4 Decades Among Participants in the Dunedin Birth Cohort Study', *Journal of the American Medical Association Network Open*, **3**(4): e203221. Available at: www.ncbi.nlm.nih.gov/pmc/articles/PMC7175086/. The figure for anxiety and depression, which are referred to as 'internalising disorders', is provided in Figure 3.
6 Priest, R.G.; Vize, C.; Roberts, A.; Roberts, M.; & Tylee, A. (1996). 'Lay People's Attitudes to Treatment of Depression: Results of Opinion Poll for Defeat Depression Campaign Just Before its Launch', *British Medical Journal*, **313**(7061): 858–59. Available at: www.ncbi.nlm.nih.gov/pmc/articles/PMC2359082.
7 Several such critiques are reviewed in this essay: Sharpe, K. (2015). 'The Silence of Prozac', *Lancet Psychiatry*, **2**(10): 871–73.
8 Keefe, P.R. (2021). *Empire of Pain: The Secret History of the Sackler Dynasty* (London: Picador).

Chapter 2

1 In the year April to April 2010–11, 43.4 million prescriptions of antidepressants were issued in England. In 2021–22, 83.4 million prescriptions were issued. In 1990, less than 10 million prescriptions were issued. Sources: Batty, D. (2011), 'Antidepressant Use in England Soars', *The Guardian*, www.theguardian.com/society/2011/dec/30/antidepressant-use-england-soars (accessed 1 May 2023); Burns, C. (2022), 'Antidepressant Prescribing Increases by 35% in Six Years', *The Pharmaceutical Journal* (8 July 2022), https://pharmaceutical-journal.com/article/news/antidepressant-prescribing-increases-by-35-in-six-years (accessed 1 May 2023); Middleton, N., Gunnell, D., Whitley, E. et al. (2001), 'Secular Trends in Antidepressant Prescribing in the UK, 1975–1998', *Journal of Public Health Medicine*, 23: 262–67.
2 Data on the number of people and adults taking antidepressants in England in the year April 2022 to April 2023 is from www.nhsbsa.nhs.uk/statistical-collections/medicines-used-mental-health-england/medicines-used-mental-health-england-201516-202223 (accessed 13 March 2024). The percentage of the adult population taking antidepressants was calculated using latest figures on the population of England, https://lginform.local.gov.uk/reports/lgastandard?mod-area=E92000001&mod-group=AllRegions_England&mod-metric=173&mod-type=namedComparisonGroup (accessed 13 March 2024). The percentage of adult women taking antidepressants comes from www.

england.nhs.uk/long-read/optimising-personalised-care-for-adults-prescribed-medicines-associated-with-dependence-or-withdrawal-symptoms/ (accessed 13 March 2024).

3 Perlis, R.H., Ramachandiran, A.K., Verhaak, P.F., Santillana, M., Baum, M.A. et al. (2026), 'Antidepressant use among American adults in a 50-state survey', *BMJ Mental Health* **29**(1): e302287.

4 Mojtabai, R., & Olfson, M. (2014). 'National Trends in Long-Term Use of Antidepressant Medications: Results from the U.S. National Health and Nutrition Examination Survey', *Journal of Clinical Psychiatry*, **75**(2): 169–77, doi:10.4088/JCP.13m08443.

5 Taylor, S.; Annand, F.; Burkinshaw, P.; Greaves, F.; Kelleher, M.; Knight, J. et al. (2019). *Dependence and Withdrawal Associated with Some Prescribed Medicines: An Evidence Review* (London: Public Health England) (for the 18% figure), and www.england.nhs.uk/long-read/optimising-personalised-care-for-adults-prescribed-medicines-associated-with-dependence-or-withdrawal-symptoms/ (for the two-thirds figure), accessed 13 March 2024.

6 Including drugs for bipolar disorder, antipsychotics and stimulants. See Ilyas, S., & Moncrieff, J. (2012). 'Trends in Prescriptions and Costs of Drugs for Mental Disorders in England, 1998–2010', *British Journal of Psychiatry*, **200**(5): 393–98. Available at: www.cambridge.org/core/journals/the-british-journal-of-psychiatry/article/trends-in-prescriptions-and-costs-of-drugs-for-mental-disorders-in-england-19982010/2F552E3BFF33EC63C302D86CFE1A1097.

7 Available here: www.nature.com/articles/s41380-022-01661-0 (full reference in notes to Preface).

8 www.altmetric.com/details/132834624. Altmetric (alternative metrics) tracks the online attention a publication receives.

9 This was said by Alison Hammond during *This Morning*'s coverage of the serotonin paper on 21 July 2022.

10 See Chapters 9 and 15 for more details. Sources include: Science Media Centre (2022), 'Expert Reaction to a Review Paper on the "Serotonin Theory of Depression"', www.sciencemediacentre.org/expert-reaction-to-a-review-paper-on-the-serotonin-theory-of-depression/ (accessed 1 May 2023); article in *The Conversation*, McIntosh, A.M., & Lewis, C. (2022), https://theconversation.com/depression-low-serotonin-may-not-be-the-cause-but-antidepressants-still-work-187477 (accessed 1 May 2023); Jauhar S.; Arnone, D.; Baldwin, D.; Bloomfield, M.; Browning, M. et al. (2023), 'A Leaky Umbrella has Little Value: Evidence Clearly Indicates the Serotonin System is Implicated in Depression', *Molecular Psychiatry*, **28**(8): 3149–152.

11 Kendrick, T., & Collinson, S. (2022). 'Antidepressants and the Serotonin Hypothesis of Depression', *British Medical Journal*, *378*, 1993, doi:10.1136/bmj.o199. The accusation about causing suicide is from a tweet by Dr James Rucker, 6 December 2023 (accessed 10 December 2023).

12 Spichak, S. (2022). 'How the Debate Over Antidepressants Puts Millions in Danger', *Daily Beast* (20 September 2022). Retrieved from www.thedailybeast.com/the-debate-over-how-antidepressants-work-is-putting-millions-of-

people-in-danger; Dickson, E. (2022), 'Who is the Psychiatrist Behind the Antidepressant Study Taking Over Right-Wing Media?', *Rolling Stone*. Retrieved from www.rollingstone.com/culture/culture-news/ssri-right-wing-attack-joanna-moncrieff-1388067/.

13 Bansal, N.; Hudda, M.; Payne, R.A.; Smith, D.J.; Kessler, D.; & Wiles, N. (2022), 'Antidepressant Use and Risk of Adverse Outcomes: Population-Based Cohort Study', *British Journal of Psychiatry Open*, **8**(5): e164; Dragioti, E.; Solmi, M.; Favaro, A.; Fusar-Poli, P.; Dazzan, P.; Thompson, T. et al. (2019), 'Association of Antidepressant Use With Adverse Health Outcomes: A Systematic Umbrella Review', *JAMA Psychiatry*, **76**(12): 1241–255.

14 Mercurio, M.; de Filippis, R.; Spina, G.; De Fazio, P.; Segura-Garcia, C.; Galasso, O. et al. (2022). 'The Use of Antidepressants is Linked to Bone Loss: A Systematic Review and Metanalysis'. *Orthopedic Reviews (Pavia)*, **14**(6): 38564; Dragioti, E. et al. (2019). 'Association of Antidepressant Use With Adverse Health Outcomes: A Systematic Umbrella Review'.

15 Sharma, T.; Guski, L.S.; Freund, N.; & Gotzsche, P.C. (2016). 'Suicidality and Aggression During Antidepressant Treatment: Systematic Review and Meta-Analyses Based on Clinical Study Reports', *British Medical Journal*, **352**: i65.

16 Hengartner, M.P.; Schulthess, L.; Sorensen, A.; & Framer, A. (2020). 'Protracted Withdrawal Syndrome After Stopping Antidepressants: A Descriptive Quantitative Analysis of Consumer Narratives from a Large Internet Forum', *Therapeutic Advances in Psychopharmacology*, **10**: 2045125320980573 and Moncrieff, J.; Read, J.; & Horowitz, M. (2024). 'The Nature and Impact of Antidepressant Withdrawal Symptoms and Proposal of the Discriminatory Antidepressant Withdrawal Symptoms Scale (DAWSS)', *Journal of Affective Disorder Reports*, in press.

17 Moore, J. (2021). 'RIP: Ed White – Advocate, Researcher and Supporter', www.madinamerica.com/2021/10/rip-ed-white-advocate-researcher-supporter/ (accessed 1 May 2023). Also Levy, M. (2020). '"All hell broke loose": The truth about coming off of anti-depressants', *The Telegraph*, 8 November 2020: www.telegraph.co.uk/health-fitness/wellbeing/mental-health/broke-loose-truth-coming-anti-depressants/ (accessed 14 March 2024).

18 Healy, D.; Le Noury, J.; & Mangin, D. (2018). 'Enduring Sexual Dysfunction After Treatment with Antidepressants, 5alpha-Reductase Inhibitors and Isotretinoin: 300 Cases', *International Journal of Risk & Safety in Medicine*, **29**(3–4): 125–34; Goldsmith, L.; & Moncrieff, J. (2011). 'The Psychoactive Effects of Antidepressants and Their Association With Suicidality', *Current Drug Safety*, **6**(2): 115–21.

19 Quotations from www.pssdnetwork.org/picture-awareness-campaign (accessed 1 May 2023).

20 Jelen, L.A., Stone, J.M., Young, A.H. & Mehta, M.A. (2022), 'The opioid system in depression', *Neuroscience & Biobehavioral Reviews* **140**: 104800.

21 France, C.M.; Lysaker, P.H.; & Robinson, R.P. (2007). 'The "Chemical Imbalance" Explanation for Depression: Origins, Lay Endorsement, and Clinical Implications', *Professional psychology: Research and Practice*: 411–20; Pilkington,

P.D.; Reavley, N.J.; & Jorm, A.F. (2013). 'The Australian Public's Beliefs About the Causes of Depression: Associated Factors and Changes over 16 Years', *Journal of Affective Disorders,* **150**(2): 356–62.

22 Cited in Moncrieff, J. (2014). 'The Chemical Imbalance Theory of Depression: Still Promoted But Still Unfounded' at https://joannamoncrieff.com/2014/05/01/the-chemical-imbalance-theory-of-depression-still-promoted-but-still-unfounded/ (accessed 1 May 2023).

23 Cited in Conneely, M.; Higgs, P.; & Moncrieff, J. (2021). 'Medicalising the Moral: The Case of Depression as Revealed in Internet Blogs', *Social Theory and Health,* **19**: 380–98.

24 This statement was prefaced by 'while the cause [of depression] is unknown', but the latter was said in a rapid-fire 'terms and conditions' tone that is difficult to catch. The advert is cited in Lacasse, J.R., & Leo, J. (2005). 'Serotonin and Depression: A Disconnect between the Advertisements and the Scientific Literature', *PLoS.Medicine,* **2**(12): e392. Also available at www.youtube.com/watch?v=twhvtzd6gXA&list=PLTvBonT9IGLswtvolxp9MmsI_Xqo4nWlU&index=1 (accessed 4 March 2024).

25 Cited in Lacasse & Leo (2005), 'Serotonin and Depression', from www.celexa.com/Celexa/faq.aspx (accessed 17 October 2005).

26 American Psychiatric Association (2024). 'What is Depression?', www.psychiatry.org/patients-families/depression/what-is-depression (accessed 8 February 2024).

27 Brendel, R. (2023). www.youtube.com/watch?v=b2Gbjbj8FOg&t=689s (accessed 28 February 2024).

28 https://blogs.bmj.com/bmj/2020/09/25/wendy-burn-medical-community-must-ensure-that-those-needing-support-to-come-off-anti-depressants-can-get-it/ (accessed 19 December 2023).

29 www.rcpsych.ac.uk/mental-health/treatments-and-wellbeing/antidepressants (accessed 29 April 2023).

30 Lacasse & Leo (2005). 'Serotonin and Depression: A Disconnect Between the Advertisements and the Scientific Literature', *PLoS.Medicine,* **2**(12): e392. Available at: https://journals.plos.org/plosmedicine/article?id=10.1371/journal.pmed.0020392.

31 Anonymous (2005). 'Television Adverts for Antidepressants Cause Anxiety', *New Scientist,* **2525**, available at https://institutions.newscientist.com/article/mg18825252-500-television-adverts-for-antidepressants-cause-anxiety/; Meek, C. (2006). 'SSRI Ads Questioned', *Canadian Medical Association Journal News,* **174:** 754 www.cmaj.ca/cgi/content/full/174/6/754-a (accessed 1 May 2023).

32 Pies, R.W. (2011). 'Psychiatry's New Brain-Mind and the Legend of the "Chemical Imbalance"', *Psychiatric Times,* 11 July 2011, www.psychiatrictimes.com/view/psychiatrys-new-brain-mind-and-legend-chemical-imbalance (accessed 1 May 2023).

33 Biogenic amine is another term for a monoamine and the monoamine theory is the original version of the chemical imbalance theory of depression as explained in Chapter 5. Monoamines (or biogenic amines) include serotonin.

34 The two blogs are these: Pies, R.W. (2011). 'Psychiatry's New Brain-Mind and the Legend of the "Chemical Imbalance"', *Psychiatric Times*, 11 July 2011, www.psychiatrictimes.com/view/psychiatrys-new-brain-mind-and-legend-chemical-imbalance (accessed 1 May 2023) and Pies, R.W. (2011). 'Doctor, Is My Mood Disorder Due to a Chemical Imbalance?', *Psychiatric Times*, 12 August 2011, www.psychiatrictimes.com/view/doctor-my-mood-disorder-due-chemical-imbalance (accessed 8 February 2024).

Chapter 3

1 Nutt, D.J., & Malizia, A.L. (2008). 'Why does the world have such a "down" on antidepressants?', *Journal of Psychopharmacology*, **22**(3): 223–26.

2 'Naked Scientist', 18 July 2023: www.thenakedscientists.com/podcasts/naked-scientists-podcast/antidepressants-ongoing-debate.

3 Pariente, C. (2023). 'The Drugs do Work', *New Humanist*, Winter 2023, 22–25 (accessed 20 December 2023).

4 You can read Cathy's own account here: https://cathywield.com/about-2/ (accessed 29 May 2024).

5 www.madinamerica.com/2023/12/escaping-the-shackles-of-psychiatry-what-ive-seen-and-survived-as-both-doctor-and-patient/ (posted 1 December 2023; accessed 12 January 2024).

6 *Ibid.*

7 There is more detail about such claims with some examples in Chapter 8.

8 https://z-p3.www.instagram.com/p/CJWeUmDgU4U/ (Posted on 20 December 2020; accessed 12 January 2024). Note the name 'serotonin' does not derive from 'serenity' but from 'serum', meaning blood.

9 Bennett, M.R., & P.M.S. Hacker (2003). *Philosophical Foundations of Neuroscience* (Oxford: Blackwell Publishing). The quote is from Patterson, D. (2003). 'Philosophical Foundations of Neuroscience: A Review', *Notre Dame Philosophical Reviews*, https://ndpr.nd.edu/reviews/philosophical-foundations-of-neuroscience/ (accessed 8 March 2024). Bennett and Hacker's new book, *The Representational Fallacy in Neuroscience and Psychology: A Critical Analysis* (Palgrave Macmillan), is due out in 2025.

10 In the following account, I have particularly drawn from Hacker, P.M.S. (1997). *Wittgenstein* (London: Phoenix); Hacker, P.M.S. (2010), *Human Nature: The Categorial Framework* (Oxford: Wiley-Blackwell) and Hacker, P.M.S. (2017). *The Passions: A Study of Human Nature* (Oxford: Wiley Blackwell).

11 Hacker (2017), p. 17.

12 Johnstone, L.B., & Boyle, M., with Cromby, J.; Dillon, J.; Harper, D.; Kinderman, P.; Longden, E.; Pilgrim, D. & Read, J. (2018). *The Power Threat Meaning Framework: Towards the identification of patterns in emotional distress, unusual experiences and troubled or troubling behaviour, as an alternative to functional psychiatric diagnosis* (Leicester: British Psychological Society) p. 14.

13 The meaning of diagnosis in mental health is well described in Johnstone et al. (2018).

14 American Psychiatric Association (2013). *Diagnostic and Statistical Manual of Mental Disorders (5th edition)* (Washington DC: American Psychiatric Association).

15 Kennis, M.; Gerritsen, L.; van Dalen, M.; Williams, A.; Cuijpers, P.; & Bockting, C. (2020). 'Prospective Biomarkers of Major Depressive Disorder: A Systematic Review and Meta-Analysis', *Molecular Psychiatry,* **25**(2): 321–38. Quotation p. 321. Available at: www.ncbi.nlm.nih.gov/pmc/articles/PMC6974432/.

16 Brown, G.W.; Andrews, B.; Harris, T.; Adler, Z.; & Bridge, L. (1986). 'Social Support, Self-Esteem and Depression', *Psychological Medicine,* **16**(4): 813–31.

17 Brown, G.W., & Harris, T.O. (1978). *Social Origins in Depression: A Study of Psychiatric Disorder in Women* (New York: Free Press).

18 Remes, O.; Mendes, J.F.; & Templeton, P. (2021). 'Biological, Psychological, and Social Determinants of Depression: A Review of Recent Literature', *Brain Sciences,* **11**(12); and Pevalin, D.J.; Reeves, A.; Baker, E.; & Bentley, R. (2017). 'The Impact of Persistent Poor Housing Conditions on Mental Health: A Longitudinal Population-Based Study', *Preventive Medicine,* **105**: 304–10.

19 Kim, Y.; Park, A.; Murphy, J. (2023). 'Patterns of Adverse Childhood Experiences and Mental Health: Evidence From College Students in Korea', *Journal of Interpersonal Violence,* **38**(3–4): 3011–29; and Cheong, E.V.; Sinnott, C.; Dahly, D.; & Kearney, P.M. (2017). 'Adverse Childhood Experiences (ACEs) and Later-Life Depression: Perceived Social Support as a Potential Protective Factor', *British Medical Journal Open,* **7**(9): e013228.

20 LaNoue, M.; Graeber, D.; de Hernandez, B.U.; Warner, T.D.; & Helitzer, D.L. (2012). 'Direct and Indirect Effects of Childhood Adversity on Adult Depression', *Community Mental Health Journal,* **48**(2): 187–92.

21 World Health Organization and the United Nations (represented by the Office of the United Nations High Commissioner for Human Rights) (2023). *Mental Health, Human Rights and Legislation. Guidance and Practice*. Geneva, quote on p. xvii. Available at: www.who.int/publications/i/item/9789240080737.

22 Moncrieff, J. (2020). '"It Was the Brain Tumor That Done It!": Szasz and Wittgenstein on the Importance of Distinguishing Disease from Behavior and Implications for the Nature of Mental Disorder', *Philosophy, Psychiatry, and Psychology,* **27**: 169–81. Available at https://discovery.ucl.ac.uk/id/eprint/10105606/.

23 E.g. psychiatrists, including Thomas Szasz and R.D. Laing, medical sociologists, such as Peter Conrad, and philosophers, including Michel Foucault.

24 Bowden, G.; Shankar, R.; Cooke, A.; & Kinderman, P. (2020). *Understanding Depression: Why Adults Experience Depression and What Can Help* (Leicester: British Psychological Society). Available at https://explore.bps.org.uk/content/report-guideline/bpsrep.2020.rep133. Quote from p. 16.

25 Puras, D. (2019). 'Report of the Special Rapporteur on the Right of Everyone to the Enjoyment of the Highest Attainable Standard of Physical and Mental Health', United Nations Human Rights Council, 24–12 June. Quote from p. 11. Retrieved from: www.ohchr.org/en/documents/thematic-reports/ahrc4134-right-everyone-enjoyment-highest-attainable-standard-physical (accessed 12 January 2024).

26 Hari, J. (2018). *Lost Connections: Uncovering the Real Causes of Depression and the Unexpected Solutions* (London: Bloomsbury).
27 WHO-UN (2023), p. xvii.
28 Parker, G. (2005). 'Melancholia', *American Journal of Psychiatry,* **162**(6): 1066.
29 Mundt, C.; Reck, C.; Backenstrass, M.; Kronmuller, K.; & Fiedler, P. (2000), 'Reconfirming the Role of Life Events for the Timing of Depressive Episodes. A Two-Year Prospective Follow-Up Study', *Journal of Affective Disorders,* **59**(1): 23–30; Harkness, K.L., & S.M. Monroe (2002), 'Childhood Adversity and the Endogenous Versus Nonendogenous Distinction in Women with Major Depression', *American Journal of Psychiatry,* **159**(3): 387–93.
30 www.madinamerica.com/2023/12/escaping-the-shackles-of-psychiatry-what-ive-seen-and-survived-as-both-doctor-and-patient/.
31 Kemp, J.J.; Lickel, J.J.; & Deacon, B.J. (2014). 'Effects of a chemical imbalance causal explanation on individuals' perceptions of their depressive symptoms', *Behavior Research & Therapy,* **56**: 47–52: www.sciencedirect.com/science/article/pii/S0005796714000308?via%3Dihub.
32 Schroder, H.S.; Duda, J.M.; Christensen, K.; Beard, C.; & Bjorgvinsson, T. (2020). 'Stressors and Chemical Imbalances: Beliefs About the Causes of Depression in an Acute Psychiatric Treatment Sample', *Journal of Affective Disorders,* **276**: 537–45.
33 Email received from Cathy Wield, 12 December 2023.

Chapter 4

1 www.independent.co.uk/voices/antidepressants-study-new-research-depression-medication-a8223801.html.
2 My work on models of drug action includes Moncrieff, J., & Cohen, D. (2005), 'Rethinking Models of Psychotropic Drug Action', *Psychotherapy & Psychosomatics,* **74**(3): 145–53 (available at: www.criticalpsychiatry.co.uk/wp-content/uploads/docs/rethinking-models-of-psychotropic-drug-action.pdf); Moncrieff, J., & Cohen, D. (2006), 'Do Antidepressants Cure or Create Abnormal Brain States?', *PLoS.Medicine,* **3**(7): e240; www.ncbi.nlm.nih.gov/pmc/articles/PMC1472553/#:~:text=The%20term%20antidepressant%20refers%20to,to%20the%20symptoms%20of%20depression; Moncrieff, J. (2008). *The Myth of the Chemical Cure: A Critique of Psychiatric Drug Treatment* (Basingstoke, UK: Palgrave Macmillan); and Moncrieff, J. (2020). *A Straight Talking Introduction to Psychiatric Drugs: The truth About How They Work and How to Come Off Them* (Monmouth: PCCS Books).
3 See glossary.
4 For the unpleasant nature of antidepressants, see Goldsmith, L., & Moncrieff, J. (2011). 'The Psychoactive Effects of Antidepressants and Their Association With Suicidality', *Current Drug Safety,* **6**(2): 115–21. For antipsychotics see: Moncrieff, J.; Cohen, D.; & Mason, J.P. (2009). 'The Subjective Experience of Taking Antipsychotic Medication: A Content Analysis of Internet Data', *Acta Psychiatrica Scandinavica,* **120**(2): 102–11.

5 He, Q.; Chen, X.; Wu, T.; Li, L.; & Fei, X. (2019), 'Risk of Dementia in Long-Term Benzodiazepine Users: Evidence from a Meta-Analysis of Observational Studies', *Journal of Clinical Neurology,* **15**(1): 9–19; Reid Finlayson, A.J.; Macoubrie, J.; Huff, C.; Foster, D.E.; & Martin, P.R. (2022). 'Experiences with Benzodiazepine Use, Tapering, and Discontinuation: An Internet Survey', *Therapeutic Advances in Psychopharmacology,* **12**: 20451253221082386.

6 Spurny, B.; Vanicek, T.; Seiger, R.; Reed, M.B.; Klobl, M. et al. (2021), 'Effects of SSRI Treatment on GABA and Glutamate Levels in an Associative Relearning Paradigm', *Neuroimage,* **232**: 117913; Duman, E.N.; Kesim, M.; Kadioglu, M.; Yaris, E.; Kalyoncu, N.I.; & Erciyes, N. (2004), 'Possible Involvement of Opioidergic and Serotonergic Mechanisms in Antinociceptive Effect of Paroxetine in Acute Pain', *Journal of Pharmacological Science,* **94**(2): 161–65.

7 https://patient.info/forums/discuss/no-emotions-29959.

8 Aitken, C. (2019). '3 Myths About Bupropion', *Psychiatric Times,* 4 April, 2019, www.psychiatrictimes.com/view/3-myths-about-bupropion (accessed 16 March 2024).

9 www.askapatient.com/viewrating.asp?drug=204447&name=TRINTELLIX.

10 D'Agostino, A.; English, C.D.; & Rey, J.A. (2015). 'Vortioxetine (Brintellix): A New Serotonergic Antidepressant', *Pharmacy & Therapeutics T,* **40**(1): 36–40.

11 Corruble, E.; de Bodinat, C.; Belaidi, C.; Goodwin, G.M.; & Agomelatine Study Group (2013). 'Efficacy of agomelatine and escitalopram on depression, subjective sleep and emotional experiences in patients with major depressive disorder: a 24-wk randomized, controlled, double-blind trial', *International Journal of Neuropsychopharmacology,* **16**(10): 2219–34.

12 From Goldsmith, L., & Moncrieff, J. (2011). 'The Psychoactive Effects of Antidepressants and Their Association with Suicidality', *Current Drug Safety,* **6**(2): 115–21, p. 117. Available at https://openaccess.city.ac.uk/id/eprint/31252/3/Goldsmith%20and%20Moncrieff%202011%20The%20Psychoactive%20Effects%20of%20Antidepressants%20and%20their%20Association%20with%20Suicidality%20Protected.pdf.

13 www.mayoclinic.org/diseases-conditions/depression/in-depth/antidepressants/art-20049305#:~:text=Fatigue%2C%20drowsiness,of%20treatment%20with%20an%20antidepressant (accessed 16 January 2024).

14 Alberti, S.; Chiesa, A.; Andrisano, C.; & Serretti, A. (2015). 'Insomnia and Somnolence Associated with Second-Generation Antidepressants During the Treatment of Major Depression: A Meta-Analysis', *Journal of Clinical Psychopharmacology,* **35**(3): 296–303.

15 Gafoor, R.; Booth, H.P.; & Gulliford, M.C. (2018). 'Antidepressant Utilisation and Incidence of Weight Gain During 10 Years' Follow-Up: Population Based Cohort Study', *British Medical Journal,* **361**: k1951.

16 Read, J.; Grigoriu, M.; Gee, A.; Diggle, J.; & Butler, H. (2020). 'The Positive and Negative Experiences of 342 Antidepressant Users', *Community Mental Health Journal,* **56**(4): 744–52, p. 748 (available at https://repository.uel.ac.uk/item/87673).

17 Breggin, P.R. (1993). *Toxic Psychiatry* (London: Fontana) p. 21.

18 An example is a critique by Tufts University psychiatrist, Nassir Ghaemi: Ghaemi, S.N. (2022). 'Symptomatic Versus Disease-Modifying Effects of Psychiatric Drugs', *Acta Psychiatrica Scandinavica,* **146**(3): 251–57, https://pubmed.ncbi.nlm.nih.gov/35653111/.
19 For example, in Crombie, J.; Harper, D.; & Reavey, P. (2013). *Psychology, Mental Health and Distress* (London: Red Globe Press).
20 Moreton, A.; Adam, M.; & Huda, A.S. (2018), 'Psychiatrists Use an Outcome Centered Prescribing Model', available at www.researchgate.net/publication/331400365_Psychiatrists'_use_an_outcome_centered_prescribing_model.

Chapter 5

1 'Discussion on Benzedrine: Uses and Abuses', *Proceedings of the Royal Society of Medicine,* **XXXII** (1938) 385–98, p. 391, www.ncbi.nlm.nih.gov/pmc/articles/PMC1997460/pdf/procrsmed00670-0135.pdf.
2 Adverts reproduced in Rasmussen, N. (2008). 'America's First Amphetamine Epidemic 1929–1971: A Quantitative and Qualitative Retrospective with Implications for the Present', *American Journal of Public Health,* **98**(6): 974–85.
3 For example, the advert for phenobarbital by Lakeside, available at www.pharmacytechs.net/blog/old-school-medicine-ads/ (accessed 16 February 2024).
4 Healy, D. (1997). *The Antidepressant Era* (New York, Harvard University Press), p. 62.
5 I have described the evolution antidepressants and views about depression in more detail in this paper: Moncrieff, J. (2008). 'The Creation of the Concept of the Antidepressant: An Historical Analysis', *Social Science and Medicine,* **66**: 2346–55, available at www.researchgate.net/publication/5529987_The_creation_of_the_concept_of_an_antidepressant_An_historical_analysis.
6 Crane, G.E. (1956). 'Further Studies on Iproniazid Phosphate', *Journal of Nervous and Mental Disease,* **124**: 322–31; Pare, C.M. & Sandler, M. (1959). 'A Clinical and Biochemical Study of a Trial of Iproniazid in the Treatment of Depression', *Journal of Neurology, Neurosurgery & Psychiatry,* **22**(3): 247–51.
7 Lehmann, H.E., et al. (1958). 'The Treatment of Depressive Conditions with Imipramine (G 22355)', *Canadian Psychiatric Association Journal,* **3**(4): 155–64 (p. 155).
8 See my accounts of this in Moncrieff, J. (2013). *The Bitterest Pills: The Troubling Story of Antipsychotic Drugs* (London: Palgrave Macmillan) and Moncrieff, J. (2013). 'Magic Bullets for Mental Disorders: The Emergence of the Concept of an "Antipsychotic" Drug', *Journal of the History of Neuroscience,* **22**(1): 30–46.
9 Crane, G.E. (1957). 'Iproniazid (Marsilid) Phosphate, a Therapeutic Agent for Mental Disorders and Debilitating Diseases', *Psychiatric Research Reports of the American Psychiatric Association,* **8**: 142–52.
10 Kline, N.S. (1958). 'Clinical Experience with Iproniazid (Marsilid)', *Journal of Clinical & Experimental Psychopathology,* **19**(2, Suppl. 1): 72–78 and discussion

78–79; Loomer, H.P.; Saunders, J.C.; & Kline, N.S. (1957). 'A Clinical and Pharmacodynamic Evaluation of Iproniazid as a Psychic Energizer', *Psychiatric Research Reports of the American Psychiatric Association*, **8**: 129–41.

11 Kuhn, R. (1957). '[Treatment of depressive states with an iminodibenzyl derivative (G 22355).]', *Schweizerische Medizinische Wochenschrift*, **87**(35–36): 1135–40; Kuhn, R. (1958) (in German). 'The Treatment of Depressive States with G 22355 (Imipramine Hydrochloride)', *American Journal of Psychiatry*, **115**(5): 459–64. Quotes from Kuhn (1958), on pp. 459 and 464.

12 Interview with Roland Kuhn in Healy, D. (1999), *The Psychopharmacologists. Volume II* (London: Arnold) pp. 93–118. Interview with Alan Broadhurst in Healy, D. (1996). *The Psychopharmacologists. Interviews by David Healy. Volume I* (London: Chapman & Hall) pp. 111–34.

13 Kuhn (1958), 'The Treatment of Depressive States with G 22355', p. 460.

14 Kuhn, R. (1970). 'The Imipramine Story', *Discoveries in Biological Psychiatry* (F. Ayd and B. Blackwell. Philadelphia, JB Lippincott Company) pp. 205–17 (p. 214).

15 Interview with David Healy in Healy (1999), *The Psychopharmacologists*, p. 99.

16 Hare, E.H.; McCance, C.; & McCormick, W.O. (1964). 'Imipramine and Drinamyl in Depressive Illness: a Comparative Trial', *British Medical Journal*, **1**: 818–20 (p. 819).

17 Overall, J.E.; Hollister, L.E.; Meyer, F.; Kimbell Jr, I.; & Shelton, J. (1964). 'Imipramine and Thioridazine in Depressed and Schizophrenic Patients. Are There Specific Antidepressant Drugs?' *Journal of the American Medical Association (JAMA)*, **189**: 605–08.

18 Jacobsen, E. (1964). 'The Theoretical Basis of the Chemotherapy of Depression', *Depression: Proceedings of the Symposium held at Cambridge 22 to 26 September 1959* (Cambridge: Cambridge University Press) 208–13 (p. 210).

19 Deniker, P., & Lemperiere, T. (1964). 'Drug Treatment of Depression', *Depression: Proceedings of the Symposium held at Cambridge 22 to 26 September 1959* (Cambridge: Cambridge University Press) 214–34 (p. 230).

20 Dally, P. (1967). *Chemotherapy of Psychiatric Disorders* (London: Logos Press Ltd) p. 10.

21 See Moncrieff, J. (2008), 'The Creation of the Concept of the Antidepressant'.

22 Henderson, D., & Gillespie, R.D. (1927). *Henderson and Gillespie's Textbook of Psychiatry* (Oxford: Oxford University Press) p. 254.

23 Rasmussen, N. (2015). 'Amphetamine-Type Stimulants: The Early History of their Medical and Non-Medical Uses', *International Review of Neurobiology*, **120**: 9–25.

24 I have written more about the links between the physical treatment procedures like ECT and newly emerging drug treatments in this paper: Moncrieff, J. (1999). 'An Investigation into the Precedents of Modern Drug Treatment in Psychiatry', *History of Psychiatry*, **10**(40 Pt 4): 475–90. Available at: www.researchgate.net/publication/11727695_An_investigation_into_the_precedents_of_modern_drug_treatment_in_psychiatry.

25 Healy, D. (1997). *The Antidepressant Era* (Cambridge, MA: Harvard University Press).

26 David Healy has also conducted research on the pharmacology of psychiatric drugs and campaigns to draw attention to unrecognised side-effects of prescribed medicines through his website, https://rxisk.org/. His book on the history of antidepressants is Healy, D. (1997). *The Antidepressant Era.*

27 Bayer, R., & Spitzer, R.L. (1985). 'Neurosis, Psychodynamics, and DSM-III: A History of the Controversy', *Archives of General Psychiatry,* **42**(2): 187–96.

28 The term 'sympathetic' derived from the idea of connection between different parts of the body. A history of the term is provided by Barboi, A. (2013). 'Sympathy, Sympathetic: Evolution of a Concept and Relevance to Current Understanding of Autonomic Disorders', *Neurology,* **80**, Supplement 7, www.neurology.org/doi/10.1212/wnl.80.7_supplement.s57.005 (accessed 7 February 2024).

29 Churchill-Davidson, H.C., & Swan, H.J.C. (1952). 'Noradrenaline and Methedrine: A Comparison of Their Circulatory Actions', *Anaesthesia,* **7**: 4. Also see Rasmussen, 2015.

30 This view is put forward tentatively in a symposium held in 1959: Jacobsen, E. (1964). 'The Theoretical Basis of the Chemotherapy of Depression', *Depression: Proceedings of the Symposium held at Cambridge 22 to 26 September 1959* (Cambridge: Cambridge University Press) 208–13, and then more assertively in the seminal paper on the noradrenaline theory of depression by Joseph Schildkraut: Schildkraut, J.J. (1965). 'The Catecholamine Hypothesis of Affective Disorders: A Review of Supporting Evidence', *American Journal of Psychiatry,* **122**(5): 509–22.

31 Larkin Jr, J.C.; Stevick, C.P.; Flanagan, J.B.; & Phillips, S. (1959). 'Stimulatory Effects of Iproniazid in Active Pulmonary Tuberculosis', *Geriatrics,* **14**(2): 89–93.

32 Zeller, E.A., & Barsky, J. (1952). 'In Vivo Inhibition of Liver and Brain Monoamine Oxidase by 1-Isonicotinyl-2-Isopropyl Hydrazine', *Proceedings of the Society for Experimental Biology & Medicine,* **81**(2): 459–61.

33 Interview in Healy, D. (1996). *The Psychopharmacologists. Interviews by David Healy. Volume I* (London: Chapman & Hall) pp. 29–50.

34 Axelrod, J., et al. (1961). 'Effect of Psychotropic Drugs on the Uptake of H3-norepinephrine by Tissues', *Science,* **133**(3450): 383–84.

35 Glowinski, J., & Axelrod, J. (1964). 'Inhibition of Uptake of Tritiated-Noradrenaline in the Intact Rat Brain by Imipramine and Structurally Related Compounds', *Nature* **204**: 1318–19.

36 Khan, S.A.; Mehta, M.C.; & Kade, A. (2011). 'Acute Effects of Citalopram and Imipramine on Psychomotor Performance in Healthy Volunteers: A Comparative Study', *Journal of Pharmaceutical Sciences and Research,* **3**: 1269–75.

37 Schildkraut, J.J.; Winokur, A.; & Applegate, C.W. (1970). 'Norepinephrine Turnover and Metabolism in Rat Brain After Long-Term Administration of Imipramine', *Science,* **168**(933): 867–69; Frazer, A., & Mendels, J. (1977). 'Do Tricyclic Antidepressants Enhance Adrenergic Transmission?', *American Journal of Psychiatry,* **134**(9): 1040–42; Heydorn, W.; Frazer, A.; & Mendels, J. (1980). 'Do Tricyclic Antidepressants Enhance Adrenergic Transmission? An Update', *American Journal of Psychiatry,* **137**(1): 113–14.

38 Lahti, R.A., & Maickel, R.P. (1971). 'The Tricyclic Antidepressants – Inhibition of Norepinephrine Uptake as Related to Potentiation of Norepinephrine and Clinical Efficacy', *Biochemical Pharmacology*, **20**: 482–86.
39 Khan, A.U. (1999). 'How do Psychotropic Drugs Really Work?' *Psychiatric Times*, **16**.
40 See, for example, this essay about Axelrod's work: Snyder, S.H. (2006). 'Turning Off Neurotransmitters', *Cell*, **125**(1): 13–15.
41 Schildkraut, J.J. (1965). 'The Catecholamine Hypothesis of Affective Disorders: A Review of Supporting Evidence', *American Journal of Psychiatry*, **122**(5): 509–22 (quote p. 509), https://ajp.psychiatryonline.org/doi/abs/10.1176/ajp.122.5.509.
42 Marano, M. (2023). 'Reserpine Induced Parkinsonism: A Hidden Threat of Herbal Medicine', *Neurological Sciences*, **44**(4): 1425–27.
43 Schildkraut (1965) quotes pp. 509 & 512.
44 *Ibid.*, p. 511.
45 See Lees, A.J.; Tolosa, E.; & Olanow, C.W. (2015). 'Four Pioneers of L-Dopa Treatment: Arvid Carlsson, Oleh Hornykiewicz, George Cotzias, and Melvin Yahr', *Movement Disorders*, **30**(1): 19–36; also Healy (1997), p. 151. The early experiment to suggests dopamine was the key neurotransmitter involved in reserpine's effects is this one: Carlsson, A.; Lindqvist, M.; & Magnusson, T. (1957). '3,4-Dihydroxyphenylalanine and 5-Hydroxytryptophan as Reserpine Antagonists', *Nature* **180**(4596): 1200.

Chapter 6

1 Whitaker-Azmitia, P. (1999). 'The Discovery of Serotonin and its Role in Neuroscience', *Neuropsychopharmacology*, **21**: 2–8.
2 Green, A.R. (2008). 'Gaddum and LSD: The Birth and Growth of Experimental and Clinical Neuropharmacology Research on 5-HT in the UK', *British Journal of Pharmacology*, **154**(8): 1583–99.
3 Twarog, B.M., & Page, I.H. (1953). 'Serotonin Content of Some Mammalian Tissues and Urine and a Method for its Determination', *American Journal of Physiology*, **175**: 157–61.
4 Green (2008).
5 Aghajanian, G.K., & Marek, G.J. (1999). 'Serotonin and Hallucinogens', *Neuropsychopharmacology*, **21**(2 Suppl): 16S–23S.
6 Woolley, D.W., & Shaw, E. (1954). 'A Biochemical and Pharmacological Suggestion About Certain Mental Disorders', *Proceedings of the National Academy of Sciences, USA*, **40**(4): 228–31. Quote from p. 230 and Gaddum, J.H., &. Hameed, K.A. (1954). 'Drugs Which Antagonize 5-Hydroxytryptamine', *British Journal of Pharmacology & Chemotherapy*, **9**(2): 240–48.
7 Pare, C.M., & Sandler, M. (1959). 'A Clinical and Biochemical Study of a Trial of Iproniazid in the Treatment of Depression', *Journal of Neurology, Neurosurgery & Psychiatry*, **22**(3): 247–51.
8 Shore, P.A.; Pletscher, A.; Tomich, E.G.; Carlsson, A.; Kuntzman, R.; & Brodie, B.B. (1957). 'Role of Brain Serotonin in Reserpine Action', *Annals of the New York Academy of Sciences*, **66**(3): 609–15 (discussion, p. 615); Brodie, B.B.; Pletscher,

A.; & Shore, P.A. (1955). 'Evidence that Serotonin has a Role in Brain Function', *Science*, **122**(3177): 968; Brodie, B.B.; Comer, M.S.; Costa, E.; & Dlabac, A. (1966). 'The Role of Brain Serotonin in the Mechanism of the Central Action of Reserpine', *Journal of Pharmacology & Experimental Therapeutics*, **152**(2): 340–49. Also see Healy, D. (1997). *The Antidepressant Era* (New York: Harvard University Press).

9 Healy, D. (1997).

10 Coppen, A.; Shaw, D.M.; & Farrell, J.P. (1963). 'Potentiation of the Antidepressive Effect of a Monoamine-Oxidase Inhibitor by Tryptophan', *Lancet*, **1**(7272): 79–81.

11 Kline, N.S.; Sacks, W.; & Simpson, G.M. (1964). 'Further Studies On: One Day Treatment of Depression with 5-Htp', *American Journal of Psychiatry*, **121**: 379–81; Coppen, A.; Shaw, D.M.; Malleson, A.; Eccleston, E.; & Gundy, G. (1965). 'Tryptamine Metabolism in Depression', *British Journal of Psychiatry*, **111**(479): 993–98.

12 Coppen, A. (1967). 'The Biochemistry of Affective Disorders', *British Journal of Psychiatry*, **113**(504): 1237–64: www.cambridge.org/core/journals/the-british-journal-of-psychiatry/article/biochemistry-of-affective-disorders/1CB6D7B69D1E60F5731D4B8FBC02CE84; Coppen, A.J. (1968). 'Depressed States and Indolealkylamines', *Advances in Pharmacology* (1968) **6**(Pt B): 283–91, www.sciencedirect.com/science/article/pii/S1054358908603282.

13 Coppen (1967), p. 1237.

14 *Ibid.*, p. 1244.

15 *Ibid.*, p. 1243.

16 *Ibid.*, p. 1258.

17 Coppen (1968), p. 290.

18 Yeragani, V.K.; Tancer, M.; Chokka, P.; & Baker, G.B. (2010). 'Arvid Carlsson, and the Story of Dopamine', *Indian Journal of Psychiatry*, **52**(1): 87–88. Available at: www.ncbi.nlm.nih.gov/pmc/articles/PMC2824994/.

19 Kielholz, P., & Poeldinger, W. (1968). 'Pharmacotherapy of Endogenous Depression', *Comprehensive Psychiatry*, **9**(3): 179–86, https://pubmed.ncbi.nlm.nih.gov/5653730/.

20 Interview with Arvid Carlsson in Healy, D. (1996). *The Psychopharmacologists. Interviews by David Healy. Volume I* (London: Chapman) pp. 51–80 (p. 60).

21 https://pubchem.ncbi.nlm.nih.gov/compound/Zimeldine.

22 A useful history of zimelidine is provided in the following article: Mulinari, S. (2015). 'Divergence and Convergence of Commercial and Scientific Priorities in Drug Development: The Case of Zelmid, the First SSRI Antidepressant', *Social Science & Medicine*, **138**: 217–24. Available at https://pubmed.ncbi.nlm.nih.gov/26123880/.

23 Wong, D.T.; Horng, J.S.; Bymaster, F.P.; Hauser, K.L.; & Molloy, B.B. (1974). 'A Selective Inhibitor of Serotonin Uptake: Lilly 110140, 3-(p-trifluoromethylphenoxy)-N-methyl-3-phenylpropylamine', *Life Sciences*, **15**(3): 471–79 (p. 471).

24 *Ibid.*, p. 478.

25 Strawbridge, R.; Javed, R.R.; Cave, J.; Jauhar, S.; & Young, A.H. (2023). 'The Effects of Reserpine on Depression: A Systematic Review', *Journal of Psychopharmacology,* **37**(3): 248–60.
26 Interview with Arvid Carlsson in Healy, D. (1996), p. 60.
27 Healy highlighted how contradictory evidence was ignored or reinterpreted to fit the theory in the manner of a failing Kuhnian paradigm (after the philosopher of science Thomas Kuhn): Healy, D. (1987). 'The Structure of Psychopharmacological Revolutions', *Psychiatric Developments,* **5**(4): 349–76.
28 Maas, J.W.; Koslow, S.H.; Davis, J.M.; Katz, M.M.; Mendels, J.; Robins, E. et al. (1980). 'Biological Component of the NIMH Clinical Research Branch Collaborative Program on the Psychobiology of Depression: I. Background and Theoretical Considerations', *Psychological Medicine,* **10**(4): 759–76.
29 Maas, J.W.; Koslow, S.H.; Katz, M.M.; Bowden, C.L.; Gibbons, R.L.; Stokes, P.E. et al. (1984). 'Pretreatment Neurotransmitter Metabolite Levels and Response to Tricyclic Antidepressant Drugs', *American Journal of Psychiatry,* **141**(10): 1159–71. Also see Healy, D. (1997). *The Antidepressant Era* (New York: Harvard University Press) p. 159.
30 Healy, D. (1987). 'The Structure of Psychopharmacological Revolutions', *Psychiatric Developments,* **5**(4): 349–76 (quote p. 367).

Chapter 7

1 Miltown advertisement, 1960s, available at https://www.goretro.com/2014/08/mothers-little-helper-vintage-drug-ads.html (third advert image down on page, accessed 13 January 2024).
2 Butisol advertisement, 1969, available from https://www.goretro.com/2014/08/mothers-little-helper-vintage-drug-ads.html (first advert image on page, accessed 13 January 2024).
3 Miltown advertisement, 1960.
4 Serax advertisement, 1967. Available from www.huffingtonpost.co.uk/entry/antidepressants-advertisements-women_n_7276906 (accessed 13 January 2024).
5 Miltown advertisement, 1960s.
6 Butisol advert, 1969.
7 Serax advertisement, 1967.
8 Butisol advert, 1969.
9 Tone, A. (2009). *The Age of Anxiety: A History of America's Turbulent Affair With Tranquilizers* (Philadelphia, PA: Basic Books).
10 *Ibid.*
11 Parry, H.J.; Balter, M.B.; Mellinger, G.D.; Cisin, I.H.; & Manheimer, D.I. (1973). 'National Patterns of Psychotherapeutic Drug Use', *Archives of General Psychiatry,* **28**(6): 18–74.
12 Roche is the sixth-largest pharmaceutical company in the world as of 2024 www.visualcapitalist.com/cp/worlds-50-largest-pharmaceutical-companies/. On the link with the Sacklers, see Keefe, P.R. (2021). *Empire of Pain: The Secret History of the Sackler Dynasty* (London: Picador).

13 Hollister, L.E.; Motzenbecker, F.P.; & Degan, R.O. (1961). 'Withdrawal Reactions from Chlordiazepoxide ("Librium")', *Psychopharmacologia*, **2**: 63–68.

14 Lader, M. (1991). 'History of Benzodiazepine Dependence', *Journal of Substance Abuse Treatment*, **8**(1–2): 53–59.

15 WHO (1992). *International Classification of Diseases 10th Revision (ICD-10)* (Geneva: World Health Organization) p. 75.

16 Margolin, L.; Cope, D.K.; Bakst-Sisser, R.; & Greenspan, J. (2007). 'The Steroid Withdrawal Syndrome: A Review of the Implications, Etiology, and Treatments', *Journal of Pain Symptom Management*, **33**(2): 224–28; Karachalios, G.N.; Charalabopoulos, A.; Papalimneou, V.; Kiortsis, D.; Dimicco, P. (2005). 'Withdrawal Syndrome Following Cessation Of Antihypertensive Drug Therapy', *International Journal of Clinical Practice*, **59**(5): 562–70.

17 Cited in Tone, 2009, note 10, p. 267.

18 *New York Times*, 7 September 1979, 'Senate Panel is Told of Dangers of Valium Abuse'.

19 http://news.bbc.co.uk/1/hi/programmes/panorama/tranquillisers/1312511.stm.

20 Trethowan, W.H. (1975). 'Pills for Personal Problems', *British Medical Journal*, **3**(5986): 749–51 (p. 749); Tyrer, P. (1974). 'The Benzodiazepine Bonanza', *Lancet*, **2**(7882): 709–10 (p. 710).

21 Gabe, J., & Bury, M. (1988). 'Tranquillisers as a Social Problem', *The Sociological Review*, **36**.

22 *Ibid.*; Tone (2009).

23 See David Healy's account of the transformation of anxiety into depression in Healy, D. (2004). 'Shaping the Intimate: Influences on the Experience of Everyday Nerves', *Social Studies in Science*, **34**(2): 219–45. Available at www.researchgate.net/publication/8413121_Shaping_the_Intimate_Influences_on_the_Experience_of_Everyday_Nerves.

24 Horwitz, A.V. (2010). 'How an Age of Anxiety Became an Age of Depression', *Milbank Quarterly*, **88**(1): 112–38. Available at www.ncbi.nlm.nih.gov/pmc/articles/PMC2888013/.

25 Fenichel, O. (1945). *The Psychoanalytic Theory of Neurosis* (New York: W.W. Norton & Co.).

26 Popper, K.R. (1963). *Conjectures and Refutations: The Growth of Scientific Knowledge* (New York: Routledge & Kegan Paul), pp. 43–86; Gellner, E. (1985). *The Psychoanalytic Movement* (London: Palladin).

27 Regier, D.A.; Hirschfeld, R.M.; Goodwin, F.K.; Burke Jr, J.D.; Lazar, J.B.; & Judd, L.L. (1988). 'The NIMH Depression Awareness, Recognition, and Treatment Program: Structure, Aims, and Scientific Basis', *American Journal of Psychiatry* **145**(11): 1351–57.

28 Cited in Herzberg, D. (2009). *Happy Pills in America. From Miltown to Prozac* (Baltimore, MA: The Johns Hopkins University Press) p. 269.

29 Cited in Shorter, E. (2021). *The Rise and Fall of the Age of Psychopharmacology*, Chapter 16 (Oxford: Oxford Medicine Online).

30 Wurtzel, E. (1994). *Prozac Nation: Young and Depressed in America* (New York: Penguin Books).

31 Cowley, G. (1990). 'The Promise of Prozac', *Newsweek*, 26 March 1990: 38–41 (quotes pp. 39 and 40).
32 Kramer, P. (1993). *Listening to Prozac: A Psychiatrist Explores Antidepressants Drugs and the Re-Making of the Self* (New York: Penguin Books Ltd).
33 Cited in Herzberg, D. (2009), p. 183.
34 Kramer, P. (1993). *Listening to Prozac: A Psychiatrist Explores Antidepressants Drugs.*
35 'The Culture of Prozac', *Newsweek*, 6 Februaty 1994. Available at www.newsweek.com/culture-prozac-190328. Accessed 14 January 2024.
36 Huguette Martel, *New Yorker* cartoon, 8 November 1993. Cited in Wurtzel (1994) and *Newsweek* (1994).
37 'With Millions Taking Prozac, A Legal Drug Culture Arises', *New York Times*, 13 December 1993. Available at www.nytimes.com/1993/12/13/us/with-millions-taking-prozac-a-legal-drug-culture-arises.html (accesssed 14 January 2024).
38 Wurtzel (1994), p. 304.
39 Herzberg, D. (2009). *Happy Pills in America. From Miltown to Prozac* (Baltimore, MA: The Johns Hopkins University Press) quotes on p. 180.
40 *Ibid.*
41 Cited in Healy (2004), p. 224.
42 *Ibid.*, p. 222.
43 Valenstein's book provides a valuable record of promotional materials of the time: Valenstein, E. (1988). *Blaming the Brain* (New York: Free Press).
44 *Ibid.*, p. 182.
45 *Ibid.*, p. 181.
46 Cited in Herzberg (2009), p. 185.
47 www.youtube.com/watch?v=twhytzd6gXA&list=PLTvBonT9IGLswtvolxp9MmsI_Xqo4nWlU&index=1 (accessed 4 March 2024).
48 Letter to Charles Medawar from President Robert Kendell, 28 November 1997.
49 'Breakdown of funding obtained for the Defeat Depression Campaign – draft', 1997.
50 'Defeat Depression campaign 1992–97' (no date).
51 'The Future of the Defeat Depression Campaign' – a brainstorming session, held on 11 September 1996 at Lilly House, 13, Hanover Square, London W1R 0PA.
52 'Down with Gloom' presented in 'How to defeat depression', available at https://holeousia.com/in-the-world/a-sunshine-act-for-scotland/british-psychiatry-marketing-as-education/the-defeat-depression-campaign/how-to-defeat-depression/ (accessed 14 January 2024).
53 In 'Defeat Depression Campaign Action Week 3–11 March 1994. Notes for Campaign Lectures'.
54 'UK Campaign to Defeat depression launched', *Thepharmaletter*, 22 August 1993. Available at www.thepharmaletter.com/article/uk-campaign-to-defeat-depression-launched (accessed 14 January 2024).
55 'Attitudes Towards Depression'. Research study conducted for the Defeat Depression Campaign, January 1992.

56 Priest, R.G.; Vize, C.; Roberts, A.; Roberts, M.; & Tylee, A. (1996). 'Lay People's Attitudes to Treatment of Depression: Results of Opinion Poll for Defeat Depression Campaign Just Before its Launch', *British Medical Journal*, **313**(7061): 858–59 (p. 858). Available at: www.ncbi.nlm.nih.gov/pmc/articles/PMC2359082/.

57 Paykel, E.S.; Hart, D.; & Priest, R.G. (1998). 'Changes in Public Attitudes to Depression During the Defeat Depression Campaign', *British Journal of Psychiatry*, **173**: 519–22: www.cambridge.org/core/journals/the-british-journal-of-psychiatry/article/changes-in-public-attitudes-to-depression-during-the-defeat-depression-campaign/2B86001C8570A9E9F610417BA763120A.

58 'Attitudes Towards Depression'. Research study conducted for the Defeat Depression Campaign, January 1992.

59 'Down with Gloom'.

60 'Attitudes Towards Depression'. Research study conducted for the Defeat Depression Campaign, January 1992; results also presented in Paykel et al. (1998).

61 'Down with Gloom'.

62 Priest et al. (1996).

63 Paykel, E.S., & Priest, R.G. (1992). 'Recognition and Management of Depression in General Practice: Consensus Statement', *British Medical Journal*, **305**(6863): 1198–202 (p. 1200); www.ncbi.nlm.nih.gov/pmc/articles/PMC1883802/.

64 'Down with Gloom', capital letters in the original.

65 Priest et al. (1996) p. 859.

66 Letter to Charles Medawar from President Robert Kendell, 28 November 1997.

67 Reproduced in Valenstein, E. (1988), p. 178.

68 *Ibid.*, p. 177.

69 'Depression: A Guide to its Recognition and Management in General Practice', produced by Neurolink, funded by Wyeth Laboratories.

70 www.theguardian.com/politics/2009/feb/09/ecstasy-horse-riding#:~:text=Jacqui%20Smith%20today%20hit%20out,families%20of%20victims%22%20of%20ecstasy.

71 Paykell et al. (1998).

72 National Institute for Health & Clinical Excellence (2004). 'Depression: Management of Depression in Primary and Secondary Care', Clinical Practice Guideline Number 23 (London: NICE).

73 Mukherjee, S. (2012). 'Post-Prozac Nation', *New York Times*, www.nytimes.com/2012/04/22/magazine/the-science-and-history-of-treating-depression.html.

74 Murray, C.J.L., & Lopez, A.D. (1996). *Global Health Statistics: A Compendium of Mortality and Disability from Diseases, Injuries, and Risk Factors in 1990 and Projected to 2020* (Cambridge, MA: Harvard University Press).

75 United Nations (2017). 'UN Health Agency Reports Depression Now "Leading Cause of Disability Worldwide"', *UN News*. Available at https://news.un.org/en/story/2017/02/552062 (accessed 14 January 2024).

76 Roser, M. (2016). 'Proof That Life is Getting Better for Humanity, in 5 Charts', *Vox,* 23 December 2016: www.vox.com/the-big-idea/2016/2012/2023/14062168/history-global-conditions-charts-life-span-poverty (accessed 4 March 2024).
77 See for example: Moynihan, R.; Heath, I.; & Henry, D. (2002). 'Selling Sickness: The Pharmaceutical Industry and Disease Mongering', *British Medical Journal,* **324**(7342): 886–91.
78 Meeting organised by the British Medical Association in 2016. The recommendations from the meeting are reported here: www.gponline.com/bma-calls-new-support-prescription-drug-dependency/article/1413165.
79 Healy, D. (2004), p. 223.

Chapter 8

1 Jones, B.E. (2020). 'Arousal and Sleep Circuits', *Neuropsychopharmacology,* **45**(1): 6–20.
2 Examples include: www.psychologytoday.com/gb/blog/your-neurochemical-self/201802/the-neurochemistry-love (accessed 14 January 2024); www.reuters.com/article/us-depression-serotonin-idUSL0579946320080605/; www.bbc.co.uk/news/uk-wales-14467942 (accessed 14 January 2024).
3 www.news-medical.net/health/What-is-Serotonin.aspx#:~:text=Chemistry%20of%20Serotonin&text=It%20was%20first%20discovered%20by,the%20Cleveland%20Clinic%20in%201948 (accessed 14 January 2024).
4 Choi, W.; Moon, J.H.; & Kim, H.(2020). 'Serotonergic Regulation of Energy Metabolism in Peripheral Tissues', *Journal of Endocrinology,* **245**(1): R1–R10.
5 Li, M.F., & Cheung, B.M. (2011). 'Rise and Fall of Anti-Obesity Drugs', *World Journal of Diabetes,* **2**(2): 19–23.
6 Faraone, S.V. (2018). 'The Pharmacology of Amphetamine and Methylphenidate: Relevance to the Neurobiology of Attention-Deficit/Hyperactivity Disorder and Other Psychiatric Comorbidities', *Neuroscience & Biobehavioral Reviews,* **87**: 255–70.
7 Hull, E.M., & Dominguez, J.M. (2007). 'Sexual Behavior in Male Rodents', *Hormones & Behavior,* **52**(1): 45–55.
8 Hull, E. M.; Muschamp, J.W.; & Sato, S. (2004). 'Dopamine and Serotonin: Influences on Male Sexual Behavior', *Physiology & Behavior,* **83**(2): 291–307.
9 Yilmaz, U.; Tatlisen, A.; Turan, H.; Arman, F.; & Ekmekcioglu, O. (1999). 'The Effects of Fluoxetine on Several Neurophysiological Variables in Patients With Premature Ejaculation', *Journal of Urology,* **161**(1): 107–11; Kara, H.; Aydin, S.; Yucel, M.; Agargun, M.Y.; Odabas, O.; & Yilmaz, Y. (1996). 'The Efficacy of Fluoxetine in the Treatment of Premature Ejaculation: A Double-Blind Placebo-Controlled Study', *Journal of Urology,* **156**(5): 1631–32.
10 Roberts, C.; Sahakian, B.J.; & Robbins, T.W. (2020). 'Psychological Mechanisms and functions of 5-HT and SSRIs in Potential Therapeutic Change: Lessons from the Serotonergic Modulation of Action Selection, Learning, Affect, and Social Cognition', *Neuroscience and Biobehavioral Reviews,* **119**: 138–67. https://pubmed.ncbi.nlm.nih.gov/32931805/.

11 Roberts et al. (2020), p. 140.
12 *Ibid.*, p. 142.
13 Berger, M.; Gray, J.A.; & Roth, B.L. (2009). 'The expanded biology of serotonin' *Annual Review of Medicine*, 60, 355–66, p. 356.
14 Renoir, T. (2013). 'Selective Serotonin Reuptake Inhibitor Antidepressant Treatment Discontinuation Syndrome: A Review of the Clinical Evidence and the Possible Mechanisms Involved', *Frontiers in Pharmacology*, **4**: 45; and Gray, N.A.; Milak, M.S.; DeLorenzo, C.; Ogden, R.T.; Huang, Y.Y.; Mann, J.J.; & Parsey, R.V. (2013). 'Antidepressant Treatment Reduces Serotonin-1A Autoreceptor Binding in Major Depressive Disorder', *Biological Psychiatry* ,**74**(1): 26–31.
15 In case you can't find the earlier reference to it: Moncrieff, J.; Cooper, R.E.; Stockmann, T.; Amendola, S.; Hengartner, M.P.; & Horowitz, M.A. (2022). 'The Serotonin Theory of Depression: A Systematic Umbrella Review of the Evidence', *Molecular Psychiatry*, doi:10.1038/s41380-022-01661-0. Available at: www.nature.com/articles/s41380-022-01661-0.
16 Cowen, P.J., & Browning, M. (2015). 'What has Serotonin to do with Depression?', *World Psychiatry*, **14**(2): 158–60.
17 Richard, D.M.; Dawes, M.A.; Mathias, C.W.; Acheson, A.; Hill-Kapturczak, N.; & Dougherty, D.M. (2009). 'L-Tryptophan: Basic Metabolic Functions, Behavioral Research and Therapeutic Indications', *International Journal of Tryptophan Research*, **2**: 45–60.
18 Young, S.N. (2013). 'Acute Tryptophan Depletion in Humans: A Review of Theoretical, Practical and Ethical Aspects', *Journal of Psychiatry & Neuroscience*, **38**(5): 294–305 (p. 295).
19 Ruhe, H.G.; Mason, N.S.; & Schene, A.H. (2007). 'Mood is Indirectly Related to Serotonin, Norepinephrine and Dopamine Levels in Humans: A Meta-Analysis of Monoamine Depletion Studies', *Molecular Psychiatry*, **12**(4): 331–59.
20 Moreno, F.A.; Erickson, R.P.; Garriock, H.A.; Gelernter, J.; Mintz, J.; Oas-Terpstra, J. et al. (2015). 'Association Study of Genotype by Depressive Response During Tryptophan Depletion in Subjects Recovered from Major Depression', *Molecular Neuropsychiatry*, **1**(3): 165–74.
21 Le Poul, E.; Boni, C.; Hanoun, N.; Laporte, A.M.; Laaris, N.; & Chauveau, J. (2000). 'Differential Adaptation of Brain 5-HT1A and 5-HT1B Receptors and 5-HT Transporter in Rats Treated Chronically with Fluoxetine', *Neuropharmacology*, **39**(1): 110–22.
22 Collier, D.A.; Stober, G.; Li, T.; Heils, A.; Catalano, M.; Di Bella, D. et al. (1996). 'A Novel Functional Polymorphism Within the Promoter of the Serotonin Transporter Gene: Possible Role in Susceptibility to Affective Disorders', *Molecular Psychiatry*, **1**(6): 453–60.
23 The paper is Caspi, A.; Sugden, K.; Moffitt, T.E.; Taylor, A.; Craig, I.W.; Harrington, H. et al. (2003). 'Influence of Life Stress on Depression: Moderation by a Polymorphism in the 5-HTT Gene', *Science*, **301**(5631): 386–89, https://pubmed.ncbi.nlm.nih.gov/12869766/. See also a historical account of this research: Ocklenburg, S. (2019). 'The Serotonin Transporter Gene and Depression', *Psychology Today*, 13 May 2019. Available at www.psychologytoday.

com/gb/blog/the-asymmetric-brain/201905/the-serotonin-transporter-gene-and-depression (accessed 14 January 2024).

24 Border, R.; Johnson, E.C.; Evans, L.M.; Smolen, A.; Berley, N.; Sullivan, P.F.; & Keller, M.C. (2019). 'No Support for Historical Candidate Gene or Candidate Gene-by-Interaction Hypotheses for Major Depression Across Multiple Large Samples', *American Journal of Psychiatry*, **176**(5): 376–87; Culverhouse, R.C.; Saccone, N.L.; Horton, A.C.; Ma, Y.; Anstey, K.J.; Banaschewski, T. et al. (2018). 'Collaborative Meta-Analysis Finds No Evidence of a Strong Interaction Between Stress and 5-HTTLPR Genotype Contributing to the Development of Depression', *Molecular Psychiatry*, **23**(1): 133–42.

25 None of the studies that looked at this distinguished between SSRIs and other types of antidepressants, but we can assume that most participants using antidepressants in modern studies would be taking SSRIs. Other antidepressants also affect the serotonin system, however, so findings may also apply to other types of antidepressants.

26 Figure 3 in the paper illustrates how serotonin and some other body chemicals are different from normal among people taking antidepressants, rather than people with depression per se. See Huang, T.; Balasubramanian, R.; Yao, Y.; Clish, C.B.; Shadyab, A.H.; Liu, B. et al. (2021). 'Associations of Depression Status with Plasma Levels of Candidate Lipid and Amino Acid Metabolites: A Meta-Analysis of Individual Data from Three Independent Samples of US Postmenopausal Women', *Molecular Psychiatry*, **26**(7): 3315–27. Available at: www.ncbi.nlm.nih.gov/pmc/articles/PMC7914294/.

27 Huang, T.; Balasubramanian, R., Yao, Y., Clish, C. B., Shadyab, A. H., Liu, B. et al. (2021). 'Associations of depression status with plasma levels of candidate lipid and amino acid metabolites: a meta-analysis of individual data from three independent samples of US postmenopausal women.' *Molecular Psychiatry* **26**(7): 3315–27.

28 Yoon, H.S.; Hattori, K.; Ogawa, S.; Sasayama, D.; Ota, M.; Teraishi, T.; & Kunugi, H. (2017). 'Relationships of Cerebrospinal Fluid Monoamine Metabolite Levels with Clinical Variables in Major Depressive Disorder', *Journal of Clinical Psychiatry*, **78**(8): e947–e956. The study is highlighted in the review by Pech, J.; Forman, J.; Kessing, L.V.; & Knorr, U. (2018). 'Poor Evidence for Putative Abnormalities in Cerebrospinal Fluid Neurotransmitters in Patients with Depression Versus Healthy Non-Psychiatric Individuals: A Systematic Review and Meta-Analyses of 23 Studies', *Journal of Affective Disorders*, **240**: 6–16.

29 Bosker, F.J.; Tanke, M.A.; Jongsma, M.E.; Cremers, T.I.; Jagtman, E.; Pietersen, C.Y. et al. (2010). 'Biochemical and Behavioral Effects of Long-Term Citalopram Administration and Discontinuation in Rats: Role of Serotonin Synthesis', *Neurochemistry International*, **57**(8): 948–57. Also Carpenter, L.L.; Anderson, G.M.; Siniscalchi, J.M.; Chappell, P.B.; & Price, L.H. (2003). 'Acute Changes in Cerebrospinal Fluid 5-HIAA Following Oral Paroxetine Challenge in Healthy Humans', *Neuropsychopharmacology*, **28**(2): 339–47, which also cites many other studies.

30 Velayudhan, A.; Bellingham, G.; & Morely-Forster, P. (2014). 'Opioid-Induced Hyperalgesia', *Continuing Education in Anaesthesia, Critical Care and Pain*, **14**(3): 125–29.

31 Healy, D. (2015). 'Serotonin and Depression', *British Medical Journal*, **350**: h1771.

32 Chou, R.; Cantor, A.; Dana, T.; Wagner, J.; Ahmed, A.Y.; Fu, R.; & Ferencik, M. (2022). 'Statin Use for the Primary Prevention of Cardiovascular Disease in Adults: Updated Evidence Report and Systematic Review for the US Preventive Services Task Force', *Journal of the American Medical Association (JAMA)*, **328**(8): 754–71.

Chapter 9

1 https://theconversation.com/depression-low-serotonin-may-not-be-the-cause-but-antidepressants-still-work-187477; https://theconversation.com/the-chemical-imbalance-theory-of-depression-is-dead-but-that-doesnt-mean-antidepressants-dont-work-187769.

2 Posternak, M.A., & Zimmerman, M. (2007). 'Therapeutic Effect of Follow-Up Assessments on Antidepressant and Placebo Response Rates in Antidepressant Efficacy Trials: Meta-Analysis,' *British Journal of Psychiatry*, **190**: 287–92.

3 An effect or difference is said to be 'statistically significant' when it is unlikely to occur by chance. By convention, a less than 5 per cent probability that the effect is a random or chance effect is considered a 'statistically significant' result, although in some circumstances, the threshold is set at less than 1 per cent or 0.1 per cent.

4 Hamilton, M. (1960). 'A Rating Scale for Depression', *Journal of Neurology, Neurosurgery & Psychiatry*, **23**: 56–62.

5 Stone, M.B.; Yaseen, Z.S.; Miller, B.J.; Richardville, K.; Kalaria, S.N.; & Kirsch, I. (2022). 'Response to Acute Monotherapy for Major Depressive Disorder in Randomized, Placebo Controlled Trials Submitted to the US Food and Drug Administration: Individual Participant Data Analysis', *British Medical Journal*, **378**: e067606. Available at: www.bmj.com/content/378/bmj-2021-067606.

6 See Chapter 10 for a discussion of this paper.

7 Hieronymus, F.; Emilsson, J.F.; Nilsson, S.; & Eriksson, E. (2016). 'Consistent Superiority of Selective Serotonin Reuptake Inhibitors Over Placebo in Reducing Depressed Mood in Patients With Major Depression', *Molecular Psychiatry*, **21**(4): 523–30.

8 Montgomery, S.A., & Åsberg, M. (1979). 'A New Depression Scale Designed to be Sensitive to Change', *British Journal of Psychiatry*, **134**: 382–89.

9 Hengartner, M.P.; Jakobsen, J.C.; Sorensen, A.; & Ploderl, M. (2020). 'Efficacy of New-Generation Antidepressants Assessed With the Montgomery–Asberg Depression Rating Scale, the Gold Standard Clinician Rating Scale: A Meta-Analysis of Randomised Placebo-Controlled Trials', *PLoS One*, **15**(2): e0229381.

10 Guy, W. (1976). 'The Clinical Global Impression Scale', *ECDEU Assessment Manual for Psychopharmacology – Revised* (Rockville, MD: US Department of Education, Health and Welfare) 218–22.

11 The original paper is Leucht, S.; Fennema, H.; Engel, R.; Kaspers-Janssen, M.; Lepping, P.; & Szegedi, A. (2013). 'What Does the HAMD Mean?', *Journal of Affective Disorders*, **148**(2–3): 243–48, https://pubmed.ncbi.nlm.nih.gov/23357658/. Irving Kirsch and I applied their data to antidepressant-placebo differences in Moncrieff, J., & Kirsch, I. (2015). 'Empirically Derived Criteria Cast Doubt on the Clinical Significance of Antidepressant–Placebo Differences', *Contemporary Clinical Trials*, **43**: 60–62. Available at www.sciencedirect.com/science/article/pii/S1551714415300033?via%3Dihub.

12 Hengartner, M.P., & Ploderl, M. (2022). 'Estimates of the Minimal Important Difference to Evaluate the Clinical Significance of Antidepressants in the Acute Treatment of Moderate-to-Severe Depression', *British Medical Journal Evidence Based Medicine*, **27**(2): 69–73.

13 Thomson, R. (1982). 'Side Effects and Placebo Amplification', *British Journal of Psychiatry*, **140**: 64–68, https://pubmed.ncbi.nlm.nih.gov/7037102/.

14 Moncrieff, J.; Wessely, S.; & Hardy, R. (1998). 'Meta-Analysis of Trials Comparing Antidepressants With Active Placebos', *British Journal of Psychiatry*, **172**: 227–31.

15 Faria, V.; Gingnell, M.; Hoppe, J.M.; Hjorth, O.; Alaie, I.; & Frick, A. et al. (2017). 'Do You Believe It? Verbal Suggestions Influence the Clinical and Neural Effects of Escitalopram in Social Anxiety Disorder: A Randomized Trial', *EBioMedicine*, **24**: 179–88. Available at www.sciencedirect.com/science/article/pii/S2352396417303857?via%3Dihub.

16 Chen, J.A.; Papakostas, G.I.; Youn, S.J.; Baer, L.; Clain, A.J.; Fava, M.; Mischoulon, D. (2011). 'Association Between Patient Beliefs Regarding Assigned Treatment and Clinical Response: Reanalysis of Data from the Hypericum Depression Trial Study Group', *Journal of Clinical Psychiatry*, **72**(12): 1669–76, https://pubmed.ncbi.nlm.nih.gov/22053942/.

17 Scott, A.J.; Sharpe, L.; & Colagiuri, B. (2022). 'A Systematic Review and Meta-Analysis of the Success of Blinding in Antidepressant RCTs', *Psychiatry Research*, **307**: 114297.

18 Kranzler, H.R.; Burleson, J.A.; Korner, P.; Del Boca, F.K.; Bohn, M.J.; Brown, J.; & Liebowitz, N. (1995). 'Placebo-Controlled Trial of Fluoxetine as an Adjunct to Relapse Prevention in Alcoholics', *American Journal of Psychiatry*, **152**(3): 391–97.

19 March, J.; Silva, S.; Petrycki, S.; Curry, J.; Wells, K.; Fairbank, J. et al. (2004). 'Fluoxetine, Cognitive-Behavioral Therapy, and their Combination for Adolescents With Depression: Treatment for Adolescents With Depression Study (TADS) Randomized Controlled Trial', *Journal of the American Medical Academy (JAMA)*, **292**(7): 807–20.

20 The paper is Jureidini, J.; Moncrieff, J.; Klau, J.; Aboustate, N.; & Raven, M. (2023). 'Treatment Guesses in the Treatment for Adolescents with Depression Study: Accuracy, Unblinding and Influence on Outcomes', *Australian and New*

Zealand Journal of Psychiatry, 48674231218623. Available at www.ncbi.nlm.nih.gov/pmc/articles/PMC10960316/.

21 Quitkin, F.M.; Rabkin, J.G.; Gerald, J.; Davis, J.M.; & Klein, D.F. (2000). 'Validity of Clinical Trials of Antidepressants', *American Journal of Psychiatry*, **157**(3): 327–37.

22 Randomised trials of other sorts of drugs for depression are set out in a table in my previous book, Moncrieff, J. (2009). *The Myth of the Chemical Cure: A Critique of Psychiatric Drug Treatment*, Revised Edition (Basingstoke, UK) pp. 145–46. Also see Chapter 5 for a description of early trials comparing antidepressants with chlorpromazine and purple hearts (Drinamyl).

23 Wagstaff, A.J.; Ormrod, D.; & Spencer, C.M. (2001). 'Tianeptine: A Review of its Use in Depressive Disorders', *CNS Drugs*, **15**(3): 231–59.

24 Slee, A.; Nazareth, I.; Bondaronek, P.; Liu, Y.; Cheng, Z.; & Freemantle, N. (2019). 'Pharmacological Treatments for Generalised Anxiety Disorder: A Systematic Review and Network Meta-Analysis', *Lanceti*, **393**(10173): 768–77. Available at https://discovery.ucl.ac.uk/id/eprint/10070219/1/Freemantle_Slee_GAD_Meta_Text%20R1_20180627%20clean.pdf.

25 Soomro, G.M.; Altman, D.; Rajagopal, S.; & Oakley-Browne, M. (2008). 'Selective Serotonin Re-Uptake Inhibitors (SSRIs) Versus Placebo for Obsessive Compulsive Disorder (OCD)', *Cochrane Database Systematic Reviews* (1): CD001765. Available at www.ncbi.nlm.nih.gov/pmc/articles/PMC7025764/.

26 Soomro, G.M.; Altman, D.; Rajagopal, S.; & Oakley-Browne, M. (2008). 'Selective Serotonin Re-Uptake Inhibitors (SSRIs) Versus Placebo for Obsessive Compulsive Disorder (OCD)', *Cochrane Database Systematic Reviews* (1): CD001765.

27 Bourin, M.; Fiocco, A.J.; & Clenet, F. (2001). 'How Valuable are Animal Models in Defining Antidepressant Activity?', *Human Psychopharmacology*, **16**(1): 9–21.

28 www.understandinganimalresearch.org.uk/news/researching-new-antidepressants-with-swimming-mice (accessed 8 March 2024).

29 NICE (2022). 'Depression in Adults: Treatment and Management NICE Guideline [NG 222]' (London: National Institute for Health and Care Excellence).

Chapter 10

1 This analysis revealed a 1.7 point difference between antidepressants and placebo on the Hamilton Depression Rating Scale. Kirsch, I.; Moore, T.J.; Scoboria, A.; & Nicholls, S.S. (2002). 'The Emperor's New Drugs: An Analysis of Antidepressant Medication Data Submitted to the US Food and Drug Administration', *Prevention and Treatment*, **5**, available at https://psycnet.apa.org/record/2002-14079-003 and for free at www.researchgate.net/publication/228550299_The_Emperor's_New_Drugs_An_Analysis_of_Antidepressant_Medication_Data_Submitted_to_the_US_Food_and_Drug_Administration (accessed 8 February 2024).

2 Scott, A.J.; Sharpe, L.; Colagiuri, B. (2022). 'A Systematic Review and Meta-Analysis of the Success of Blinding in Antidepressant RCTs', *Psychiatry Research*, **307**: 114297.

3 Turner, E.H.; Matthews, A.M.; Linardatos, E.; Tell, R.A.; & Rosenthal, R. (2008). 'Selective Publication of Antidepressant Trials and its Influence on Apparent Efficacy', *New England Journal of Medicine*, **358**(3): 252–60. Available at www.nejm.org/doi/full/10.1056/NEJMsa065779.

4 Ioannidis, J.P. (2008). 'Effectiveness of Antidepressants: An Evidence Myth Constructed from a Thousand Randomized Trials?', *Philosophy, Ethics and Humanities in Medicine*, **3**: 14.

5 This material has been summarised by David Healy (2014) in 'Zoloft Efficacy', report compiled 30 July 2014: https://samizdathealth.org/wp-content/uploads/2020/2012/Holmes-Appendix-2021-Efficacy-Data.pdf (accessed 13 March 2024).

6 The main study publication is Keller, M.B.; Ryan, N.D.; Strober, M.; Klein, R.G.; Kutcher, S.P.; Birmaher, B. et al. (2001). 'Efficacy of Paroxetine in the Treatment of Adolescent Major Depression: A Randomized, Controlled Trial', *Journal of the American Academy of Child and Adolescent Psychiatry*, **40**(7): 762–72. The ghost writer claim was made by Peter Doshi, associate editor of the *British Medical Journal*, among others: Doshi, P. (2015). 'No Correction, No Retraction, No Apology, No Comment: Paroxetine Trial Reanalysis Raises Questions About Institutional Responsibility', *British Medical Journal*, **351**: h4629.

7 The campaign was described in Doshi (2015).

8 This process is described in Jureidini, J.N.; McHenry, L.B.; & Mansfield, P.R. (2008). 'Clinical Trials and Drug Promotion: Selective Reporting of Study 329', *International Journal of Risk and Safety in Medicine*, **20**: 73–81. Available at: www.researchgate.net/publication/228649054_Clinical_Trials_and_Drug_Promotion_Selective_Reporting_of_Study_329.

9 Le Noury, J.; Nardo, J.M.; Healy, D.; Jureidini, J.; Raven, M.; Tufanaru, C.; & Abi-Jaoude, E. (2015). 'Restoring Study 329: Efficacy and Harms of Paroxetine and Imipramine in Treatment of Major Depression in Adolescence', *British Medical Journal*, **351**: h4320.

10 The headline is from *The Guardian*: Boseley, S. (2018). 'The Drugs Do Work: Antidepressants Are Effective, Study Shows', 21 February 2018: www.theguardian.com/science/2018/feb/2021/the-drugs-do-work-antidepressants-are-effective-study-shows (accessed 12 March 2024). The publication is Cipriani, A.; Furukawa, T.A.; Salanti, G.; Chaimani, A.; Atkinson, L.Z., Ogawa, Y. et al. (2018). 'Comparative Efficacy and Acceptability of 21 Antidepressant Drugs for the Acute Treatment of Adults with Major Depressive Disorder: A Systematic Review and Network Meta-Analysis', *Lancet*, **391**(10128): 1357–66. Available at www.ncbi.nlm.nih.gov/pmc/articles/PMC5889788/.

11 Odds (as in betting) are preferred over proportions in many studies because they have good statistical properties.

12 The following paper explains this in more detail: Kirsch, I., & Moncrieff, J. (2007). 'Clinical Trials and the Response Rate Illusion', *Contemporary Clinical*

Trials, **28**: 348–51. Available at www.researchgate.net/publication/6618603_Clinical_trials_and_the_response_rate_illusion.

13 E.g. Royston, P.; Altman, D.G.; & Sauerbrei, W. (2006). 'Dichotomizing Continuous Predictors in Multiple Regression: A Bad Idea', *Statistics in Medicine*, **25**(1): 127–41.

14 Munkholm, K.; Paludan-Muller, A.S.; & Boesen, K. (2019). 'Considering the Methodological Limitations in the Evidence Base of Antidepressants for Depression: A Reanalysis of a Network Meta-Analysis', *British Medical Journal Open*, **9**(6): e024886. Available at https://bmjopen.bmj.com/content/9/6/e024886.

15 Furukawa, T.A.; Maruo, K.; Noma, H.; Tanaka, S.; Imai, H.; Shinohara, K. et al. (2018). 'Initial Severity of Major Depression and Efficacy of New Generation Antidepressants: Individual Participant Data Meta-Analysis', *Acta Psychiatrica Scandinavica*, **137**(6): 450–58.

16 Stone, M.B.; Yaseen, Z.S.; Miller, B.J.; Richardville, K.; Kalaria, S.N. & Kirsch, I. (2022). 'Response to Acute Monotherapy for Major Depressive Disorder in Randomized, Placebo Controlled Trials Submitted to the US Food and Drug Administration: Individual Participant Data Analysis', *British Medical Journal*, **378**: e067606.

17 Chen, J.A.; Papakostas, G.I.; Youn, S.J.; Baer, L.; Clain, A.J.; Fava, M.; & Mischoulon, D. (2011). Association Between Patient Beliefs Regarding Assigned Treatment and Clinical Response: Reanalysis of Data From the Hypericum Depression Trial Study Group', *Journal of Clinical Psychiatryi*, **72**(12): 1669–76.

18 Medical Research Council (1965). 'Clinical Trial of the Treatment of Depressive Illness', *British Medical Journal*, **1**: 881–86.

19 Joyce, P.R., & Paykel, E.S. (1989). 'Predictors of Drug Response in Depression', *Archives of General Psychiatry*, **46**(1): 89–99.

20 I cover ECT in Chapter 3 of my book: Moncrieff, J. (2008). *The Myth of the Chemical Cure: A Critique of Psychiatric Drug Treatment* (Basingstoke, UK, Palgrave Macmillan). Also see Read, J., & Moncrieff, J. (2022). 'Depression: Why Drugs and Electricity Are Not the Answer', *Psychological Medicine* **52**(8): 1401–10. Available at https://discovery.ucl.ac.uk/id/eprint/10149120/.

21 Zhang, Y.; Yang, H.; Yang, S.; Liang, W.; Dai, P.; Wang, C.; & Zhang, Y. (2013). 'Antidepressants for Bipolar Disorder: A Meta-Analysis of Randomized, Double-Blind, Controlled Trials', *Neural Regeneration Research*, **8**(31): 2962–74; and Sidor, M.M., & Macqueen, G.M. (2011). 'Antidepressants for the Acute Treatment of Bipolar Depression: A Systematic Review and Meta-Analysis', *Journal of Clinical Psychiatry*, **72**(2): 156–67.

22 Cavendish, L. (2023). 'You can't just cheer up people who have depression. There's a key role for antidepressants', *The Guardian*, 5 March 2023: www.theguardian.com/commentisfree/2023/mar/05/you-cant-just-cheer-up-people-who-have-depression-theres-a-key-role-for-antidepressants.

23 Cipriani et al. (2018).

24 Geddes, J.R.; Carney, S.M.; Davies, C.; Furukawa, T.A.; Kupfer, D.J.; Frank, E.; & Goodwin, G.M. (2003). 'Relapse Prevention With Antidepressant Drug Treatment in Depressive Disorders: A Systematic Review', *Lancet,* **361**(9358): 653–61.

25 Horowitz, M.A., & Taylor, D. (2022). 'Distinguishing Relapse From Antidepressant Withdrawal: Clinical Practice and Antidepressant Discontinuation Studies', *British Journal of Psychiatry Advances,* **28**: 297–311.

26 Lewis, G.; Marston, L.; Duffy, L.; Freemantle, N.; Gilbody, S.; Hunter, R. et al. (2021). 'Maintenance or Discontinuation of Antidepressants in Primary Care', *New England Journal of Medicine,* **385**(14): 1257–67. Available at www.nejm.org/doi/full/10.1056/NEJMoa2106356.

27 See Horowitz, M.A., & Taylor, D. (2019). 'Tapering of SSRI Treatment to Mitigate Withdrawal Symptoms', *Lancet Psychiatry,* **6**(6): 538–46 and Horowitz & Taylor (2022).

28 www.bbc.co.uk/news/health-58735841.

29 The letters are Liang, C.S.; Tseng, P.T.; & Chen, M.H. (2021). *New England Journal of Medicine,* **385**(27): 2586–87; Kuschpel, M.S. (2021). *New England Journal of Medicine* **385**(27): 2587. Available (with the authors' reply) at www.nejm.org/doi/10.1056/NEJMc2117168?url_ver=Z39.88-2003&rfr_id=ori:rid:crossref.org&rfr_dat=cr_pub%20%20pubmed.

30 From an interview with Allen Frances by CNN, reproduced in www.behaviorismandmentalhealth.com/2018/10/30/allen-frances-and-the-increasing-use-of-antidepressants/ (accessed 12 March 2024).

31 Rush, A.J.; Trivedi, M.H.; Wisniewski, S.R.; Nierenberg, A.A.; Stewart, J.W.; Warden, D. et al. (2006). 'Acute and Longer-Term Outcomes in Depressed Outpatients Requiring One or Several Treatment Steps: A STAR*D Report', *American Journal of Psychiatry,* **163**(11): 1905–17: https://pubmed.ncbi.nlm.nih.gov/17074942/.

32 Pigott, H.E.; Kim, T.; Xu, C.; Kirsch, I.; & Amsterdam, J. (2023). 'What are the Treatment Remission, Response and Extent of Improvement Rates After up to Four Trials of Antidepressant Therapies in Real-World Depressed Patients? A Reanalysis of the STAR*D Study's Patient-Level Data With Fidelity to the Original Research Protocol', *British Medical Journal Open,* **13**(7): e063095. Available at www.ncbi.nlm.nih.gov/pmc/articles/PMC10373710/.

33 Pigott (2011), 'An Introduction: The Story of Bias in the STAR*D Trial and More'. Available at www.madinamerica.com/2011/03/%EF%BB%BFan-introduction-the-story-of-bias-in-the-stard-trial-more/ (accessed 16 January 2024).

34 The paper is: Pigott, H.E.; Leventhal, A.M.; Alter, G.S.; & Boren, J. J. (2010). 'Efficacy and Effectiveness of Antidepressants: Current Status Of Research', *Psychotherapy and Psychosomatics,* **79**(5): 267–79. Available at www.researchgate.net/publication/45114131_Efficacy_and_Effectiveness_of_Antidepressants_Current_Status_of_Research. You can read a detailed account of all the problems with this study in Pigott's blog: Pigott (2011).

35 Pigott et al. (2023).

36 Posternak, M.A.; Solomon, D.A.; Leon, A.C.; Mueller, T.I.; Shea, M.T.; Endicott, J.; & Keller, M. B. (2006). 'The Naturalistic Course of Unipolar Major Depression in the Absence of Somatic Therapy', *Journal of Nervous & Mental Diseases,* **194**(5): 324–29.

37 Wang, J. (2004). 'A Longitudinal Population-Based Study of Treated and Untreated Major Depression', *Medical Care,* **42**(6): 543–50.

38 Pigott et al. (2023).

39 Hengartner, M.P.; Angst, J.; & Rossler, W. (2018). 'Antidepressant Use Prospectively Relates to a Poorer Long-Term Outcome of Depression: Results from a Prospective Community Cohort Study over 30 Years', *Psychotherapy & Psychosomatics,* **87**(3): 181–83. Available at www.researchgate.net/profile/Michael-Hengartner/publication/324729020_Antidepressant_Use_Prospectively_Relates_to_a_Poorer_Long-Term_Outcome_of_Depression_Results_from_a_Prospective_Community_Cohort_Study_over_30_Years/links/5b8e3b0045851540d1c44f48/Antidepressant-Use-Prospectively-Relates-to-a-Poorer-Long-Term-Outcome-of-Depression-Results-from-a-Prospective-Community-Cohort-Study-over-30-Years.pdf.

40 See Fishwick, C. (2013). 'Your Experiences of Antidepressants', *The Guardian,* www.theguardian.com/society/2013/nov/21/your-experiences-antidepressants-responses.

41 The placebos were a placebo tablet and a fake acupuncture procedure. The paper is Wechsler, M.E.; Kelley, J.M.; Boyd, I.O.; Dutile, S.; Marigowda, G.; Kirsch, I. et al. (2011). 'Active Albuterol or Placebo, Sham Acupuncture, Or No Intervention in Asthma', *New England Journal of Medicine,* **365**(2): 119–26. Available at www.ncbi.nlm.nih.gov/pmc/articles/PMC3154208/.

42 NHS information suggests one to two weeks for antidepressants overall: www.nhs.uk/mental-health/talking-therapies-medicine-treatments/medicines-and-psychiatry/antidepressants/overview/#:~:text=Antidepressants%20usually%20need%20to%20be,effects%20usually%20wear%20off%20quickly (accessed 7 February 2024); and tow to four weeks for SSRIs: www.nhs.uk/mental-health/talking-therapies-medicine-treatments/medicines-and-psychiatry/ssri-antidepressants/overview/#:~:text=Doses%20and%20duration%20of%20treatment&text=SSRIs%20usually%20need%20to%20be,t%20stop%20taking%20the%20medicine (accessed 7 February 2024). WebMD suggests four to six weeks: www.webmd.com/depression/ssris-myths-and-facts-about-antidepressants (accessed 7 February 2024).

43 This scenario is loosely based on a number of people I have known professionally and personally, but does not refer to any particular individual.

44 Kirsch, I.; Moore, T.J.; Scoboria, A.; & Nicholls, S. S. (2002). 'The Emperor's New Drugs: An Analysis of Antidepressant Medication Data Submitted to the US Food and Drug Administration', *Prevention and Treatment,* **5**(1), Article 23: https://doi.org/10.1037/1522-3736.5.1.523a. Also, the renowned epidemiologist, John Ioannidis (2008). 'Effectiveness of Antidepressants: An Evidence Myth Constructed From a Thousand Randomized Trials?', *Philosophy, Ethics & Humanities in Medicine,* **3**: 14.

45 It was one of several factors mentioned by GPs in this study: Hyde, J.; Calnan, M.; Prior, L.; Lewis, G.; Kessler, D.; & Sharp, D. (2005). 'A Qualitative Study Exploring How GPs Decide to Prescribe Antidepressants', *British Journal of General Practice,* **55**(519): 755–62.

Chapter 11

1 Moncrieff, J.; Cohen, D.; & Mason, J.P. (2009). 'The Subjective Experience of Taking Antipsychotic Medication: A Content Analysis of Internet Data', *Acta Psychiatrica Scandinavica,* **120**(2): 102–11.

2 Goldsmith, L., & Moncrieff, J. (2011). 'The Psychoactive Effects of Antidepressants and Their Association With Suicidality', *Current Drug Safety,* **6**(2): 115–21. The paper is available here: https://openaccess.city.ac.uk/id/eprint/31252/3/Goldsmith%20and%20Moncrieff%202011%20The%20Psychoactive%20Effects%20of%20Antidepressants%20and%20their%20Association%20with%20Suicidality%20Protected.pdf.

3 Price, J.; Cole, V.; & Goodwin, G.M. (2009). 'Emotional Side-Effects of Selective Serotonin Reuptake Inhibitors: Qualitative Study', *British Journal of Psychiatry,* **195**(3): 211–17 (quote from p. 211). Available at www.cambridge.org/core/journals/the-british-journal-of-psychiatry/article/emotional-sideeffects-of-selective-serotonin-reuptake-inhibitors-qualitative-study/88C72E9EA0961C-DE777C2FDCDBCE1CA9.

4 *Ibid.*, quotes from p. 213.

5 *Ibid.*

6 Read, J.; Grigoriu, M.; Gee, A.; Diggle, J.; & Butler, H. (2020). 'The Positive and Negative Experiences of 342 Antidepressant Users', *Community Mental Health Journal,* **56**(4): 744–52 (quote p. 749).

7 Padala, P.R.; Padala, K.P.; Majagi, A.S.; Garner, K.K.; Dennis, R.A.; & Sullivan, D.H. (2020). 'Selective Serotonin Reuptake Inhibitors-Associated Apathy Syndrome: A Cross-Sectional Study', *Medicine (Baltimore),* **99**(33): e21497. Available at www.ncbi.nlm.nih.gov/pmc/articles/PMC7437849/ (accessed 17 January 2024).

8 Read, J.; Cartwright, C.; & Gibson, K. (2014). 'Adverse Emotional and Interpersonal Effects Reported by 1,829 New Zealanders While Taking Antidepressants', *Psychiatry Research,* **216**(1): 67–73 (quote p. 70). Available at www.sciencedirect.com/science/article/pii/S0165178114000833.

9 Figures from Read et al., (2014).

10 The proportion of people experiencing numbing was reported as 46 per cent in the paper, but people using more than one antidepressant were excluded for unclear reasons. Of the whole group, the proportion is 47 per cent. The paper is Goodwin, G.M.; Price, J.; De Bodinat, C.; & Laredo, J. (2017). 'Emotional Blunting With Antidepressant Treatments: A Survey Among Depressed Patients', *Journal of Affective Disorders,* **221**: 31–35 (quote p. 32). Available at https://ora.ox.ac.uk/objects/uuid:8a7067a3-7b21-481f-ac80-32f1929d3ff7/files/m36d35fac5273c3389dfd4036795d061d.

11 Opbroek A; Delgado P.L.; Laukes C; McGahuey, C.; Katsanis, J., et al. (2002), 'Emotional blunting associated with SSRI-induced sexual dysfunction. Do SSRIs inhibit emotional responses?' *Int. J. Neuropsychopharmacol,* **5(2)**: 147–51; Goldsmith & Moncrieff (2011).

12 Langley, C.; Armand, S.; Luo, Q.; Savulich, G.; Segerberg, T.; Sondergaard, A. et al. (2023). 'Chronic Escitalopram in Healthy Volunteers has Specific Effects on Reinforcement Sensitivity: A Double-Blind, Placebo-Controlled Semi-Randomised Study', *Neuropsychopharmacology,* **48**(4): 664–70. Available at www.nature.com/articles/s41386-022-01523-x.

13 Masdrakis, V.G.; Markianos, M.; & Baldwin, D.S. (2023). 'Apathy Associated With Antidepressant Drugs: A Systematic Review', *Acta Neuropsychiatrica,* **35**(4): 189–204 (quotes p. 189). Apathy is defined as a 'decrease in emotional responsiveness to circumstances which would have triggered intense mood reactions prior to pharmacotherapy' (p. 189). Available at www.cambridge.org/core/journals/acta-neuropsychiatrica/article/apathy-associated-with-antidepressant-drugs-a-systematic-review/438BB4416FA8A4D7C83A8EC9 7DA477F9.

14 'Do Antidepressants Dull Emotions?' An interview with Ron Pies, M.D. Available at www.beliefnet.com/columnists/beyondblue/2009/05/when-does-grief-turn-into-depr.html (accessed 17 January 2024).

15 Dawson, G., & Pies, R.W. (2022). 'Antidepressants Do Not Work by Numbing Emotions', *Psychiatric Times,* www.psychiatrictimes.com/view/antidepressants-do-not-work-by-numbing-emotions (accessed 17 January 2024).

16 Price et al. (2009).

17 Fornaro, M.; Anastasia, A.; Valchera, A.; Carano, A.; Orsolini, L.; Vellante, F. et al. (2019). 'The FDA "Black Box" Warning on Antidepressant Suicide Risk in Young Adults: More Harm Than Benefits?' *Frontiers in Psychiatry,* **10**: 294; Soumarai, S., & Koppel, R. (2018). 'FDA's Continuing Use of "Black Box" for Antidepressants Ignores the Harms of this Warning', *Statnews,* 29 August 2018. Available at www.statnews.com/2018/08/29/fda-antidepressants-black-box-warnings-harms/ (accessed 17 January 2024).

18 Healy describes the early evidence in *Let Them Eat Prozac: The Unhealthy Relationship between the Pharmaceutical Industry and Depression* (New York: New York University Press, 2004) quote p. 15.

19 *Ibid.*

20 Healy, D. (2000). 'Emergence of Antidepressant Induced Suicidality', *Primary Care Psychiatry,* **6**: 23–28.

21 http://news.bbc.co.uk/1/hi/programmes/panorama/2310197.stm (accessed 17 January 2024).

22 Noel, C. (2015). 'Antidepressants and Suicidality: History, the Black-Box Warning, Consequences, and Current Evidence', *Mental Health Clinician,* **5**: 202–11. Available at https://meridian.allenpress.com/mhc/article/5/5/202/127720/Antidepressants-and-suicidality-History-the-black (accessed 17 January 2024).

23 *Ibid.*

24 For example, Dubicka, B.; Hadley, S.; & Roberts, C. (2006). 'Suicidal Behaviour in Youths With Depression Treated with New-Generation Antidepressants: Meta-Analysis', *British Journal of Psychiatry*, **189**: 393–98 and Sharma, T.; Guski, L.S.; Freund, N.; & Gotzsche, P.C. (2016). 'Suicidality and Aggression During Antidepressant Treatment: Systematic Review and Meta-Analyses Based on Clinical Study Reports', *British Medical Journal*, **352**: i65. Available at www.ncbi.nlm.nih.gov/pmc/articles/PMC4729837/.

25 *Ibid.*

26 For example, Lagerberg, T.; Fazel, S.; Molero, Y.; Franko, M.A.; Chen, Q.; Hellner, C.; Lichtenstein, P.; & Chang, Z. (2020). 'Associations Between Selective Serotonin Reuptake Inhibitors and Violent Crime in Adolescents, Young, and Older Adults: A Swedish Register-Based Study', *European Neuropsychopharmacology*, **36**: 1–9.

27 Sharma et al. (2016).

28 Spear, L.P. (2000). 'The Adolescent Brain and Age-Related Behavioral Manifestations', *Neuroscience & Biobehavioral Reviews*, **24**(4): 417–63.

29 Safer, D.J., & Zito, J.M. (2006). 'Treatment-Emergent Adverse Events From Selective Serotonin Reuptake Inhibitors by Age Group: Children Versus Adolescents', *Journal of Child and Adolescent Psychopharmacology*, **16**(1–2): 159–69.

30 Garcia, F.D.; Delavenne, H.G.; Assumpcao Ade, F.; & Thibaut, F. (2013). 'Pharmacologic Treatment of Sex Offenders With Paraphilic Disorder', *Current Psychiatry Reports*, **15**(5): 356.

31 Healy, D.; Le Noury, J.; & Mangin, D. (2018). 'Enduring Sexual Dysfunction After Treatment With Antidepressants, 5alpha-Reductase Inhibitors and Isotretinoin: 300 Cases', *International Journal of Risk and Safety in Medicine*, **29**(3–4): 125–34. Available at www.ncbi.nlm.nih.gov/pmc/articles/PMC6004900/.

32 Healy, D. (2020). 'Antidepressants and Sexual Dysfunction: A History', *Journal of the Royal Society of Medicine*, **113**(4): 133–35. Available at www.ncbi.nlm.nih.gov/pmc/articles/PMC7160790/.

33 This was one of the first papers on persistent sexual dysfunction: Csoka, A.B.; Bahrick, A.; & Mehtonen, O.P. (2008). 'Persistent Sexual Dysfunction After Discontinuation of Selective Serotonin Reuptake Inhibitors', *Journal of Sexual Medicine*, **5**(1): 227–33. Available at www.researchgate.net/publication/5675798_Persistent_Sexual_Dysfunction_after_Discontinuation_of_Selective_Serotonin_Reuptake_Inhibitors.

34 Farnsworth, K.D., & Dinsmore, W.W. (2009). 'Persistent Sexual Dysfunction in Genitourinary Medicine Clinic Attendees Induced by Selective Serotonin Reuptake Inhibitors', *International Journal of STD and AIDS*, **20**(1): 68–69 (quotes p. 69).

35 Healy, D. (2024). 'Post-SSRI Sexual Dysfunction (PSSD)'. Available at https://rxisk.org/post-ssri-sexual-dysfunction-pssd/ (accessed 17 January 2024).

36 Healy, D. (2020).

37 *Ibid.*

38 De Jong, T.R.; Snaphaan, L.J.; Pattij, T.; Veening, J.G.; Waldinger, M.D.; Cools, A.R.; & Olivier, B. (2006). 'Effects of Chronic Treatment With Fluvoxamine and

Paroxetine During Adolescence on Serotonin-Related Behavior in Adult Male Rats', *European Neuropsychopharmacology*, **16**(1): 39–48; Iniguez, S.D.; Warren, B.L.; & Bolanos-Guzman, C.A. (2010). 'Short- and Long-Term Functional Consequences of Fluoxetine Exposure During Adolescence in Male Rats', *Biological Psychiatry*, **67**(11): 1057–66.

39 Maciag, D.; Simpson, K.L.; Coppinger, D.; Lu, Y.; Wang, Y.; Lin, R.C.; & Paul, I.A. (2006). 'Neonatal Antidepressant Exposure has Lasting Effects on Behavior and Serotonin Circuitry', *Neuropsychopharmacology*, **31**(1): 47–57.

40 Simonsen, A.L.; Danborg, P.B.; & Gotzsche, P.C. (2016). 'Persistent Sexual Dysfunction After Early Exposure to SSRIs: Systematic Review of Animal Studies', *International Journal of Risk and Safety in Medicine*, **28**(1): 1–12.

41 Healy, D.; Le Noury, J.; & Mangin, D. (2018). 'Enduring Sexual Dysfunction After Treatment With Antidepressants, 5alpha-Reductase Inhibitors and Isotretinoin: 300 Cases', *International Journal of Risk and Safety in Medicine*, **29**(3–4): 125–34.

42 Pirani, Y., Delgado-Ron, J.A., Marinho, P., Gupta, A., Grey, E. et al. (2025), 'Frequency of self-reported persistent post-treatment genital hypoesthesia among past antidepressant users: a cross-sectional survey of sexual and gender minority youth in Canada and the US', *Soc Psychiatry Psychiatr Epidemiol*, **60**(7): 1771–79.

43 Peleg, L.C.; Rabinovitch, D.; Lavie, Y.; Rabbie, D.M.; Horowitz, I.; Fruchter, E.; & Gruenwald, I. (2022). 'Post-SSRI Sexual Dysfunction (PSSD): Biological Plausibility, Symptoms, Diagnosis, and Presumed Risk Factors', *Sex Med Rev*, **10**(1): 91–98 (p. 94).

44 www.pssdnetwork.org/patient-spotlight/roy (accessed 9 February 2024).

45 Ghorayshi, A. (2023). 'After Antidepressants a Loss of Sexuality', *New York Times*, 9 November 2023: www.nytimes.com/2023/11/09/health/antidepressants-ssri-sexual-dysfunction.html (accessed 17 January 2024).

46 BBC *Panorama*, 2023, www.bbc.co.uk/programmes/m001n39z.

47 *Ibid.*

48 https://www.pssdnetwork.org/patient-spotlight/roy.

49 It has now been covered in the *New York Times*, on the BBC's *Panorama*, the *Daily Mail*, *The Telegraph* and *The Guardian*, among other outlets in the UK.

50 Healy, D.; Le Noury, J.; & Mangin, D. (2019). 'Post-SSRI Sexual Dysfunction: Patient Experiences of Engagement With Healthcare Professionals', *International Journal of Risk and Safety in Medicine*, **30**(3): 167–78 (quotes p. 172). Available at https://rxisk.org/wp-content/uploads/2019/09/PSSD-Patient-Experiences-2019-Manuscript.pdf.

51 Ghorayshi, A. (2023). 'After Antidepressants a Loss of Sexuality'.

52 https://real-psychiatry.blogspot.com/2023/07/post-ssri-sexual-dysfunction-pssd.html?spref=tw (accessed 17 January 2024).

53 Evans-Hoeker, E.A.; Eisenberg, E.; Diamond, M.P.; Legro, R.S.; Alvero, R.; Coutifaris, C. et al. (2018), 'Major Depression, Antidepressant Use, and Male and Female Fertility', *Fertility & Sterility*, **109**(5): 879–87; Chang, Q.; Ma, X.Y.; Xu, X.R.; Su, H.; Wu, Q.J.; & Zhao, Y.H. (2020), 'Dose-dependent increase in risk of bleeding and bleeding complications in relation to SSRI

use at delivery', *Eur J Obstet Gynecol Reprod Biol*, **296**: 265–69; Toh, S., Mitchell, A.A., Louik, C., Werler, M.M., Chambers, C.D. & Hernandez-Diaz, S. (2009), 'Selective serotonin reuptake inhibitor use and risk of gestational hypertension', *Am J Psychiatry*, **166**(3): 320–28; Huang, H., Coleman, S., Bridge, J.A., Yonkers, K. & Katon, W. (2014), 'A meta-analysis of the relationship between antidepressant use in pregnancy and the risk of preterm birth and low birth weight', *Gen Hosp Psychiatry*, **36**(1): 13–18; 'Antidepressant Use in Depressed Women During Pregnancy and the Risk of Preterm Birth: A Systematic Review and Meta-Analysis of 23 Cohort Studies', *Frontiers in Pharmacology*, **11**: 659; Ondemark, M., Nordstrom, L. & Lindqvist, P.G.; Desaunay, P., Eslier, M., Alexandre, J., Dreyfus, M., Chretien, B., Guenole, F. (2024), 'Antidepressants and fetal death: A systematic review and disproportionality analysis in the WHO safety database (VigiBase(®))', *Psychiatry Res*, **339**: 116048.

54 Animal studies are summarised in Domingues, R.R., et al. (2023), 'Maternal serotonin: implications for the use of selective serotonin reuptake inhibitors during gestation', *Biol Reprod*, **109**(1): 17–28.

55 The immediate complications for the baby are detailed in Hendson, L.; Shah, V.; & Trkulja, S. (2021), 'Selective Serotonin Reuptake Inhibitors Or Serotonin-Norepinephrine Reuptake Inhibitors in Pregnancy: Infant and Childhood Outcomes', *Paediatric Child Health*, **26**(5): 321–22.

56 Ulbrich, K.A., Zumpf, K., Ciolino, J.D., Shah, M., Miller, E.S. et al. (2021), 'Acute Delivery Room Resuscitation of Neonates Exposed to Selective Serotonin Reuptake Inhibitors', *J Pediatr*, **232**: 103–108 e102.

57 Huang, W., Page, R.L., Morris, T., Ayres, S., Ferdinand, A.O. et al. (2023), 'Maternal exposure to SSRIs or SNRIs and the risk of congenital abnormalities in offspring: A systematic review and meta-analysis', *PLoS One*, **18**(11): e0294996.

58 Anderson, K.N., Lind, J.N., Simeone, R.M., Bobo, W.V., Mitchell, A.A. et al. (2020), 'Maternal Use of Specific Antidepressant Medications During Early Pregnancy and the Risk of Selected Birth Defects', *JAMA Psychiatry*, **77**(12): 1246–55.

59 Johnson, K.C., Smith, A.K., Stowe, Z.N., Newport, D.J., Brennan, P.A. (2016), 'Preschool outcomes following prenatal serotonin reuptake inhibitor exposure: differences in language and behavior, but not cognitive function', *J Clin Psychiatry*, **77**(2): e176–182; Rai, D., Lee, B.K., Dalman, C., Newschaffer, C., Lewis, G. et al. (2017), 'Antidepressants during pregnancy and autism in offspring: population based cohort study', *BMJ*, **358**: j2811; Man, K.K.C., Chan, E.W., Ip, P., Coghill, D., Simonoff, E. et al. (2017). "Prenatal antidepressant use and risk of attention-deficit/hyperactivity disorder in offspring: population based cohort study." BMJ 357: j2350.

60 Ramsteijn, A.S., et al. (2020), 'Perinatal selective serotonin reuptake inhibitor exposure and behavioral outcomes: A systematic review and meta-analyses of animal studies', *Neurosci Biobehav Rev*, **114**: 53–69; Chen, M.X., Cheng, S., Lei, L., Zhang, X.F., Liu, Q. et al. (2021), 'The effects of maternal SSRI

exposure on the serotonin system, prefrontal protein expression and behavioral development in male and female offspring rats', *Neurochem Int*, **146**: 105041.

61 Gaspar, P., et al. (2003), 'The developmental role of serotonin: news from mouse molecular genetics', *Nat Rev Neurosci*, **4**(12): 1002–12.

62 Martin, F.Z., Sharp, G.C., Easey, K.E., Madley-Dowd, P., Bowen, L. et al. (2026), 'Patterns of antidepressant prescribing around pregnancy: a descriptive analysis using Clinical Practice Research Datalink GOLD', *Br J Gen Pract*, **76**(762): e918–e928.

63 The 'public health emergency' quotation is from Urato, A. (2012), 'A New Epidemic: Antidepressants During Pregnancy', https://davidhealy.org/a-new-epidemic/ (9 July 2012: accessed 28 May 2024). The second quotation is from Dr Urato's testimony to the FDA panel, which can be read here: https://rxisk.org/antidepressants-and-pregnancy-adam-urato/#:~:text=The%20public%20needs%20better%20information,brain%2C%20and%20has%20chemical%20effects (accessed 7 April 2026).

64 The panel hearing can be viewed in full here: www.fda.gov/patients/fda-expert-panels/fda-expert-panel-selective-serotonin-reuptake-inhibitors-ssris-and-pregnancy-07212025 (accessed 7 April 2026).

65 https://womensmentalhealth.org/posts/fda-expert-panel-on-ssris-and-pregnancy/ (accessed 7 April 2026).

66 Studies that report an association between pregnancy complications and depression have mostly not accounted for the effects of antidepressants themselves; for example, Simonovich, S.D., Nidey, N.L., Gavin, A.R., Pineros-Leano, M., Hsieh, W.J. et al. (2021), 'Meta-Analysis Of Antenatal Depression and Adverse Birth Outcomes in US Populations, 2010–20', *Health Affairs (Millwood)*, **40**(10): 1560–65.

67 Animal studies include: Beeder, L.A., & Samplaski, M.K. (2020), 'Effect of Antidepressant Medications on Semen Parameters and Male Fertility', *International Journal of Urology*, **27**(1): 39–46; Bataineh, H.N., & Daradka, T. (2007), 'Effects of Long-Term Use of Fluoxetine on Fertility Parameters in Adult Male Rats', *NeuroEndocrinology Letters*, **28**(3): 321–25. Human studies include: Akasheh, G.; Sirati, L.; Noshad Kamran, A.R.; & Sepehrmanesh, Z. (2014), 'Comparison of the Effect of Sertraline with Behavioral Therapy on Semen Parameters in Men with Primary Premature Ejaculation', *Urology*, **83**(4): 800–04; Koyuncu, H.; Serefoglu, E.C.; Yencilek, E.; Atalay, H.; Akbas, N.B.; & Sarica, K. (2011), 'Escitalopram Treatment for Premature Ejaculation has a Negative Effect on Semen Parameters', *International Journal of Impotence Research*, **23**(6): 257–61.

68 https://rxisk.org/wp-content/uploads/2024/01/Fertility-Labels-0502012.pdf (accessed 10 February 2024).

69 Willingham, E. (2022). 'People Have Been Having Less Sex—Whether They're Teenagers or 40-Somethings', *Scientific American,* 3 January 2022, www.scientificamerican.com/article/people-have-been-having-less-sex-whether-theyre-teenagers-or-40-somethings/ (accessed 2 March 2024).

Chapter 12

1 Healy, D. (2019). 'Post-SSRI Sexual Dysfunction & Other Enduring Sexual Dysfunctions', *Epidemiology and Psychiatric Science* **29**: e55.

2 Waddington, J.L.; Youssef, H.A.; & Kinsella, A. (1990). 'Cognitive Dysfunction in Schizophrenia Followed Up Over 5 Years, and its Longitudinal Relationship to the Emergence of Tardive Dyskinesia', *Psychological Medicine,* **20**(4): 835–42.

3 Gardos, G.; Cole, J.O.; Haskell, D.; Marby, D.; Paine, S.S.; & Moore, P. (1988). 'The Natural History of Tardive Dyskinesia', *Journal of Clinical Psychopharmacology,* **8**(4 Suppl): 31S–37S.

4 Carey, B. (2018). 'Many People Taking Antidepressants Discover They Cannot Quit', *New York Times*, 7 April 2018, www.nytimes.com/2018/04/07/health/antidepressants-withdrawal-prozac-cymbalta.html (accessed 17 January 2024).

5 Carey, B. (2018). 'Antidepressants and Withdrawal: Readers Tell Their Stories', *New York Times,* 17 April 2018, www.nytimes.com/2018/04/17/health/antidepressants-withdrawal-readers.html (accessed 17 January 2024).

6 James Davies is the author of *Cracked: Why Psychiatry is Doing More Harm Than Good* (London: Icon Books, 2013), among other titles.

7 American Psychiatric Association (2010). *American Psychiatric Association Practice Guideline for the Treatment of Patients with Major Depressive Disorder*, 3rd Edition (Washington, DC: APA) p. 39, https://psychiatryonline.org/pb/assets/raw/sitewide/practice_guidelines/guidelines/mdd.pdf (accessed 17 January 2024).

8 National Institute for Health and Clinical Excellence (2009). 'Depression: Management of Depression in Primary and Secondary Care', Revised Clinical Practice Guideline Number 23 (London: National Institute for Health and Clinical Excellence) www.nice.org.uk/page.aspx?o=235213 (accessed June 2018).

9 Cowan, P.J. (2020). 'Management and Treatment of Depressive Disorders' in Geddes, J.R.; Andreasen, N.C.; & Goodwin, G.M., *New Oxford Textbook of Psychiatry* (Oxford: Oxford University Press) Chapter 77, p. 812.

10 The review is Davies, J., & Read, J. (2019). 'A Systematic Review Into the Incidence, Severity and Duration of Antidepressant Withdrawal Effects: Are Guidelines Evidence-Based?', *Addictive Behaviors,* **97**: 111–21. Available at www.sciencedirect.com/science/article/pii/S0306460318308347?via%3Dihub.

11 Read, J.; Cartwright, C.; & Gibson, K. (2014). 'Adverse Emotional and Interpersonal Effects Reported by 1,829 New Zealanders While Taking Antidepressants', *Psychiatry Research,* **216**(1): 67–73.

12 Horowitz, M.A.; Buckman, J.; Saunders, R.; Aguirre, E.; Davies, J;. & Moncrieff, J. (2024). 'Withdrawal Effects From Antidepressants Reported by Patients Enrolled in a Primary Care Psychotherapy Service' (manuscript in preparation).

13 Dilsaver, S.C., & J.F. Greden (1984). 'Antidepressant Withdrawal Phenomena', *Biological Psychiatry,* **19**(2): 237–56.

14 Luo, Y.; Kataoka, Y.; Ostinelli, E.G.; Cipriani, A.; & Furukawa, T.A. (2020). 'National Prescription Patterns of Antidepressants in the Treatment of Adults With Major Depression in the US Between 1996 and 2015: A Population Representative Survey Based Analysis', *Frontiers in Psychiatry,* **11**: 35.

15 Framer, A. (2021). 'What I Have Learnt From Helping Thousands of People Taper Off Antidepressants and Other Psychotropic Medications', *Therapeutic Advances in Psychopharmacology*, **11**: 2045125321991274.
16 Pope, C. (2022). 'Drug Half-Life Explained', www.drugs.com/article/drug-half-life.html (accessed 22 January 2024).
17 Ashton, C.H. (2002). *Benzodiazepines: How They Work and How to Withdraw* (Newcastle upon Tyne: Newcastle University). Available at https://benzo.org.uk/manual/ (accessed 22 January 2024).
18 Ashton, H. (1991). 'Protracted Withdrawal Syndromes From Benzodiazepines', *Journal of Substance Abuse Treatment*, **8**(1–2): 19–28 (quotes p. 19), https://pubmed.ncbi.nlm.nih.gov/1675688/.
19 Center for Substance Abuse Treatment (2010). 'Protracted Withdrawal', *Substance Abuse Treatment Advisory*, **9**(1): 1–8.
20 Read Moncrieff, J., & Horowitz, M.A. (2023). 'Designing Withdrawal Support Services for Antidepressant Users: Patients' Views on Existing Services and What They Really Need', *Journal of Psychiatric Research*, **161**: 298–306.
21 Moncrieff, J.; Read, J.; & Horowitz, M. (2024). 'The Nature and Impact of Antidepressant Withdrawal Symptoms and Proposal of the Discriminatory Antidepressant Withdrawal Symptoms Scale (DAWSS)', *Journal of Affective Disorder Reports*, in press. Available at www.sciencedirect.com/science/article/pii/S2666915324000519.
22 Taylor, S.; Annand, F.; Burkinshaw, P.; Greaves, F.; Kelleher, M.; Knight, J. et al. (2019). *Dependence and Withdrawal Associated With Some Prescribed Medicines: An Evidence Review* (London: Public Health England).
23 Vine, S. (2018). 'My Agony Hooked on Anxiety Pills', *Daily Mail*, 3 October 2018; Carey, B., & Gebeloff, R. (2018). 'Many People Taking Antidepressants Discover They Cannot Quit', *New York Times*, 7 April 2018.
24 Royal College of Psychiatrists (2020). 'Stopping Antidepressants'. Available at www.rcpsych.ac.uk/mental-health/treatments-and-wellbeing/stopping-antidepressants (accessed 22 January 2024).
25 Hayes, J., & Jauhar, S. (2019). 'Antidepressants Withdrawal: Reviewing the Paper Behind the Headlines', *Mental Elf* (18 October 2018). Available at www.nationalelfservice.net/treatment/antidepressants/antidepressant-withdrawal-reviewing-the-paper-behind-the-headlines/ (accessed 22 January 2024). Also Jauhar, S., & Hayes, J. (2019). 'The War on Antidepressants: What We Can and Can't Conclude from the Systematic Review of Antidepressant Withdrawal Effects by Davies and Read', *Addictive Behaviors*, **97**: 122–25. Available at www.ncbi.nlm.nih.gov/pmc/articles/PMC7613096/. Quotes are from the blog.
26 Davies, J., & Read, J. (2019). 'Authors' Response to a Critique by Jauhar and Hayes of "A systematic review into the incidence, severity and duration of antidepressant withdrawal effects: Are guideline evidence-based?"', *Addictive Behaviors* **97**: 127–30 (available at https://repository.uel.ac.uk/item/844x2).
27 Personal account provided by one of the people involved.

28 The paper is Henssler, J.; Schmidt, Y.; Schmidt, U.; Schwarzer, G.; Bschor, T.; & Baethge, C. (2024). 'Incidence of Antidepressant Discontinuation Symptoms: A Systematic Review and Meta-Analysis', *Lancet Psychiatry,* 10.1016/S2215-0366(24)00133-0. Our response is Horowitz, M., & Moncrieff, J. (2024). 'Study Claiming Antidepressant Withdrawal is Less Common Than Thought Fails to Account for Risks in Long-Term Users', *The Conversation.* Available at https://theconversation.com/study-claiming-antidepressant-withdrawal-is-less-common-than-thought-fails-to-account-for-risks-in-long-term-users-231728 (accessed 11 June 2024).

29 Jauhar and Keedwell quotes from 'Expert Reaction to Systematic Review and Meta-Analysis of Discontinuation Symptoms After Stopping Antidepressants', 5 June 2024, www.sciencemediacentre.org/expert-reaction-to-systematic-review-and-meta-analysis-of-discontinuation-symptoms-after-stopping-antidepressants/ (accessed 11 June 2024).

30 Pariante, C. (2024). 'The Myth That Antidepressants are Addictive has been Debunked – They are a Vital Tool in Psychiatry', *The Guardian,* www.theguardian.com/commentisfree/article/2024/jun/08/antidepressants-addictive-has-been-debunked-psychiatry-depression-withhdrawal-symptoms (accessed 11 June 2024).

31 See for example, @lauradelano's post on X on 6 June, which reads: 'The way I see it, reviews like this new one in Lancet Psychiatry are reminders that we current and former psychiatric drug-takers need to look inwards to one another to deepen the trust we have in the reality – and the deep wisdom – of our personal and collective experiences with these pharmaceutical products. Our stories of iatrogenic harm (both from taking and from getting off these drugs) are the best – and, IMO, the most reliable – evidence there is. ONWARDS!'

32 Schraer, R.; Hix, C.; & Harris, L. (2023). 'Antidepressants: Two Million Taking Them for Five Years or More', *BBC News,* www.bbc.co.uk/news/uk-65825012 (accessed 11 June 2024).

33 Brown, M.; Lewis, S. (2021). 'The Patient Voice: Antidepressant Withdrawal, Medically Unexplained Symptoms, and Functional Neurological Disorders'. *Journal of Critical Psychology, Counselling, and Psychotherapy,* **20**: 14–20.

34 See Chapter 2.

35 White, E. (2021). 'Antidepressant Withdrawal: Avoid Doctors?', 15 February 2021. Available at https://rxisk.org/antidepressant-withdrawal-avoid-doctors/ (accessed 22 January 2024).

36 Ashton, H. (1991) p. 19.

37 Horowitz, M., & Talor, D.M. (2024). *The Maudsley Deprescribing Guidelines: Antidepressants, Benzodiazepines, Gabapentinoids and Z-drugs,* The Maudsley Prescribing Guidelines Series (Oxford: Wiley Blackwell). This is not freely available, but if you are having problems with withdrawal, you could ask your doctor to get a copy.

Chapter 13

1 www.sciencemediacentre.org/about-us/funding/.
2 Science Media Centre (2022). 'Expert Reaction to a Review Paper on the "Serotonin Theory of Depression"', 20 July 2022, www.sciencemediacentre.org/expert-reaction-to-a-review-paper-on-the-serotonin-theory-of-depression/ (accesssed on 14 January 2024).
3 Freud, S. (1911). *The Interpretation of Dreams*, 3rd Edition. Available in English translation at https://psychclassics.yorku.ca/Freud/Dreams/dreams.pdf (accessed 2 March 2024) p. 42.
4 All quotations from Science Media Centre (2022).
5 American Psychiatric Association (2024). 'What is Depression?', www.psychiatry.org/patients-families/depression/what-is-depression (accessed 8 February 2024).
6 Pies, R.W. (2011). 'Doctor, Is My Mood Disorder Due to a Chemical Imbalance?', *Psychiatric Times*, 12 August 2011, www.psychiatrictimes.com/view/doctor-my-mood-disorder-due-chemical-imbalance (accessed 1 May 2023).
7 Pies, R., & Dawson, G. (2022). 'The Serotonin Fixation: Much Ado About Nothing New', *Psychiatric Times*, 3 August 2022, www.psychiatrictimes.com/view/the-serotonin-fixation-much-ado-about-nothing-new (accessed 14 January 2024).
8 Quoted in Dickson, E. (2022). 'Who is the Psychiatrist Behind the Antidepressant Study Taking Over Right-Wing Media?', *Rolling Stone*, 30 July 2022, www.rollingstone.com/culture/culture-news/ssri-right-wing-attack-joanna-moncrieff-1388067/.
9 As we documented in this paper: Ang, B.; Horowitz, M.; & Moncrieff, J. (2022). 'Is the Chemical Imbalance an "Urban Legend"? An Exploration of the Status of the Serotonin Theory of Depression in the Scientific Literature', *Social Science & Medicine – Mental health*, **2**: 1–9, available at www.sciencedirect.com/science/article/pii/S266656032200038X (accessed 8 February 2024).
10 See Appendix 1 and American Psychiatric Association (2024).
11 Kirkey, S. (2022). 'Doctors Have Stopped Believing that "Chemical Imbalance" Causes Depression. They Didn't Tell Us', *National Post*, 16 September 2022, https://nationalpost.com/health/serotonin-chemical-imbalance-depression (accessed 8 February 2024).
12 See Chapter 2.
13 Pies, R.W., & Dawson, G. (2022). 'Serotonin or Not, Antidepressants Work', *Psychiatric Times*, 6 September 2022, www.psychiatrictimes.com/view/serotonin-or-not-antidepressants-work (accessed 14 January 2024).
14 Pies, R., & Dawson, G. (2022). 3 August 2022.
15 Science Media Centre (2022).
16 *Ibid.*
17 Rihmer, Z.; Dome, P.; & Katona, C. (2022). 'Serotonin and Depression – A Riposte to Moncrieff et al. (2022)', *Neuropsychopharmacologia Hungarica*, **24**(3): 120–25.
18 Bartova, L.; Lanzenberger, R.; Rujescu, D.; & Kasper, S. (2023). 'Reply to: "The serotonin theory of depression: a systematic umbrella review of the evidence"

published by Moncrieff J, Cooper RE, Stockmann T, Amendola S, Hengartner MP, Horowitz MA in *Molecular Psychiatry* (20 July 2022. doi: 10.1038/s41380-022-01661-0)', *Molecular Psychiatry*, **28**(8): 3153–54.

19 Arnone, D.; Wise, T.; Fitzgerald, P.B.; Harmer, C.J. (2024). 'The Involvement of Serotonin in Major Depression: Nescience in Disguise?', *Molecular Psychiatry*, 19 February 2024, doi: 10.1038/s41380-024-02459-y. Online ahead of print.

20 More detail and references to individual studies on antidepressants and emotion processing can be found in our second 'authors' reply' to letters about the serotonin paper: Moncrieff, J.; Cooper, R.E.; Stockmann, T.; Amendola, S.; Hengartner, M.P.; & Horowitz, M.A. (2024). 'Difficult Lives Explain Depression Better Than Broken Brains', *Molecular Psychiatry*, **29**(1): 206–09. Available at www.nature.com/articles/s41380-024-02462-3.

21 Hamish McAllister-Williams on Naked Scientist, 18 July 2023, www.thenaked-scientists.com/podcasts/naked-scientists-podcast/antidepressants-ongoing-debate.

22 Devlin, H. (2022). 'Study Claims to Find First Direct Evidence of a Link Between Low Serotonin and Depression', *The Guardian*, 5 November 2022: www.theguardian.com/society/2022/nov/05/study-finds-first-evidence-of-link-between-low-serotonin-levels-and-depression.

23 Erritzoe, D.; Godlewska, B.R.; Rizzo, G.; Searle, G.E.; Agnorelli, C. et al. (2023). 'Brain Serotonin Release Is Reduced in Patients With Depression: A [(11)C] Cimbi-36 Positron Emission Tomography Study With a d-Amphetamine Challenge', *Biological Psychiatry*, **93**(12): 1089–98. Quotes from p. 5, italics added. www.sciencedirect.com/science/article/pii/S0006322322017048?via%3Dihub.

24 The study involved eleven pigs in all, but only four contributed to this particular analysis. The paper is Jorgensen, L.M.; Weikop, P.; Villadsen, J.; Visnapuu, T.; Ettrup, A.; Hansen, H.D. et al. (2017). 'Cerebral 5-HT Release Correlates With [(11)C]Cimbi36 PET Measures of 5-HT2A Receptor Occupancy in the Pig Brain', *Journal of Cerebral Blood Flow & Metabolism*, **37**(2): 425-–34.

25 Politis, M., & Niccolini, F. (2015). 'Serotonin in Parkinson's Disease', *Behavioral Brain Research*, **277**: 136–45.

26 A one-sided statistical test assumes the effect can only go in one direction: i.e. serotonin can only be lower. This is only acceptable in rare situations in which we are sure the effect cannot be the reverse. This was clearly not the case in this study, where there are no precedents in humans and scant data in animals. A two-sided test is the norm.

27 This blog provides a detailed critique of the study: Fried, E. (2022). '"Clear evidence" for serotonin hypothesis of depression?' Available at https://eiko-fried.com/clear-evidence-for-serotonin-hypothesis-of-depression/ (accessed 15 January 2024).

28 Hengartner, M.P., & Ploderl, M. (2023). 'No Clear Evidence of Reduced Brain Serotonin Release Capacity in Patients With Depression', *Biological Psychiatry*, **93**(12): e61.

29 https://twitter.com/dawsoo07/status/1549784664566628360, posted on 20 July 2022 (accessed 12 January 2024).

30 E.g. Awais Aftab, cited in Spichak, S. (2022). 'How the Debate Over Antidepressants Puts Millions in Danger', *The Daily Beast*, www.thedailybeast.com/the-debate-over-how-antidepressants-work-is-putting-millions-of-people-in-danger#:~:text=While%20the%20psychiatrists%20who%20spoke,has%20fostered%20downsides%20over%20time (accessed 26 January 2024).

31 Johns Hopkins Drug Discovery receives funding from Janssen, https://drugdiscovery.jhu.edu/about-us/funding/ (accessed 8 February 2024) and Adam Kaplin, Assistant Professor of Psychiatry at Johns Hopkins, received funding from Janssen, www.hopkinsmedicine.org/news/newsroom/news-releases/2019/07/ketamine-isnt-an-opioid-and-treats-depression-in-a-unique-way (accessed 8 February 2024).

32 www.hopkinsmedicine.org/health/treatment-tests-and-therapies/esketamine-for-treatment-resistant-depression (accessed 15 January 2024).

33 Eriksson, P.S.; Perfilieva, E.; Bjork-Eriksson, T.; Alborn, A.M.; Nordborg, C.; Peterson, D.A.; & Gage, F.H. (1998). 'Neurogenesis in the Adult Human Hippocampus', *Nature Medicine*, **4**(11): 1313–17.

34 Malberg, J.E.; Eisch, A.J.; Nestler, E.J.; & Duman, R.S. (2000). 'Chronic Antidepressant Treatment Increases Neurogenesis in Adult Rat Hippocampus', *Journal of Neuroscience*, **20**(24): 9104–10.

35 Geerlings, M.I., & Gerritsen, L. (2017). 'Late-Life Depression, Hippocampal Volumes, and Hypothalamic-Pituitary-Adrenal Axis Regulation: A Systematic Review and Meta-analysis', *Biological Psychiatry*, **82**(5): 339–50.

36 Teicher, M.H.; Anderson, C.M.; Ohashi, K.; Khan, A.; McGreenery, C.E.; Bolger, E.A. et al. (2018). 'Differential Effects of Childhood Neglect and Abuse During Sensitive Exposure Periods on Male and Female Hippocampus', *Neuroimage*, **169**: 443–52; Lu, H.; Li, X.; Wang, Y.; Song, Y.; & Liu, J. (2018). 'The Hippocampus Underlies the Association Between Self-Esteem and Physical Health', *Scientific Reports*, **8**(1): 17141. Antidepressant effects are shown in this study: Geerlings, M.I.; Brickman, A.M.; Schupf, N.; Devanand, D.P.; Luchsinger, J.A.; Mayeux, R.; & Small, S.A. (2012). 'Depressive Symptoms, Antidepressant Use, and Brain Volumes on MRI in a Population-Based Cohort of Old Persons Without Dementia', *Journal of Alzheimers Disease*, **30**(1): 75–82.

37 Winter, N.R.; Leenings, R.; Ernsting, J.; Sarink, K.; Fisch, L.; Emden, D. et al. (2022). 'Quantifying Deviations of Brain Structure and Function in Major Depressive Disorder Across Neuroimaging Modalities', *JAMA Psychiatry*, **79**(9): 879–88 (quotes p. 879). Available at www.ncbi.nlm.nih.gov/pmc/articles/PMC9330277/.

38 The authors' interpretation was that the evidence was 'more nuanced': Lino de Oliveira, C.; Bolzan, J.A.; Surget, A.; & Belzung, C. (2020). 'Do Antidepressants Promote Neurogenesis in Adult Hippocampus? A Systematic Review and Meta-Analysis on Naive Rodents', *Pharmacology & Therapeutics*, **210**: 107515, https://pubmed.ncbi.nlm.nih.gov/32109488/.

39 Choe, Y.M.; Kim, K.W.; Jhoo, J.H.; Ryu, S.H.; Seo, E.H.; Sohn, B.K. et al. (2016). 'Multicenter, Randomized, Placebo-Controlled, Double-Blind Clinical Trial

of Escitalopram on the Progression-Delaying Effects in Alzheimer's Disease', *International Journal of Geriatric Psychiatry,* **31**(7): 731–39; Chataway, J.; De Angelis, F.; Connick, P.; Parker, R.; Plantone, D.; Doshi, A. et al. (2020). 'Efficacy of Three Neuroprotective Drugs in Secondary Progressive Multiple Sclerosis (MS-SMART): A Phase 2b, Multiarm, Double-Blind, Randomised Placebo-Controlled Trial', *Lancet Neurology,* **19**(3): 214–25.

40 Zamproni, L.N.; Mundim, M.T.V.V.; & Porcionatto, M.A. (2021). 'Neurorepair and Regeneration of the Brain: A Decade of Bioscaffolds and Engineered Microtissue', *Front in Cell & Developmental Biology,* **9**: 649891.

41 Conventionally, this is interpreted as evidence that ECT is correcting an underlying abnormality in neurogenesis in people with depression and assumed to provide support for the idea that such an abnormality exists. See An, X., & Wang, Y. (2022). 'Electroconvulsive Shock Increases Neurotrophy and Neurogenesis: Time Course and Treatment Session Effects', *Psychiatry Research* **309**: 114390, www.sciencedirect.com/science/article/pii/S016517812200004X?via%3Dihub.

42 This study found a lack of evidence for neurogenesis in adult humans: Sorrells, S.F.; Paredes, M.F.; Cebrian-Silla, A.; Sandoval, K.; Qi, D.; Kelley, K.W. et al. (2018). 'Human Hippocampal Neurogenesis Drops Sharply in Children to Undetectable Levels in Adults', *Nature,* **555**(7696): 377–81. This paper is a discussion of the evidence overall: Snyder, J.S. (2019). 'Recalibrating the Relevance of Adult Neurogenesis', *Trends in Neuroscience,* **42**(3): 164–78.

43 Bullmore, E. (2018). *The Inflamed Mind: A Radical New Approach to Depression* (London: Short Books Ltd).

44 O'Connor, M.F.; Bower, J.E.; Cho, H.J.; Creswell, J.D.; Dimitrov, S.; Hamby, M.E. et al. (2009). 'To Assess, to Control, to Exclude: Effects of Biobehavioral Factors on Circulating Inflammatory Markers', *Brain Behavior & Immunity,* **23**(7): 887–97. On antidepressants: Mosiolek, A.; Pieta, A.; Jakima, S.; Zborowska, N.; Mosiolek, J.; & Szulc, A. (2021). 'Effects of Antidepressant Treatment on Peripheral Biomarkers in Patients with Major Depressive Disorder (MDD)', *Journal of Clinical Medicine* **10**(8).

45 Horowitz, M.A.; Wertz, J.; Zhu, D.; Cattaneo, A.; Musaelyan, K.; Nikkheslat, N. et al. (2014). 'Antidepressant Compounds Can Be Both Pro- and Anti-Inflammatory in Human Hippocampal Cells', *International Journal of Neuropsychopharmacology,* **18**(3).

46 Miller, J.J. (2019). 'Depression's Journey From Monoamines to Glutamate', *Psychiatric Times,* **36**(5): 21 May, www.psychiatrictimes.com/view/esketamine-depressions-journey-monoamines-glutamate (accessed 8 February 2024).

47 www.hopkinsmedicine.org/health/treatment-tests-and-therapies/esketamine-for-treatment-resistant-depression.

48 Moriguchi, S.; Takamiya, A.; Noda, Y.; Horita, N.; Wada, M.; Tsugawa, S. et al. (2019). 'Glutamatergic Neurometabolite Levels in Major Depressive Disorder: A Systematic Review and Meta-Analysis of Proton Magnetic Resonance Spectroscopy Studies', *Molecular Psychiatry,* **24**(7): 952–64.

49 Iro, C.M.; Hamati, R.; El Mansari, M.; & Blier, P. et al. (2021). 'Repeated but Not Single Administration of Ketamine Prolongs Increases of the Firing Activity of Norepinephrine and Dopamine Neurons', *International Journal of Neuropsychopharmacology*, **24**(7): 570–79; Liebe, T.; Li, M.; Colic, L.; Munk, M.H.J.; Sweeney-Reed, C.M.; Woelfer, M. et al. (2018). 'Ketamine Influences the Locus Coeruleus Norepinephrine Network, With a Dependency on Norepinephrine Transporter Genotype – A Placebo-Controlled Fmri Study', *Neuroimage: Clinical*, **20**: 715–23.

50 This response is Moncrieff, J.; Cooper, R.E.; Stockmann, T.; Amendola, S.; Hengartner, M.P.; Ploderl, M.; & Horowitz, M.A. (2023). 'The Serotonin Hypothesis of Depression: Both Long Discarded and Still Supported?', *Molecular Psychiatry*, **28**(8): 3160–63 (quote p. 3160). Available at www.nature.com/articles/s41380-023-02094-z.

Chapter 14

1 From a conversation held on 22 July 2022.

2 Email received on 20 July 2022. Name changed for purposes of anonymity.

3 From emails received between 20 and 25 July 2022.

4 Cited in Love, S. (2022). 'The New Study on Serotonin and Depression Isn't About Antidepressants', *Vice*, 22 July 2022: www.vice.com/en/article/88qge4/the-new-study-on-serotonin-and-depression-isnt-about-antidepressants-chemical-imbalance (accessed 28 January 2024).

5 It was covered by *Sky News*: https://news.sky.com/story/antidepressants-called-into-question-as-researchers-find-no-convincing-evidence-depression-is-caused-by-chemical-imbalance-12655342 (accessed 7 June 2023); the BBC *Today* programme and BBC Scotland, among other places.

6 A right of centre TV channel in the UK.

7 An organisation set up to bring underrepresented perspectives in the mental health field into the media, www.safelyheldspaces.org/.

8 *The Conversation* piece about the study is Moncrieff, J., & Horowitz, M. (2022). 'Depression is Probably Not Caused By a Chemical Imbalance in the Brain – New Study', 20 July 2022, https://theconversation.com/depression-is-probably-not-caused-by-a-chemical-imbalance-in-the-brain-new-study-186672 (accessed 28 January 2024). The figures for readership are provided in a second article we wrote for *The Conversation*: Horowitz, M., & Moncrieff, J. (2022). 'Chemical Imbalance Theory of Depression: Clearing Up Some Misconceptions', 23 August 2022, https://theconversation.com/chemical-imbalance-theory-of-depression-clearing-up-some-misconceptions-188921 (accessed 28 January 2024). Figures were derived from the Altmetric site in July 2022: www.altmetric.com/details/132834624?src=bookmarklet#score.

9 You can nevertheless view it here: www.youtube.com/watch?v=d65J2Kqv4xQ.

10 The *Daily Mail* has a recent record of interrogating the medical orthodoxy on various issues. See, for example: www.dailymail.co.uk/health/article-2620866/

From-psychiatrist-whod-never-anti-depressants-heart-doctor-steers-clear-statins-reveal-medical-treatments-experts-refuse-themselves.html.

11 Gornall, J. (2022). 'Have millions been taking antidepressants with harmful side-effects for decades - when there's no scientific evidence they do what they claim? Some experts have suspected it for years. Now patients have been left reeling by a groundbreaking study,' *The Daily Mail*, 20 July 2022, www.dailymail.co.uk/news/article-11033517/Have-millions-taking-antidepressants-harmful-effects-decades-no-reason.html (accessed 28 January 2024); Ely, J. (2022). 'Depression "is NOT caused by low serotonin levels": Study casts doubt over widespread use of potent drugs designed to treat chemical imbalance in brain', *The Daily Mail*, 20 July 2022: www.dailymail.co.uk/health/article-11027847/Depression-NOT-caused-low-serotonin-levels-study.html (accessed 28 January 2024); Andrews, L. (2022). 'A $15 billion hustle? Expert says pill-prescribing psychiatrists KNEW that depression isn't caused by low serotonin levels – as landmark study shows that pricy drugs do little to help mental health', *The Daily Mail*, 21 July 2022: www.dailymail.co.uk/news/article-11035903/Expert-says-psychiatrists-KNOW-theory-low-serotonin-levels-cause-depression-incomplete.html (accessed 28 January 2024); Ennals, E. (2022). 'Antidepressants do work, insist top doctors as they hit back at bombshell study which found there was no "convincing evidence" of a link between low serotonin and mental illness', *Mail on Sunday*, 23 July 2022: www.dailymail.co.uk/health/article-11042143/Joanne-Moncrieff-University-College-London-disproves-link-low-serotonin-depression.html (accessed 28 January 2024).

12 www.nbcnews.com/news/us-news/epoch-times-falun-gong-growth-rcna111373.

13 Programme and transcript available at www.foxnews.com/opinion/tucker-carlson-drugs-not-answer-every-human-problem.

14 Schraer, R. (2022). 'Did we all believe a myth about depression?' BBC News website, 5 August 2022, www.bbc.co.uk/news/health-62286093 (accessed 27 May 2024).

15 Cleverley, E. (2022). 'Depression myths: "Stopping medication made me twice as bad"', BBC News website, 5 August 2022: www.bbc.co.uk/news/newsbeat-62390763 (accessed 27 May 2024).

16 WBUR On Point (2022). 'Behind the New Study Changing How Doctors View Depression', 1 August 2022. Programme and transcript available at www.wbur.org/onpoint/2022/08/01/inside-the-new-study-changing-home-doctors-view-depression (accessed 28 January 2024).

17 Weekend Prime (2022), Newsnation, 13 August 2022.

18 Dickson, E. (2022). 'Who Is the Psychiatrist Behind the Antidepressant Study Taking Over Right-Wing Media?', *Rolling Stone*, 30 July 2022: www.rollingstone.com/culture/culture-news/ssri-right-wing-attack-joanna-moncrieff-1388067/ (accessed 28 January 2024).

19 Levine, B.E. (2022). 'Behind Rolling Stone's Hatchet Job on a Psychiatrist Critical of Neoliberal Capitalism', *Counter Punch*, 11 August 2022: www.counterpunch.org/2022/2008/2011/behind-rolling-stones-hatchet-job-on-a-psychiatrist-critical-of-neoliberal-capitalism/ (accessed 16 February 2024).

20 Dickson, E. (2019). 'Marianne Williamson Is Dangerously Wrong About Antidepressants', *Rolling Stone,* 2 August 2019: www.rollingstone.com/culture/culture-news/marianne-williamson-wrong-about-antidepressants-866807/.
21 You can read my response in full here: Moncrieff, J. (2022). 'First they ignore you. Then they ridicule you. And then they attack you ...': https://joanna-moncrieff.com/2022/08/03/first-they-ignore-you-then-they-ridicule-you-and-then-they-attack-you/, 3 August 2022 (accessed 28 May 2024).
22 McKeigue, P.M.,;Kennedy, S.; Weir, A.; Bishop, J.; McGurnaghan, S.J.; McAllister, D. et al. (2021). 'Relation of Severe COVID-19 to Polypharmacy and Prescribing of Psychotropic Drugs: The REACT-SCOT Case-Control Study', *BMC Medicine,* **19**(1): 51.
23 Ruddick, G. (2017). 'Rolling Stone, rock'n'roll magazine turned liberal cheerleader, up for sale', *The Guardian,* 18 September 2017: www.theguardian.com/us-news/2017/sep/2018/rolling-stone-magazine-up-for-sale (accessed 28 January 2024).
24 Editorial: Moncrieff, J. (2016). 'Misrepresenting Harms in Antidepressant Trials', *British Medical Journal,* **352**: i217; Blog: Moncrieff, J. (2016). 'Further evidence of the adverse effects of antidepressants, and why these have taken so long to be confirmed', 2 February 2016, https://joannamoncrieff.com/2016/2002/2002/further-evidence-of-the-adverse-effects-of-antidepressants-and-why-these-have-taken-so-long-to-be-confirmed/ (accessed 28 January 2024).
25 See note 148.
26 An example by a leading psychiatrist: Frances, A. (2013). *Saving Normal: An Insider's Revolt Against Out-Of-Control Psychiatric Diagnosis, DSM-5, Big Pharma, and the Medicalization of Ordinary Life* (New York: Mariner Books).
27 Kirkey, S. (2022). 'Doctors have stopped believing that "chemical imbalance" causes depression. They didn't tell us', *National Post,* 16 September 2022, https://nationalpost.com/health/serotonin-chemical-imbalance-depression (accessed 28 January 2024).
28 Love, S. (2022).
29 Conrad, P. (1992). 'Medicalisation and Social Control', *Annual Review of Sociology,* **18**: 209–32.
30 Ratnayake, S. (2022). 'Why Has the Misleading "Chemical Imbalance" Theory of Mental Illness Persisted for So Long?', *Slate,* 4 August 2022, https://slate.com/technology/2022/2008/ssris-chemical-imbalance-depression.html (accessed 28 January 2024).
31 Jackson is cited in Love (2022); Ratnayake, S. (2022).
32 Bulik, B.S. (2019). 'Hey, big spender: Pharma's $6.6B TV ad outlay outranks most other industries, report says', *Fierce Pharma,* 15 May 2019: www.fiercepharma.com/marketing/hey-big-spenders-pharma-ranks-top-five-industries-for-tv-media-spending-says-report.
33 https://mediaradar.com/blog/medical-and-pharma-advertisers/ (accessed 2 March 2024).
34 Willis, E.; Friedel, K.; Heisten, M.; Pickett, M.; & Bhowmick, A. (2023). 'Communicating Health Literacy on Prescription Medications on Social Media:

In-depth Interviews With "Patient Influencers"', *Journal of Medical Internet Research*, **25**: e41867; see also Castronuovo, C. (2023). 'TikTokers Put Consumers at Risk as Drug Ads Go Unchecked by FDA', *Bloomberg Law*, 14 December 2023, https://news.bloomberglaw.com/health-law-and-business/tiktokers-put-consumers-at-risk-as-drug-ads-go-unchecked-by-fda (accessed 2 March 2024).

Chapter 15

1 Leading British psychiatrist Michael Shepherd was a renowned sceptic of the new drug. See for example, Shepherd, M. (1994). 'Neurolepsis and the Psychopharmacological Revolution: Myth and Reality', *Hist Psychiatry*, **5**(17 Pt 1): 89–96. See also Chapter 5, notes 15 and 16 for references to antidepressants sceptics.

2 www.ucl.ac.uk/psychiatry/research/pharmacological-treatments-depression-and-bipolar-disorder. Studies featured were the ANTLER study of antidepressant discontinuation (see Chapter 2), and the PANDA study of sertraline for depression. This found no effect on the main outcome of depressive symptoms, small effects on some other outcomes and that participants could detect what they were allocated to better than chance, suggesting the possibility of amplified placebo effects. The PANDA study is Lewis, G. et al. (2019). 'The Clinical Effectiveness of Sertraline in Primary Care and the Role of Depression Severity and Duration (PANDA): A Pragmatic, Double-Blind, Placebo-Controlled Randomised Trial', *Lancet Psychiatry*, **6**(11): 903–14. Available at www.ncbi.nlm.nih.gov/pmc/articles/PMC7029306/.

3 Pawlikowska, B. (2023). *Heal From Depression. The Mind, Body and Soul Solution: A Personal Journey* (Mysiadlo, Poland: Adventure Unlimited Beata Pawlikowska).

4 www.youtube.com/watch?v=jpUCxE2MkdM (accessed 21 February 2024).

5 www.madinamerica.com/2023/01/threatened-polish-journalist/ (accessed 21 February 2024).

6 www.youtube.com/watch?v=xjIX4rPWxiw (accessed 21 February 2024).

7 You can watch it here: www.youtube.com/watch?v=xjIX4rPWxiw.

8 www.madinamerica.com/2023/01/threatened-polish-journalist/ (accessed 21 February 2024).

9 https://socialbites.ca/politics/157982.html (accessed 21 February 2021).

10 Quotes from personal communication, 15 August 2023, reproduced with permission.

11 A Johnson & Johnson (the parent company of Janssen) press release from 5 May 2018 discussed 'the potential of esketamine nasal spray to address a significant unmet need for the more than 30 percent of people suffering from major depressive disorder who do not respond to two or more currently available antidepressants', www.jnj.com/media-center/press-releases/new-phase-3-data-show-esketamine-nasal-spray-demonstrated-rapid-improvements-in-depressive-symptoms-in-patients-with-treatment-resistant-depression (accessed 2 March 2024).

12 You can read more in Horowitz, M.A., & Moncrieff, J. (2021). 'Are We Repeating Mistakes of the Past? A Review of the Evidence for Esketamine', *British Journal of Psychiatry,* **219**(5): 614–17. Available at https://discovery.ucl.ac.uk/id/eprint/10125093/.

13 Jauhar, S., & Morrison, P. (2019). 'Esketamine for Treatment Resistant Depression', *British Medical Journal,* **366**: l5572.

14 Horowitz & Moncrieff (2021). 'Are We Repeating the Mistakes of the Past?'.

15 https://scientific-publishing.webshop.elsevier.com/research-process/paper-retraction-meaning-and-main-reasons/ (accessed 21 February 2024).

16 You can read the online versions of the letters and our reply here: www.cambridge.org/core/journals/the-british-journal-of-psychiatry/article/are-we-repeating-mistakes-of-the-past-a-review-of-the-evidence-for-esketamine/C4BDC70050164FD9D88DF40967C2853A#comments. The reference for the print version of our reply is Horowitz, M. and J. Moncrieff (2021). 'Esketamine: Uncertain Safety and Efficacy Data in Depression', *British Journal of Psychiatry,* **219**(5): 621–22, https://pubmed.ncbi.nlm.nih.gov/35048830/.

17 Ennals, E. (2023). 'Demands for "flawed" study that cast doubts on the effectiveness of antidepressants to be AXED', *The Daily Mail,* 17 June 2023, www.dailymail.co.uk/health/article-12206165/Demands-flawed-study-cast-doubts-effectiveness-antidepressants-AXED.html

18 Nutt, D.J., & Malizia, A.L. (2008). 'Why Does the World Have Such a "Down" on Antidepressants?', *Journal of Psychopharmacology,* **22**(3): 223–26; Nutt also endorsed 'Depression: A Guide to its Recognition and management in General Practise' (produced by Neurolink, funded by Wyeth Laboratories, no date).

19 Wise, J. (2023). 'Review That Questioned Serotonin Theory of Depression was', *British Medical Journal,* **381** (20 June 2023): 1419.

20 Wilkinson, R., & Jauhar, S. (2023). 'Serotonin Hypothesis of Depression: Balance (and Imbalance) is in the Eye of the Beholder', www.nationalelfservice.net/treatment/antidepressants/serotonin-hypothesis-depression/ (accessed 21 February 2024).

21 X explains, 'A hashtag – written with a # symbol – is used to index keywords or topics on X. This function was created on X, and allows people to easily follow topics they are interested in', https://help.x.com/en/using-x/how-to-use-hashtags#:~:text=A%20hashtag%E2%80%94written%20with%20a,topics%20they%20are%20interested%20in.

22 Tweet by Joanna Moncrieff, 24 June 2023.

23 Tweet by Robert Howard, 24 June 2023.

24 Tweet by Bert, 27 June 2023.

25 Tweet by Peter Sterling, 26 June 2023.

26 Tweet by Bert 27 June 2023.

27 The 'comment' is Jauhar, S.; Arnone, D.; Baldwin, D.S.; Bloomfield, M.; Browning, M.; Cleare, A.J. et al. (2023). 'A Leaky Umbrella Has Little Value: Evidence Clearly Indicates the Serotonin System is Implicated in Depression', *Molecular Psychiatry,* **28**(8): 3149–52. Available here: www.nature.com/articles/s41380-023-02095-y.

28 Our reply (which was also a reply to several other letters) is Moncrieff, J.; Cooper, R.E.; Stockmann, T.; Amendola, S.; Hengartner, M.P.; Ploderl, M.; Horowitz, M.A. (2023). 'The Serotonin Hypothesis of Depression: Both Long Discarded and Still Supported?', *Molecular Psychiatry,* **28**(8): 3160–63. Available here: www.nature.com/articles/s41380-023-02094-z.
29 GRADE stands for Grading of Recommendations, Assessment, Development, and Evaluations. Siemieniuk, R., & Guyatt, G. (2024). 'What is Grade?', *BMJ (British Medical Journal) Best Practice,* https://bestpractice.bmj.com/info/toolkit/learn-ebm/what-is-grade/#:~:text=GRADE%20has%20four%20levels%20of,data%20starts%20at%20low%20quality (accessed 2 March 2024).
30 References to this research can all be found in Moncrieff et al. (2023). 'The Serotonin Hypothesis of Depression: Both Long Discarded and Still Supported?'
31 One of these reviews claimed there was no publication bias present but used an unusual method for testing it. When we reanalysed it using the usual method, we showed publication bias was present. This is explained in Moncrieff et al. (2023). 'The Serotonin Hypothesis of Depression: Both Long Discarded and Still Supported?'
32 *Ibid.*
33 Jauhar et al. (2023) p. 3.
34 Tweets by Michael Hengartner and Sameer Jauhar, 27 June 2023.
35 E.g. tweet by Robert Howard, 20 June 2023.
36 See my account of this history in Moncrieff, J. (2009). *The Myth of the Chemical Cure: a critique of psychiatric drug treatment*, Revised Edition (Basingstoke, UK: Palgrave Macmillan) pp. 47–51.
37 *Ibid.*
38 Historian Andrew Scull's book is informative on this subject: Scull, A. (2022). *Desperate Remedies: Psychiatry and the Mysteries of Mental Illness* (London: Allen Lane).
39 Healy, D. (2004). 'Shaping the Intimate: Influences on the Experience of Everyday Nerves', *Social Studies in Science,* **34**(2): 219–45.
40 She was a signatory to this open letter, for example: Davies, J.; Horowitz, M.; Montagu, L.; Hollins, S.; Read, J.; Moncrieff, J. et al. (2023). 'The Government has a Moral Duty to Help Those Harmed by Prescribed Dependence Forming Drugs', *British Medical Journal,* **381**: 1417.
41 Bell, J. (2020). 'Big Pharma Backed Away From Brain Drugs. Is a Return in Sight?', 'BiopharmaDive', 29 January 2020: www.biopharmadive.com/news/pharma-neuroscience-retreat-return-brain-drugs/570250/ (accessed 11 March 2024).
42 Whitaker, R. (2021). 'Anatomy of an Industry: Commerce, Payments to Psychiatrists and Betrayal of the Public Good', 'Mad in America' website 18 September 2021: www.madinamerica.com/2021/2009/anatomy-industry-commerce-payments-psychiatrists-betrayal-public-good/ (accessed 29 May 2024).
43 Demasi, M. (2022). 'From FDA to MHRA: Are Drug Regulators for Hire?', *British Medical Journal,* **377**: 01538.

44 Das, S., & Ungoed-Thomas, J. (2023). 'Revealed: Drug Firms Funding UK Patient Groups That Lobby for NHS Approval of Medicines', *The Guardian*, 22 July 2023: www.theguardian.com/science/2023/jul/2022/revealed-drug-firms-funding-uk-patient-groups-that-lobby-for-nhs-approval-of-medicines (accessed 11 March 2024).

45 This is a review of studies showing doctors' behaviour is influenced by drug company inducements: Mitchell, A.P.; Trivedi, N.U.; Gennarelli, R.L.; Chimonas, S.; Tabatabai, S.M.; Goldberg, J. et al. (2021). 'Are Financial Payments From the Pharmaceutical Industry Associated With Physician Prescribing? A Systematic Review', *Annals of Internal Medicine*, **174**(3): 353–61.

Chapter 16

1 I will use the term 'psychedelics' loosely to include classical psychedelics, such as LSD and psylocibin, and drugs such ketamine and MDMA (commonly known as ecstasy) that produce some psychedelic-like effects.

2 Professor Arthur Christopoulos of Monash University, www.monash.edu/pharm/about/news/alchemy/issue-34/antibiotics-for-the-mind (accessed 24 March 2026).

3 Chen, J. (2022), 'How Ketamine Drug Helps with Depression', *Yale Medicine* (9 March 2022): www.yalemedicine.org/news/ketamine-depression (accessed 14 February 2024); https://saveminds.co.uk/depression-treatment-london/ (accessed 24 March 2026).

4 https://www.cam.ac.uk/stories/psychedelic-medicine#group-section-Helping-others-heal-834CvMMAUV (accessed 24 March 2026).

5 https://theintercept.com/2022/07/26/mdma-psilocybin-fda-ptsd/ (accessed 14 February 2024).

6 https://oxfordhealth.nhs.uk/ips/ketamine-trd/ (accessed 24 March 2026).

7 www.myodysseypbc.com/welcome (accessed 24 March 2026).

8 https://mhrt.nsw.gov.au/files/mhrt/MMAPresentation/3.%20MMA%20overview%2020190805.pdf (accessed 24 March 2026).

9 Cavarra, M., Falzone, A., Ramaekers, J.G., Kuypers, K.P.C. & Mento, C. (2022), 'Psychedelic-Assisted Psychotherapy – A Systematic Review of Associated Psychological Interventions', *Frontiers in Psychology*, **13**: 887255. www.ncbi.nlm.nih.gov/pmc/articles/PMC9226617/.

10 https://time.com/6262291/psychedelics-mdma-couples-therapy/ (accessed 24 March 2026).

11 Greenberg, G. (2010), *Manufacturing Depression: The Secret History of a Modern Disease* (London: Bloomsbury).

12 www.reddit.com/r/TherapeuticKetamine/comments/17xpz1v/iv_ketamine_and_the_comedown/ (accessed 24 March 2026).

13 https://frontlinegenomics.com/one-trip-can-change-your-life-psychedelics-genetics-and-rewiring-your-brain/#:~:text=DMT%20

(N%2CN%2DDimethyltryptamine,for%20up%20to%20a%20month (accessed 24 March 2026).

14 https://mindmedicineaustralia.org.au/stories-of-suffering-and-transformation/ (accessed 24 March 2026).

15 For example, see this comprehensive critique of the methodology of psychedelic studies: van Elk, M., and Fried, E.I. (2023), 'History repeating: guidelines to address common problems in psychedelic science', *Therapeutic Advances in Psychopharmacology*, **13**: 20451253231198466, and Žuljević, M.F., Mijatović, A., Orhanović, R., Goasdoué, G. & Gujinović, D. (2026), 'Consistency of protocol and safety data reporting in clinical trial registrations and corresponding publications of interventions involving MDMA and psilocybin', *J Clin Epidemiol*, **192**: 112170.

16 https://compasspathways.com/about-us/ (accessed 24 March 2026).

17 Bogenschutz, M.P., Ross, S., Bhatt, S., Baron, T., Forcehimes, A.A. et al. (2022), 'Percentage of Heavy Drinking Days Following Psilocybin-Assisted Psychotherapy vs Placebo in the Treatment of Adult Patients With Alcohol Use Disorder: A Randomized Clinical Trial', *JAMA Psychiatry*, **79**(10): 953–62.

18 Sumner, R.L., McMillan, R., Spriggs, M.J., Campbell, D., Malpas, G., Maxwell, E. et al. (2020), 'Ketamine Enhances Visual Sensory Evoked Potential Long-term Potentiation in Patients With Major Depressive Disorder', *Biological Psychiatry: Cognitive Neuroscience & Neuroimaging* **5**(1): 45–55.

19 42 per cent of participants had tried psychedelics before in the following trial, for example: von Rotz, R., Schindowski, E.M., Jungwirth, J., Schuldt, A., Rieser, N.M. et al. (2023), 'Single-dose psilocybin-assisted therapy in major depressive disorder: A placebo-controlled, double-blind, randomised clinical trial', *EClinicalMedicine*, **56**: 101809.

20 Carhart-Harris, R., Giribaldi, B., Watts, R., Baker-Jones, M., Murphy-Beiner, A., Murphy, R. et al. (2021), 'Trial of Psilocybin versus Escitalopram for Depression', *New England Journal of Medicine*, **384**(15): 1402–11; Mertens, L.J., Koslowski, M., Betzler, F., Brand, M., Evens, R. et al. (2026), 'Efficacy and Safety of Psilocybin in Treatment-Resistant Major Depression: The EPISODE Randomized Clinical Trial', *JAMA Psychiatry*, Mar 18:e260132. doi: 10.1001/jamapsychiatry.2026.0132. Online ahead of print.

21 Goodwin, G.M., Aaronson, S.T., Alvarez, O., Arden, P.C., Baker, A., Bennett, J.C. et al. (2022), 'Single-Dose Psilocybin for a Treatment-Resistant Episode of Major Depression', *New England Journal of Medicine*, **387**(18): 1637–48.

22 Mertens et al. (2026), see note 21.

23 Marcantoni, W.S., Akoumba, B.S., Wassef, M., Mayrand, J., Lai, H., Richard-Devantoy, S. & Beauchamp, S. (2020), 'A systematic review and meta-analysis of the efficacy of intravenous ketamine infusion for treatment resistant depression: January 2009–January 2019', *Journal of Affective Disorders*, **277**: 831–41.

24 Plöderl, M., Cooper, R., Walker, T., Shah, V., Horowitz, M. et al. (2025), 'Effects of ketamine and esketamine on death, suicidal behaviour, and suicidal ideation in

psychiatric disorders: A systematic review and meta-analysis', preprint posted at www.medrxiv.org/content/10.1101/2025.08.19.25333796v1.

25 Ketamine can also be used as an anaesthetic, incidentally, but is used infrequently because of its side effects.

26 Lii, T.R., Smith, A.E., Flohr, J.R., Okada, R.L., Nyongesa, C.A. et al. (2023), 'Randomized trial of ketamine masked by surgical anesthesia in patients with depression', *Nat Ment Health*, **1**(11): 876–86.

27 For details see: Horowitz, M., & Moncrieff, J. (2021), 'Esketamine: Uncertain Safety and Efficacy Data in Depression', *British Journal of Psychiatry*, **219**(5): 621–22. The FDA report itself is available here: www.accessdata.fda.gov/drugsatfda_docs/nda/2019/211243Orig1s000MedR.pdf (accessed 11 August 2024).

28 As reported in this discussion by leading US psychiatrists: Strakowski, S.M., Sanacora, G. & Nemeroff, C.B. (2022), 'Does Ketamine Live Up to the Hype in Depression?' *Medscape Psychiatry*, 11 August: www.medscape.com/viewarticle/976364 (accessed March 2024).

29 Busby, M. (2023), 'Ketamine clinics have emerged across the US. They're already going bust', *The Guardian* (11 April 2023): www.theguardian.com/society/2023/apr/2011/ketamine-clinics-us-business-safety-mental-health (accessed 14 February 2024).

30 Petrow, 2023.

31 Cueto, I., and O. Goldhill (2023), 'Ketamine clinics' bust serves as warning of business challenge facing psychedelic therapy', *Statnews* (16 May 2023): www.statnews.com/2023/2005/2016/ketamine-clinics-show-struggle-making-psychedelic-therapy-profitable/ (accessed 14 February 2024).

32 www.oxfordhealth.nhs.uk/ketamine/ (accessed 14 February 2024).

33 Busby, 2023.

34 Rootman, J.M., Kryskow, P., Harvey, K., Stamets, P., Santos-Brault, E. et al. (2021), 'Adults who microdose psychedelics report health related motivations and lower levels of anxiety and depression compared to non-microdosers', *Sci Rep*, **11**(1): 22479.

35 Murphy, R.J., Muthukumaraswamy, S., de Wit, H. (2024), 'Microdosing Psychedelics: Current Evidence From Controlled Studies', *Biol Psychiatry Cogn Neurosci Neuroimaging*, **9**(5): 500–11.

36 www.nbcnews.com/news/us-news/depths-matthew-perrys-addiction-6-8-shots-day-55k-month-ketamine-rcna166806.

37 www.hopkinsmedicine.org/health/treatment-tests-and-therapies/esketamine-for-treatment-resistant-depression.

38 www.cam.ac.uk/stories/psychedelic-medicine (accessed 25 March 2026).

39 https://compasspathways.com/our-work/about-psilocybin-therapy-and-treatment/ (accessed 25 March 2026).

40 Mullard, A. (2021), 'Will psychedelics be "a revolution in psychiatry"?', *Nature Reviews: Drug Discovery*, **20**(6): 418–19: www.nature.com/articles/d41573-021-00087-7.

41 Petrow, S. (2023), 'I tried ketamine to treat my depression: it was terrifying', *Washington Post* (12 February 2023): www.washingtonpost.com/wellness/2023/2002/2012/ketamine-depression-treatment-failure/ (accessed 14 February 2024).

42 www.scientificamerican.com/blog/cross-check/as-psychedelics-revival-rolls-on-don-t-downplay-bad-trips/ (accessed 27 March 2026).

43 Olofsson, M., Osika, W., Goldberg, S.B., Hendricks, P.S., Petrovic, P. et al. (2026), 'Difficulties following naturalistic psychedelic use and associations with adverse childhood experiences', *Int J Drug Policy*, **148**: 105105.

44 For references on side effects and risks of ketamine and esketamine, see: Horowitz, M.A., and Moncrieff, J. (2021), 'Are we repeating mistakes of the past? A review of the evidence for esketamine', *British Journal of Psychiatry*, **219**(5): 614–17. For further indications of an association between esketamine and suicide and suicidal ideation, see: Gastaldon, C., Raschi, E., Kane, J.M., Barbui, C. & Schoretsanitis, G. (2021), 'Post-Marketing Safety Concerns with Esketamine: A Disproportionality Analysis of Spontaneous Reports Submitted to the FDA Adverse Event Reporting System', *Psychotherapy & Psychosomatics*, **90**(1): 41–48.

45 https://nida.nih.gov/publications/drugfacts/over-counter-medicines (accessed 14 February 2024); also www.dea.gov/sites/default/files/2020-06/DXM-2020.pdf (accessed 6 March 2024). On dependence, see: www.justice.gov/archive/ndic/pubs11/11563/11563p.pdf, and Mutschler, J., Koopmann, A., Grosshans, M., Hermann, D., Mann, K., and Kiefer, F. (2010), 'Dextromethorphan withdrawal and dependence syndrome', *Deutsches Arzteblatt International*, **107**(30): 537–40.

46 This Medscape information suggests bupropion increases the concentration of DXM threefold: https://reference.medscape.com/drug/auvelity-dextromethorphan-bupropion-4000211#10 (accessed 6 March 2024). This older study suggests it may increase it much more (over thirty times): Kotlyar, M., Brauer, L.H., Tracy, T.S., Hatsukami, D.K., Harris, J., Bronars, C.A. & Adson, D.E. (2005), 'Inhibition of CYP2D6 activity by bupropion', *Journal of Clinical Psychopharmacology*, **25**(3): 226–29.

47 www.auvelity.com/how-auvelity-works (accessed 31 March 2026); www.axsome.com/wp-content/uploads/2024/11/auvelity-prescribing-information.pdf (accessed 31 March 2026).

48 Clayton, A.H., Lasser, R., Parikh, S.V., Iosifescu, D.V., Jung, J., Kotecha, M. et al. (2023), 'Zuranolone for the Treatment of Adults with Major Depressive Disorder: A Randomized, Placebo-Controlled Phase 3 Trial', *Am J Psychiatry*, **180**(9): 676–84.

49 Deligiannidis, K.M., Meltzer-Brody, S., Maximos, B., Peeper, E.Q., Freeman, M., Lasser, R. et al. (2023), 'Zuranolone for the Treatment of Postpartum Depression', *American Journal of Psychiatry*, **180**(9): 668–75.

50 https://www.drugs.com/medical-answers/how-zurzuvae-differ-traditional-antidepressants-3575176/#:~:text=Is%20Zurzuvae%20a%20controlled%20substance,Paranoia, accessed 25th Mar 2026.

51 www.pulsetoday.co.uk/news/clinical-areas/mental-health-and-addiction/esketamine-antidepressant-nasal-spray-rejected-by-nice/#:~:text=By%20Isabel%20Shaw,NHS%20in%20England%20and%20Wales (accessed 25 March 2026).
52 www.nice.org.uk/guidance/GID-TA11356/documents/draft-guidance (accessed 25 March 2026).
53 www.science.org/content/article/fda-rejected-mdma-assisted-ptsd-therapy-other-psychedelics-firms-intend-avoid-fate#:~:text=In%20the%20span%20of%20just,also%20commonly%20known%20as%20ecstasy (accessed 27 March 2026); www.psychologytoday.com/us/blog/shrink-speak/202603/the-government-exhibits-caution-about-psychedelics (accessed 24 March 2026).
54 www.precisionformedicine.com/blog/unpacking-fdas-draft-guidance-on-psychedelic-research-for-clinical-success/#:~:text=FDA%20acknowledges%20that%20the%20unique,aspects%20of%20the%20psychedelic%20experience (accessed 31 March 2026).
55 The following paper shows psychedelic-assisted psychotherapy has equal effects to antidepressants when both are openly administered: Williams, Z.J., Barnett, H. and Szigeti, B. (2026), 'Psychedelic Therapy vs Antidepressants for the Treatment of Depression Under Equal Unblinding Conditions: A Systematic Review and Meta-Analysis', *JAMA Psychiatry*; also see Žuljević, et al. (2026), note 17.
56 Tovey, D. and Tricco, A.C. (2026), 'Editors' choice April 2026', *J Clin Epidemiol*, **192**: 112223.

Chapter 17

1 The campaign is described here: Goldman, L.S., Nielsen, N.H., and Champion, H.C. (1999), 'Awareness, diagnosis, and treatment of depression', *Journal of General Internal Medicine*, **14**(9): 569–80. Merchandise is available from Etsy, among other places.
2 Loughman, A., and N. Haslam (2018), 'Neuroscientific explanations and the stigma of mental disorder: a meta-analytic study', *Cognitive Research: Principles & Implications*, **3**(1): 43.
3 Conneely, M., Higgs, P., and Moncrieff, J. (2021), 'Medicalising the Moral: The Case of Depression as Revealed in Internet Blogs', *Social Theory & Health*, **19**: 380–98 (quote on p. 391). Available at https://discovery.ucl.ac.uk/id/eprint/10104085/.
4 Kroenke, K., Spitzer, R.L., and Williams, J.B. (2001), 'The PHQ-9: Validity of a Brief Depression Severity Measure', *Journal of General Internal Medicine*, **16**(9): 606–13.
5 https://reconnectwellnessclub.com/ (accessed 14 February 2024). Some text supplied by Joe Tudor in personal communication.
6 Bowden, G., Holttum, S., Shankar, R., Cooke, A., and Kinderman, P. (eds) (2020), *Understanding Depression: Why Adults Experience Depression and What Can Help* (London: British Psychological Society).

7 www.england.nhs.uk/personalisedcare/social-prescribing/.
8 For more information on social prescribing, see www.gov.uk/government/publications/social-prescribing-applying-all-our-health/social-prescribing-applying-all-our-health (accessed 29 May 2024).
9 NICE (2022). *Depression in Adults: Treatment and Management NICE Guideline* [NG 222] (London: National Institute for Health and Care Excellence (NICE)). Available at www.nice.org.uk/guidance/ng222.
10 See, for example, Noetel, M., Sanders, T., Gallardo-Gómez, D., Taylor, P., del Pozo Cruz, B., van den Hoek, D., et al. (2024), 'Effect of Exercise for Depression: Systematic Review and Network Meta-Analysis of Randomised Controlled Trials', *British Medical Journal*, 384: e075847. Available at www.bmj.com/content/384/bmj-2023-075847.long.
11 Hari, J. (2018), *Lost Connections: Uncovering the Real Causes of Depression and the Unexpected Solutions* (London: Bloomsbury). Joe took inspiration from Hari's focus on the importance of connecting with other people.
12 See chapter 2, note 2.
13 Works by such writers include: James, O. (2006), 'Selfish Capitalism is Bad for Our Mental Health', *The Guardian*, 3 January 2008, www.theguardian.com/commentisfree/2008/jan/2003/comment.mentalhealth (accessed 14 February 2024); Davies, J. (2021), *Sedated: How Modern Capitalism Created Our Mental Health Crisis* (London: Atlantic Books); Davies, W. (2015), *The Happiness Industry: How the Government and Big Business Sold Us Well-Being* (London: Verso Books); Fisher, M. (2009), *Capitalist Realism: Is There No Alternative?* (Alresford, UK: Zero Books).
14 Davies, J. (2017), 'Political Pills: Psychopharmaceuticals and Neoliberalism as Mutually Supporting', *The Sedated Society* (London: Palgrave Macmillan), 189–225 (quote on p. 205).
15 Rose, N. (2006), 'Disorders without Borders? The Expanding Scope of Psychiatric Practice', *Biosocieties*, 1(4): 465–84 (quote on p. 479).

Chapter 18

1 I describe the interaction between powerful interests and knowledge further in my book: Moncrieff, J. (2008). *The Myth of the Chemical Cure: A Critique of Psychiatric Drug Treatment* (Basingstoke, UK: Palgrave Macmillan).
2 American Psychiatric Association (2024). 'What is Depression?', www.psychiatry.org/patients-families/depression/what-is-depression (accessed 8 February 2024). Ex-president of the APA, Rebecca Brendel, claiming depression has been shown to be due to a chemical imbalance, April 2023: www.youtube.com/watch?v=b2Gbjbj8FOg&t=689s (accessed 28 February 2024).

Epilogue

1 Neurodiversity is a concept used to refer to ADHD and 'autism spectrum disorders'. It is often taken to mean that there are differences, which should

not be thought of as defects, in the brains of people with these conditions. It is important to note that no such differences have been established, however. Further discussion and references can be found in Timimi, S. (2021). *Insane Medicine: How the Mental Health Industry Creates Damaging Treatment Traps and How You Can Escape Them* (independently published).

2 On bipolar disorder, see Moncrieff, J. (2014). 'The Medicalisation of "Ups and Downs": The Marketing of the New Bipolar Disorder', *Transcultural Psychiatry*. On adult ADHD, see Moncrieff, J.; Rapley, M; & Timimi, S. (2014). 'The Construction of Psychiatric Diagnoses: The Case of Adult ADHD' in Speed, E.; Moncrieff, J.; & Rapley; M. (eds), *De-medicalizing Misery II* (Basingstoke, UK: Palgrave Macmillan) 76–88.

Appendix 1

1 Folk, J., & Folk, M. (2021) 'Chemical Imbalance Theory False', www.anxietycentre.com/articles/chemical-imbalance/ (accessed 17 March 2024). Note that the drug company websites for this and other entries in this appendix may now be defunct.

2 *Ibid.*

3 www.prozac.com/how_prozac/how_it_works.jsp?reqNavId=2.2 (accessed 10 February 2007).

4 www.effexorxr.com/condition.asp (accessed 21 September 2006).

5 Cited in Lacasse, J.R., & Leo, J. (2005). 'Serotonin and Depression: A Disconnect between the Advertisements and the Scientific Literature', *PLoS.Med*, **2**(12): e392. Also available at www.youtube.com/watch?v=twhvtzd6gXA&list=PLTvBonT9IGLswtvolxp9MmsI_Xq04nWlU&index=1 (accessed 4 March 2024).

6 Cited in *ibid.*

7 www.hpra.ie/img/uploaded/swedocuments/2f50c532-bff8-4bfe-be8b-cfd253f09815.pdf (accessed 17 March 2024).

8 www.verywellhealth.com/what-is-serotonin-5189485 (accessed 28 April 2023).

9 https://my.clevelandclinic.org/health/articles/22572-serotonin#:~:text=When%20serotonin%20is%20at%20normal,of%20serotonin%20in%20your%20brain (accessed 17 March 2024).

10 www.nhs.uk/mental-health/talking-therapies-medicine-treatments/medicines-and-psychiatry/antidepressants/overview/#:~:text=Antidepressants%20usually%20need%20to%20be,effects%20usually%20wear%20off%20quickly (accessed 17 March 2024) and www.nhs.uk/mental-health/talking-therapies-medicine-treatments/medicines-and-psychiatry/ssri-antidepressants/overview/#:~:text=Doses%20and%20duration%20of%20treatment&text=SSRIs%20usually%20need%20to%20be,t%20stop%20taking%20the%20medicine (accessed 17 March 2024).

11 www.healthyminds.org/multimedia/depression.pdf (accessed 13 February 2006).

12 www.psychiatry.org/patients-families/depression/what-is-depression (accessed 8 February 2024).

13 www.rcpsych.ac.uk/mentalhealthinformation/mentalhealthproblems/depression/depression.aspx (accessed 22 December 2006).
14 www.rcpsych.ac.uk/healthadvice/treatmentswellbeing/antidepressants.aspx (accessed 1 May 2014).
15 www.yourhealthinmind.org/treatments-medication/medication (accessed 18 August 2022).
16 www.cdc.gov/mentalhealth/learn/index.htm (accessed 17 March 2024).

Appendix 2

1 www.rcpsych.ac.uk/mental-health/treatments-and-wellbeing/stopping-antidepressants; Horowitz, M., and Talor, D.M. (2024). *The Maudsley Deprescribing Guidelines: Antidepressants, Benzodiazepines, Gabapentinoids and Z-drugs*, The Maudsley Prescribing Guidelines Series (Oxford, Wiley Blackwell).

Index

Note: *Italicised* page references denote illustrations and tables, and those in **bold** denote glossary definitions.